TRAU
SECRETS

Second Edition

TRAUMA SECRETS

Second Edition

GIDEON P. NAUDÉ, MBChB, FRCS (Edinburgh), FRCS (Glasgow), FACS
Chief of Staff
Department of Surgery
Tuolumne General Hospital
Sonora Community Hospital
Sonora, California

FREDERIC S. BONGARD, MD, FACS
Associate Professor, Department of Surgery
University of California, Los Angeles, UCLA School of Medicine
Los Angeles, California
Chief, Division of Trauma and Critical Care
Director of Surgical Education
Harbor-UCLA Medical Center
Torrance, California

DEMETRIOS DEMETRIADES, MD, PhD, FACS
Professor of Surgery
Department of Surgery
Division of Trauma/Critical Care
Keck School of Medicine, University of Southern California
Director of Trauma and Surgical Intensive Care Unit
Los Angeles County and University of Southern California Medical Center
Los Angeles, California

HANLEY & BELFUS, INC. / Philadelphia

Publisher: HANLEY & BELFUS, INC.
              Medical Publishers
              210 South 13th Street
              Philadelphia, PA 19107
              (215) 546-7293; 800-962-1892
              FAX (215) 790-9330
              Web site: http://www.hanleyandbelfus.com

**WO
18.2** `
**T777
2003**

Note to the reader: Although the information in this book has been carefully reviewed for correctness of dosage and indications, neither the authors nor the editors nor the publisher can accept any legal responsibility for any errors or omissions that may be made. Neither the publisher nor the editors make any warranty, expressed or implied, with respect to the material contained herein. Before prescribing any drug, the reader must review the manufacturer's current product information (package inserts) for accepted indications, absolute dosage recommendations, and other information pertinent to the safe and effective use of the product described.

Library of Congress Control Number: 2002116189

TRAUMA SECRETS, 2nd edition   ISBN 1-56053-506-7

Last digit is the print number: 9   8   7   6   5   4   3   2   1

CONTENTS

DEDICATION

To my beloved wife, Pamela, my sons,
Gideon and Frans, and my daughters,
Chandré and Nicole

GPN

To my sons, Reid and Alec

FSB

To my wife, Elizabeth, my daughters,
Alexis and Stephanie, and my son,
Nicholas

DD

CONTRIBUTORS

Deirdre Anglin, M.D., M.P.H.
Assistant Professor of Emergency Medicine, Department of Emergency Medicine, Keck School of Medicine, University of Southern California; Los Angeles County and University of Southern California Medical Center, Los Angeles, California

Juan A. Asensio, M.D., F.A.C.S.
Unit Chief, Trauma Surgery Service "A," Division of Trauma/Critical Care Department of Surgery, University of Southern California, Los Angeles County and University of Southern California Medical Center; Associate Professor, Los Angeles County and University of Southern California Medical Center, Los Angeles, California

Elizabeth Beale, M.B.B.Ch., M.Med., M.R.C.P.
Research Associate, Department of Surgery, University of Southern California School of Medicine, Los Angeles, California

Howard Belzberg, M.D.
Associate Professor, Department of Surgery, Division of Trauma, University of Southern California; Associate Director, Surgical Intensive Care Unit, Los Angeles County and University of Southern California Medical Center, Los Angeles, California

Thomas V. Berne, M.D.
Professor, Department of Surgery, University of Southern California; Chief Physician, Department of Surgery, Los Angeles County and University of Southern California Medical Center, Los Angeles, California

Frederic S. Bongard, M.D., F.A.C.S.
Associate Professor, Department of Surgery, University of California, Los Angeles, UCLA School of Medicine, Los Angeles; Chief, Division of Trauma and Critical Care; Director of Surgical Education, Harbor-UCLA Medical Center, Torrance, California

Ian Carmody, M.D., F.R.C.S. (C.)
Clinical Instructor, Department of Surgery, University of California, Los Angeles, Los Angeles, California

Edward E. Cornwell III, M.D.
Associate Professor, Department of Surgery, The Johns Hopkins School of Medicine; Chief, Adult Trauma, The Johns Hopkins Hospital, Baltimore, Maryland

Demetrios Demetriades, M.D., Ph.D., F.A.C.S.
Professor of Surgery, Department of Surgery, Division of Trauma/Critical Care, Keck School of Medicine, University of Southern California; Director of Trauma and Surgical Intensive Care Unit, Los Angeles County and University of Southern California Medical Center, Los Angeles, California

Christian de Virgilio, M.D.
Assistant Professor, Department of Surgery, University of California, Los Angeles, UCLA School of Medicine, Los Angeles; Division of Vascular Surgery, Department of Surgery, Harbor-UCLA Medical Center, Torrance; Veterans Affairs Medical Center, West Los Angeles, California

Carlos E. Donayre, M.D.
Associate Professor, Division of Vascular Surgery, Department of Surgery, University of California, Los Angeles, UCLA School of Medicine, Los Angeles; Division of Vascular Surgery, Department of Surgery, Harbor-UCLA Medical Center, Torrance, California

William R. Dougherty, M.D., F.A.C.S.
Department of Surgery, University of Southern California School of Medicine; Los Angeles County—University of Southern California Medical Center, Los Angeles, California

Marc Eckstein, M.D.
Associate Professor, Department of Emergency Medicine, Keck School of Medicine, University of Southern California; Los Angeles County and University of Southern California Medical Center; Medical Director, Los Angeles Fire Department, Los Angeles, California

Dale S. Ford, R.N., M.P.H., C.I.C.
Massachusetts General Hospital, Boston, Massachusetts

Warren L. Garner, M.D.
Associate Professor of Surgery, University of Southern California; Los Angeles County and University of Southern California Medical Center, Los Angeles, California

Debra Ann Gilmore, R.N., M.S.N., A.C.N.P.
Trauma Nurse Coordinator, Department of Surgery, Harbor-UCLA Medical Center, Torrance, California

Jonathan R. Hiatt, M.D.
Professor, Department of Surgery, University of California, Los Angeles, UCLA School of Medicine; Vice Chairman, Department of Surgery, Cedars-Sinai Medical Center, Los Angeles, California

H. Range Hutson, M.D.
Instructor, Department of Emergency Medicine, Harvard Medical School; Brigham and Women's Hospital, Boston, Massachusetts

M. Margaret Knudson, M.D.
Associate Professor, Department of Surgery, University of California, San Francisco, School of Medicine; Chief, Division of Pediatric Trauma, San Francisco General Hospital, San Francisco, California

Jackson Lee, M.D.
Associate Professor of Clinical Orthopaedics, Department of Orthopaedic Surgery, University of Southern California School of Medicine; Director, Orthopaedic Trauma Service, Los Angeles County—University of Southern California Medical Center, Los Angeles, California

Diku Mandavia, M.D., F.A.C.E.P., F.R.C.P.C.
Clinical Associate Professor of Emergency Medicine, Keck School of Medicine, University of Southern California; Attending Staff Physician, Department of Emergency Medicine, Cedars-Sinai Medical Center, Los Angeles, California

Sujal Mandavia, M.D., F.A.C.E.P., F.R.C.P.(C.)
Clinical Assistant Professor of Emergency Medicine, Keck School of Medicine, University of Southern California; Attending Staff, Trauma Liaison, Emergency Department, Cedars-Sinai Medical Center, Los Angeles, California

Patricia Eubanks May, M.D., F.A.C.S.
Assistant Professor, Department of Surgery, University of Nevada School of Medicine; Veterans Affairs Sierra Nevada Health Care System, Reno, Nevada

James P. McAndrews, D.D.S.
Assistant Clinical Professor, Oral and Maxillofacial Surgery, University of Southern California School of Dentistry; Medical Staff, University of Southern California University Hospital; Medical Staff, Los Angeles County and University of Southern California Medical Center, Los Angeles, California

Duncan Q. McBride, M.D.
Associate Professor of Clinical Neurosurgery, Department of Surgery, University of California, Los Angeles, UCLA School of Medicine, Los Angeles; Chief, Division of Neurosurgery, Harbor-UCLA Medical Center, Torrance, California

Justin D. Merszei, M.D.
Department of Surgery, University of Southern California School of Medicine, Los Angeles, California

Charles Moon, M.D.
Assistant Professor, Clinical Department of Orthopaedics, University of Southern California School of Medicine, Los Angeles, California

James A. Murray, M.D.
Assistant Professor, Department of Surgery, Division of Trauma, Keck School of Medicine, University of Southern California, Los Angeles, California

Gideon P. Naudé, M.B.Ch.B., F.R.C.S.(Edin.), F.R.C.S.(Glasg.), F.A.C.S.
Chief of Staff, Department of Surgery, Tuolumne General Hospital; Sonora Community Hospital, Sonora, California

Johannes Hendrik Naudé, M.B.Ch.B., F.C.S.Urol.(S.A.)
Professor of Urology, University of Cape Town; Chief of Urology, Groote Schuur Hospital, Cape Town, South Africa

Edward Newton, M.D.
Associate Professor, Interim Chair, Department of Emergency Medicine, Keck School of Medicine, University of Southern California, Los Angeles, California

Thomas T. Noguchi, M.D.
Professor Emeritus of Forensic Pathology, Emergency Medicine and Surgery, Department of Pathology and Laboratory Medicine, University of Southern California Keck School of Medicine; Attending Staff, Los Angeles County and University of Southern California Medical Center, Los Angeles, California

Dat Tien Nguyen, M.D.
Surgical Oncological Fellow, Department of Surgery, Harbor-UCLA Medical Center, Torrance, California

Thuan T. Nguyen, M.D.
Assistant Professor, Division of Plastic and Reconstructive Surgery, Department of Surgery, University of Southern California School of Medicine, Los Angeles, California

Patrizio Petrone, M.D.
Division of Trauma/Critical Care, Department of Surgery; Chief, International Research Fellow, University of Southern California—Los Angeles County and University of Southern California Medical Center, Los Angeles, California

Mary-Anne Purtill, M.D.
Clinical Instructor, Department of Surgery, University of California, Los Angeles, UCLA School of Medicine, Los Angeles; Fellow, Division of Trauma and Critical Care, Department of Surgery, Harbor-UCLA Medical Center, Torrance, California

Jesús Ramírez, M.D.
Critical Care Fellow, Division of Trauma and Critical Care, University of Southern California; Critical Care Fellow, Los Angeles County and University of Southern California Medical Center, Los Angeles, California

Gustavo A. Roldán, M.D.
Division of Trauma/Critical Care, Department of Surgery; Chief, International Research Fellow, University of Southern California—Los Angeles County and University of Southern California Medical Center, Los Angeles, California

Javier Romeo, M.D.
Critical Care Fellow, Department of Surgery, University of Southern California Keck School of Medicine; Critical Care Fellow, Los Angeles County and University of Southern California Medical Center, Los Angeles, California

Bradley J. Roth, M.D.
Assistant Professor of Surgery, Division of Trauma/Critical Care Medicine, University of Southern California; Los Angeles County and University of Southern California Trauma Center, University of Southern California University Hospital, Los Angeles, California

Lakshmanan Sathyavagiswaran, M.D., F.A.C.P., F.C.A.P., F.R.C.P.(C.)
Chief Medical Examiner-Coroner, Los Angeles County Department of Coroner; Keck School of Medicine, University of Southern California; Geffen School of Medicine, University of California, Los Angeles; Attending Staff, Los Angeles County and University of Southern California Medical Center, Los Angeles, California

Stefan René Schirber, M.D.
Chief Surgery Resident, Department of Surgery, Santa Barbara Cottage Hospital, Santa Barbara, California

Joel Sercarz, M.D.
Associate Professor, Department of Surgery, University of California, Los Angeles, UCLA School of Medicine, Los Angeles; Harbor-UCLA Medical Center, Torrance; Attending Surgeon, UCLA Medical Center, Los Angeles, California

William C. Shoemaker, M.D.
Professor of Surgery and Anesthesia, Trauma/Critical Care, Keck School of Medicine, University of Southern California; Los Angeles County and University of Southern California Medical Center, Los Angeles, California

Barbara A. Silver, M.D.
Associate Professor of Clinical Psychiatry, Department of Psychiatry, University of California, Los Angeles, UCLA School of Medicine, Los Angeles; Director of Consultation and Liaison Psychiatry, Harbor-UCLA Medical Center, Torrance, California

Jonathan C. Song, M.D.
Assistant Professor of Ophthalmology, Keck School of Medicine, University of Southern California; Doheney Eye Institute, Los Angeles, California

Bruce E. Stabile, M.D.
Professor, Department of Surgery, University of California, Los Angeles, UCLA School of Medicine, Los Angeles; Chair, Department of Surgery; Acting Medical Director, Harbor-UCLA Medical Center, Torrance, California

Michael J. Stamos, M.D.
Associate Professor, Department of Surgery, University of California, Los Angeles, UCLA School of Medicine, Los Angeles; Chief, Section of Colon and Rectal Surgery, Department of Surgery, Harbor-UCLA Medical Center, Torrance, California

Samuel J. Stratton, M.D., F.A.C.E.P.
Associate Professor of Medicine, Department of Emergency Medicine, University of California, Los Angeles, UCLA School of Medicine, Los Angeles; Department of Emergency Medicine, Harbor-UCLA Medical Center, Torrance; Medical Director, Los Angeles County Emergency Medical Services Agency, Los Angeles, California

Areti Tillou, M.D.
Clinical Instructor, Department of Surgery, Division of Trauma and Critical Care, University of Southern California; Assistant Unit Chief, Trauma Unit B, Los Angeles County/USC Medical Center, Los Angeles, California

Francois H. Van Zyl, M.B.Ch.B.
Department of Medicine, Stellenbosch University, Stellenbosch, Cape Province, South Africa

Hernan I. Vargas, M.D.
Assistant Professor, Department of Surgery, University of California, Los Angeles, UCLA School of Medicine, Los Angeles; Chief, Division of Surgical Oncology, Harbor-UCLA Medical Center, Torrance, California

George C. Velmahos, M.D., F.A.C.S., F.R.C.S.
Associate Professor of Surgery, Division of Trauma and Critical Care, University of Southern California; Chief, Trauma Unit C, Los Angeles County/USC Medical Center, Los Angeles, California

Kenneth Waxman, M.D.
Director, Department of Surgery, Santa Barbara Cottage Hospital, Santa Barbara, California

Dennis-Duke R. Yamashita, D.D.S.
Professor, Chairman and Director, Oral and Maxillofacial Surgery, University of Southern California School of Dentistry; Section Chair, University of Southern California University Hospital; Director, Los Angeles County/USC Medical Center, Los Angeles, California

Bruce Edwin Zawacki, M.D., M.A.
Emeritus Associate Professor of Surgery, University of Southern California; Los Angeles County and University of Southern California Medical Center, Los Angeles, California

PREFACE TO THE FIRST EDITION

The efficient and proper care of the trauma patient is a complex and demanding task. Students, residents, and staff are often presented with a myriad of physiologic derangements requiring immediate attention in the shortest time. Major works have been composed on how to take care of the trauma patient. While meritorious in their own right, these works are often too detailed and too long for the medical student and the junior house staff to grasp. This becomes apparent on rounds when the answer to a simple question is either confused or completely incorrect.

The three editors of this work regularly round with medical students and house staff on trauma patients. Day after day, the simplest of concepts seem difficult to grasp. For that reason, we wrote this pocket manual to assist in reviewing the basic concepts of trauma care. It was not our intention to replace any of the textbooks or trauma care manuals that are available. Rather, we intended to create a simple reference that contains the core information that the house staff and students may ask themselves or may be asked on rounds.

To achieve this, two of the largest trauma centers in Los Angeles County divided the body of knowledge. We invited contributors from other trauma centers who had particular interest in the subject at hand. The end result, we believe, is a readable, understandable, and concise synopsis of the most important questions in trauma care. We hope that the students and house staff who use this manual will benefit from its content and will guide us in the preparation of future revisions.

PREFACE TO THE SECOND EDITION

With the first edition of *Trauma Secrets*, we hoped to provide a concise, yet substantial reference in trauma care, focusing on presenting core information in a readily accessible format with tables, lists, and mnemonics used throughout the text. The Socratic method of teaching is employed, using questions and answers that will arise on rounds, in trauma care settings, and on exams.

In the second edition, the discussions have been revised, updated, and expanded, and a new chapter on alcohol and illicit drugs provides an overview of the impact of substance abuse on the population. A comprehensive index makes the material readily accessible.

Caring for trauma patients is a challenge; they often present with numerous injuries requiring immediate intervention. We hope that *Trauma Secrets* will serve as a valuable tool in their management.

Gideon P. Naudé, M.B.Ch.B., F.R.C.S. (Edin.), F.R.C.S. (Glasg.), F.A.C.S.
Frederic S. Bongard, M.D., F.A.C.S.
Demetrios Demetriades, M.D., Ph.D., F.A.C.S.

I. Trauma Basics

1. PREHOSPITAL TRAUMA CARE

Marc Eckstein, M.D., and Samuel J. Stratton, M.D.

1. What are emergency medical services (EMS)?
EMS is a regional system of out-of-hospital and hospital emergency response. It includes emergency medical technicians (EMTs), paramedics, paramedic base stations (for radio communications between the field and on-line medical control), receiving hospitals, and specialty care centers (such as trauma centers). In most of the United States, a centralized local regional agency oversees the organization and medical quality of a community EMS system.

2. What is meant by the term *triage*?
Triage means "to sort." When there are a number of patients at an incident, it is important to sort them into groups based on the severity of their injuries. The "immediate" group consists of the most critical but potentially salvageable patients. The "delayed" group comprises patients whose injuries do not pose an immediate threat to life or limb but have the potential to do so. The "minor" group comprises patients with minor, non–life-threatening injuries. Many of the patients in the "minor" group can be either treated and released at the scene or transported in large groups to medical facilities in a nonurgent manner.

3. How are incidents involving multiple victims best managed in the field?
The S-T-A-R-T system (Simple Triage and Rapid Treatment) is an easily learned technique to methodically evaluate multiple patients very quickly. It involves assessing breathing, perfusion, and mental status to categorize patients into one of three categories: Immediate (red); Delayed (yellow); or Minor (green) (Figure 1). This system, which can be used by people with minimal training, allows rapid triaging of multiple patients in a very organized fashion.

4. What is the Incident Command System (ICS)?
A technique called the Incident Command System (ICS) is the standard method for management of multiple-victim incidents. The field medical response is one component of the ICS. The ICS organizes the medical, fire suppression, law enforcement, administrative, and other operational aspects of a multiple-victim response into a systematic approach that places responsibility for the response on the most experienced person in the field. This person is designated the "incident commander."

5. How are trauma victims triaged in the field for transport to a trauma center hospital?
Field trauma triage schemes are usually based on a combination of physical parameters and trauma mechanisms. The American College of Surgeons recommends a field triage scheme that is based on respiratory rate, systolic blood pressure, Glasgow Coma Scale, and mechanism of injury. The following injury mechanisms are high risk and should be considered for immediate transport to a trauma center:
 All penetrating injuries to head, neck, torso, and extremities proximal to the elbow and knee
 Flail chest
 Combination trauma with burns
 Two or more proximal long-bone fractures

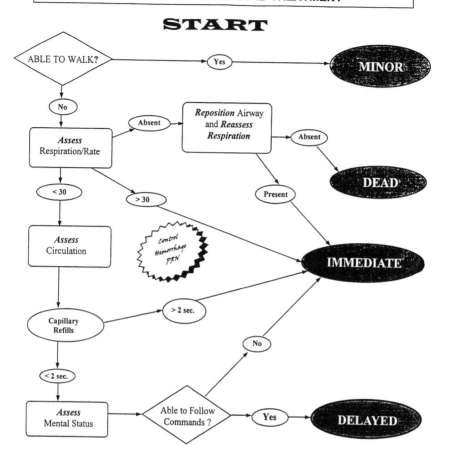

Simple Triage and Rapid Treatment

Pelvic fractures
Limb paralysis
Amputation proximal to wrist and ankle

6. What is the Trauma Score?

The Trauma Score (TS) or Revised Trauma Score (RTS) is a method of rapid scoring for triage and assessment of severity of injury in the field. The RTS is based on the respiratory rate, systolic blood pressure, and Glasgow Coma Scale (eye opening, verbal response, motor response).

7. When should spinal immobilization be considered in the out-of-hospital setting?

Initial consideration for spinal immobilization should be based on the mechanism of injury. Any blunt or penetrating injury that could lead to spinal injury should be considered an indication for spinal immobilization. Unconscious victims or those with altered mental status who cannot give a clear history of the mechanism of injury should be considered for spinal immobilization. Water sport injury victims who have dived into water are at high risk for cervical spine injury and should be immobilized. Gun-shot or high-velocity penetrating injuries of the torso may have occult thoracic or lumbar spine injury and should be considered for spinal immobilization. However, if these patients are neurologically intact in the field, they are unlikely to have any spinal cord injuries.

8. What indications are currently used by paramedics to "clear" a patient's cervical spine in the field and not place the patient in full spinal immobilization?

Patients who are awake and alert; with no evidence of intoxication with drugs or ethanol; with no major distracting injuries; with no complaints of neck pain or tenderness elicited on palpation of the neck; and with no numbness or paresthesias of the extremities do not need to be immobilized in many prehospital systems. The mechanism of injury should always be considered first, however. Even in the presence of the above criteria, patients at high risk owing to their mechanism of injury should be immobilized.

9. Is spinal immobilization of the small child different from that of the adult?

Small children have a disproportionately large cranial occiput region that requires padding to elevate the shoulders and torso to maintain spinal alignment when being placed on a flat surface. Proper alignment of the head and shoulders is also important for maintaining an open airway.

10. A victim of a motor vehicle accident who is 34 weeks pregnant is en route to a trauma center by paramedics. She is noted to have a blood pressure of 84 by palpation. What should paramedics do to address the patient's hypotension?

Place the patient in the left lateral decubitus position.

11. What is supine hypotension syndrome?

It is hypotension caused by the weight of the gravid uterus compressing the inferior vena cava, compromising venous return to the heart, and resulting in systemic hypotension. This may be avoided by placing these patients in the left lateral decubitus position, or by placing blanket rolls beneath the right side of the backboard.

12. What are three types of airway adjuncts available for paramedics to use on trauma patients?

Endotracheal tube, esophageal-tracheal combination tube (Combi-tube®), and the laryngeal mask airway (LMA).

13. What is the main advantage of the Combi-tube over an endotracheal tube?

Although the endotracheal tube is still the gold standard for airway management, its placement may be difficult in some trauma patients, particularly in the prehospital setting. The Combi-tube is inserted blindly; direct visualization of the vocal cords is not required. It therefore offers an alternative in patients whom paramedics are unable to intubate.

14. When is endotracheal intubation indicated in the field?

Out-of-hospital endotracheal intubation is indicated for management of an uncontrolled airway, including the airway of the unconscious victim or head injury victim at high risk for aspiration or loss of airway. It is also indicated for management of the hypoventilating victim with head, chest, facial, or other injury.

15. What are some factors that make intubation difficult to perform on major trauma patients in the prehospital setting?

Possible cervical spine injuries that require in-line stabilization of the neck

Inadequate suction

Poor lighting

Patients with full stomachs are prone to vomiting and aspiration

Combative patients who often require paralytic agents or other medications to facilitate intubation. Prehospital use of these agents is severely restricted or prohibited in most systems.

16. How can the potential cervical spine–injured patient be endotracheally intubated in the field?

Endotracheal intubation can be performed safely using the oral route if a second rescuer provides manual head and cervical spine immobilization during the procedure. Nasal tracheal intubation is also a method that can be considered for the potential cervical spine–injured patient.

17. What is the role of the surgical approach to an airway in the field?

Needle cricothyrotomy is the most common surgical airway approach used in the out-of-hospital setting. Although there are different techniques and devices, needle cricothyrotomy is the placement of a large-bore needle (14-gauge) into the trachea through the cricoid membrane. A field surgical airway should be considered when endotracheal intubation is indicated but cannot be accomplished, usually in the setting of severe face or neck injury.

18. What are the "absolute" indications to pronounce patients in traumatic cardiac arrest dead in the field?

Patients with who are apneic, pulseless, and without neurologic reflexes, who have any of the following physical or circumstantial conditions may be pronounced: incineration; decapitation; massive crush injury; penetrating or blunt injury with evisceration of the heart, lung, or brain; decomposition; extrication time greater than fifteen minutes, where no resuscitative measures can be performed prior to extrication; pulseless, apneic victims of a multiple victim incident where insufficient medical resources preclude initiating resuscitative measures; rigor mortis; or post-mortem lividity.

19. For patients with traumatic cardiac arrest, what factors should be strongly considered to terminate resuscitative efforts in the field?

Patients with blunt trauma with a clearly lethal mechanism of injury; and patients with penetrating injuries found in asystole.

20. What are potential complications of spinal immobilization?

Patients placed in spinal immobilization are at risk of aspiration because they are restrained and cannot clear their airway. Spinal immobilization is usually uncomfortable and can cause secondary pain, particularly if used for prolonged periods of time.

21. What is the pneumatic antishock garment (PASG), and how does it work?

The pneumatic antishock garment (PASG) or military antishock trousers (M.A.S.T.) is a device designed to encircle the legs, pelvis, and abdomen with inflatable compartments that, when fully inflated to 60–80 mmHg, applies external pressure to the areas of the body that are encircled. The PASG increases peripheral vascular resistance by external compression. The increase in peripheral vascular resistance supports the blood pressure of a hypotensive victim.

22. What are the indications for the use of the PASG?

The PASG is indicated for treatment of hypotension due to ruptured abdominal aortic aneurysm. It is acceptable to use for hypotension due to suspected pelvic fracture, otherwise uncontrollable lower extremity hemorrhage, severe (unobtainable pulse and blood pressure) traumatic hypotension, and anaphylactic shock (unresponsive to standard therapy). The PASG should not be used in the setting of diaphragmatic rupture, penetrating thoracic injury, pulmonary edema, abdominal evisceration, or cardiogenic shock. In the setting of penetrating thoracic injury, the PASG should be avoided because it can increase hemorrhage from uncontrolled bleeding sites in the chest.

23. What are the indications for field needle thoracostomy?

Needle thoracostomy is a method used to decompress a tension pneumothorax. The usual technique is to place a 14-gauge or 16-gauge needle with a plastic catheter into the pleural space through the second or third intercostal space in the midclavicular line, or through the fourth or fifth intercostal space in the anterior axillary line. Once the pleural space is entered, it is decompressed, with the plastic catheter left in place and the needle withdrawn. Indications for field needle thoracostomy are chest injury with absent or diminished breath sounds on the affected side and severe hypotension. Other findings that support performing a needle thoracostomy in the field are confusion, cyanosis, hypotension, jugular venous distention, respiratory distress, shock, subcutaneous emphysema, and tracheal deviation.

24. How should abdominal evisceration be managed in the field setting?

The eviscerated organs or tissue should be covered with gauze soaked with sterile saline, and efforts should be made to avoid reintroduction of the eviscerated parts back into the abdominal cavity. The patient should not be allowed to roll onto the area of evisceration, and the PASG should not be placed over the evisceration.

25. What is the proper prehospital treatment of a patient impaled by an object?

Leave the object in place and stabilize it with large field dressings in order to minimize further internal injuries. Removal of impaled objects in the field is contraindicated because such removal might release a tamponading effect on a blood vessel, resulting in uncontrollable hemorrhage.

26. Should a helmet worn by an injury victim be removed immediately at the scene of an injury?

Accepted out-of-hospital practice is to remove a helmet in the field to provide access to the airway, neck, and face. However, a helmet should be removed only if the cervical spine can be protected during the removal. If a helmet cannot be safely removed in the field, the victim should be immobilized and transported with the helmet left in place. Helmets removed in the field should be brought with the patient to the hospital for examination by the treating physicians to help determine the severity of head injury.

27. What are special aspects of the field management of electrical injuries?

Rescuers might ensure that the scene is safe and the risk of electrocution no longer exists prior to contact with the victim. Electrical injuries are often complicated by cardiac rhythm disturbances because of electrical flow through the heart and its conduction system. Therefore, cardiac monitoring is indicated if available in the field. Electrical shock cardiac arrest victims should be immediately evaluated for ventricular fibrillation and countershocked if indicated. Electrical burns often appear minor when, in fact, there has been significant tissue and nerve damage. All electrical injury victims should be transported from the field for medical evaluation. Identification of entrance and exit electrical burns is helpful in determining the extent of electrical injury. Rescuers should attempt to obtain information regarding the voltage and amperage of the current causing the electrical injury.

28. True or false: An adult who has sustained 60% total body surface area (TBSA) full-thickness burns in a house fire should be transported directly to the closest regional burn center.

False. This patient is at high risk for airway compromise secondary to thermal burns of the face or smoke inhalation. The patient should be transported to the nearest facility that can stabilize the airway and initiate fluid resuscitation prior to transfer to a burn center. Transporting such patients the extra distance to the regional burn center can result in a preventable death from airway or hemodynamic compromise.

29. What strategies should be used in the field for safe extrication of an entrapped injury victim?

Entrapped victims are frequently encountered in motor vehicle accidents. While extrication of the patient is underway, the airway, breathing, circulation, and spine should be assessed as done initially for any injury victim. While still entrapped, patients can often have spinal stabilization established, airway and breathing addressed, and establishment of intravenous access for fluid administration.

30. What is Waddell's triad in reference to pediatric injury?

Waddell's triad is an injury complex that can be anticipated when a child pedestrian has been struck by an automobile. When a child is struck by an automobile driven on the right side of the road, the child's femur is typically struck by the bumper while the fender strikes the spleen area. The child is usually thrown through the air, striking the opposite side of his head upon landing. This triad of femur and spleen injury on one side and head injury on the opposite side should be expected for young pedestrians struck by automobiles.

31. How does one deal with the child who is still in a car seat found at the scene of an automobile accident?

A child can be transported while still in the car seat. The car seat can be used for spinal immobilization by taping the head to the back of the car seat. If the child is in shock, the seat can be laid on its back, elevating the child's legs. Careful examination of the child while still in the car seat can be accomplished in the field.

32. When should a deformed extremity fracture be realigned in the field?

Generally, extremity fractures should be immobilized as they are found in the field. If a fracture is deformed with loss of pulse or sensation distal to the fracture site, the extremity should be realigned and immobilized to allow for possible release of compression of vessels or nerves.

33. Name three devices to immobilize a femur fracture.
1. Hare© Traction splint
2. Sager© splint
3. Pneumatic splint

34. What strategies in the field may benefit victims of severe crush injury?

Vigorous intravenous fluids will keep renal perfusion and urine flow maximized to decrease the risk of renal failure secondary to the nephrotoxic byproducts of crushed muscle. Intravenous sodium bicarbonate will alkalinize the urine and decrease precipitation of acidic muscle breakdown products in the renal tubules. Inhaled beta-agonists (such as albuterol) will cause temporary shift of potassium into the intracellular space and decrease the hyperkalemia associated with muscle injury.

35. What are the priorities in the field management of the trauma victim in shock?

Airway-ventilation management, spinal stabilization, and rapid transport to definitive care. External hemorrhage should also be controlled as rapidly as possible. Attempts to place intravenous lines and administer fluids should be initiated *while en route* to the receiving hospital. While en route, patients should be covered and efforts made to limit hypothermia.

36. List some of the disadvantages associated with the use of helicopters for transport of trauma patients.
- Added delays required to secure a landing site
- Inherent dangers associated with helicopters, both in terms of crashes and risks to by-standers near the landing site
- Difficulty in treating patients once airborne owing to the confines of the helicopter
- Need for specialized training of paramedic personnel in air ambulances

37. List three reasons why prehospital administration of large volumes of intravenous fluids might be harmful.
1. Increased hydrostatic pressure in blood vessels may promote hemorrhage through elevation of systemic arterial blood pressure
2. Dilution of existing clotting factors may decrease body's ability to stop ongoing blood loss from smaller vessels
3. Mechanical disruption of active clot formation

38. When treating a victim of a high-speed motor vehicle accident, why is it important to determine from paramedics if air bags were deployed in the vehicle?
Air bags may mask any signs suggesting a traumatic aortic rupture. Prior to the widespread availability of air bags, physicians often used physical findings such as steering wheel marks on the chest wall as indicators of possible aortic injury. Air bags make such physical findings less likely. This underscores the need for treating physicians to get an accurate history from paramedics about the mechanism of injury.

39. What other information is vital to obtain from paramedics concerning victims of motor vehicle accidents and what particular internal injuries should you suspect for each of these factors?

HISTORY ELEMENT	SUSPECTED INJURY
Deformed steering column	Traumatic aortic injury
High-speed deceleration	Traumatic aortic injury, renal artery thrombosis
Presence of a lap belt	Chance fracture of lumbar vertebrae
Single-vehicle accident	Possible involvement of drugs or ethanol
Minimal damage to vehicle despite patient's serious condition	Possible medical event causing the crash (e.g., myocardial infarction, dysrhythmia, CNS event)
Patient ejected from vehicle	Multiple internal and head injuries

BIBLIOGRAPHY

1. Bickell WH, Wall MJ, Pepe PE, et al: Immediate versus delayed fluid resuscitation for hypotensive patients with penetrating torso injuries. N Engl J Med 331:1105–1109, 1994.
2. Committee on Trauma: Resources for Optimal Care of the Injured Patient. Chicago, American College of Surgeons, 1993.
3. Domeier RM, O'Connor RF, Delbridge TR, et al: Use of the pneumatic antishock garment (PASG). Prehospital Emerg Care 1:32, 1997.
4. Schulz CH, Koenig KL: A medical disaster response to reduce immediate mortality after an earthquake. N Engl J Med 334:438–444, 1996.

2. TRAUMA SCORING SYSTEMS

Debra Ann Gilmore, R.N., M.S.N., ACNP

1. What is the purpose of trauma scoring systems?
The purpose of trauma scoring systems is threefold:
1. To develop triage protocols and systems that ensure "the right patient gets to the right hospital in the right amount of time"
2. To facilitate meaningful research comparing homogeneous groups
3. To evaluate the quality of patient care both intrainstitutionally and globally from a "trauma system" perspective

2. List several scoring systems currently available.
CRAMS (Circulation, Respiration, Abdomen, Motor, Speech Scale)
Glasgow Coma Scale (GCS)
Trauma Score (TS)
Revised Trauma Score (RTS)
Trauma Index (TI)
AIS (Abbreviated Injury Severity)
ISS (Injury Severity Score)
TRISS (RTS or TS combined with ISS)
ICD-9-CM (International Classification of Diseases, 9th Revision, Clinical Modification)
APACHE (Acute Physiology and Chronic Health Evaluation)
Pediatric Trauma Score (PTS)

3. Which systems are anatomic? Which ones are physiologic? Which ones are both?

Anatomic	Physiologic	Anatomic and Physiologic
Abbreviated Injury Score	Glasgow Coma Scale	TRISS
Injury Severity Score	Trauma Score	Pediatric Trauma Score
ICD-9-CM	Revised Trauma Score	
	CRAMS	
	APACHE	

4. Which scoring systems are most commonly used in trauma management and research?
The most commonly used scoring systems for evaluating trauma patients are the TS, RTS, AIS, and ISS. The GCS is a component of both the TS and RTS. The GCS is also the most commonly used tool for evaluating a head-injured patient's level of consciousness (see questions 9 and 10).

5. Which systems might be useful in prehospital triage and why?
The ISS system is used to evaluate outcome using severity of anatomic injury indices. The accuracy of the ISS depends on identification of all anatomic injuries, making it less useful for patient triage. The TS and the RTS are commonly used in combination with the ISS to determine the probability of survival (refer to question 19). Both the TS and RTS are based on physiologic parameters at initial evaluation in the field or emergency department and therefore may be useful as a field triage tool. CRAMS is a simple system used for patient triage and has also been used successfully in the prehospital setting.

6. What is the Trauma Score? List the five variables in the Trauma Score. How does the Trauma Score differ from the Revised Trauma Score?

The Trauma Score is a physiologic score used to identify seriously injured patients. The variables included in the TS are GCS, blood pressure, capillary refill, respiratory rate (RR), and respiratory effort. The maximum score is 16. The RTS differs in that it does not include capillary refill and respiratory effort, thus yielding a maximum score of 12. The capillary refill and respiratory effort were eliminated because they are difficult to assess objectively and frequently are not documented consistently. The RTS assigns a coded value to each variable (systolic blood pressure [SBP], RR, GCS) and is more heavily weighted for serious head injuries, thus providing a more accurate estimation of outcome than the TS.

Revised Trauma Score[a]

GCS	SBP	RR	CODED VALUE
13–15	>89	10–29	4
9–12	76–89	>29	3
6–8	50–75	6–9	2
4–5	1–49	1–5	1
3	0	0	0

[a]$RTS = 0.9368 GCS_c + 0.7326 SPP_c + 0.2908 RR_c$ where the subscript c refers to coded value.
(From Feliciano DV, Moore EE, Mattox KL (eds): Trauma, 3rd ed. Norwalk, CT, Appleton & Lange, 1996, with permission.)

7. What is a major weakness of the TS and RTS?

Although these physiologic scores offer the ease of quick tabulation for patient triage in the field, they both rely on an accurate GCS score and respiratory rate. The GCS and respiratory rate are frequently difficult to assess because of a number of conditions. For example, drugs, alcohol, hemorrhage, or airway problems can prevent an accurate GCS and respiratory rate from being obtained. Despite this limitation, the RTS continues to show good specificity and sensitivity in many studies.

8. What is the Pediatric Trauma Score (PTS)?

The PTS is a combined scoring system using both physiologic and anatomic data (weight, airway, SBP, central nervous system, open wound, skeletal). The values range from −6 to 12. Studies recommend patients with a score of 8 or less should be managed at a level I pediatric trauma center. Subsequent studies have shown that, statistically, the PTS has no predictive advantage over the RTS.

9. What is the Glasgow Coma Scale (GCS)? How is it used in trauma patient scoring?

The GCS is an instrument used to quantify a patient's level of consciousness. The components of the GCS are eye opening, verbal response, and motor response (see table). To determine the GCS, the patient's best response in each category is assessed and matched to the numeric score. The three scores are summed to obtain the GCS score. The highest possible GCS score is 15. The lowest possible score is 3. Clinically, serial assessments are frequently done to detect trends in neurologic improvement or deterioration in the patient's level of consciousness.

Glasgow Coma Scale

VARIABLE	PATIENT RESPONSE	SCORE
Eye Opening	Spontaneous	4
	To voice	3
	To pain	2
	None	1

(*continued*)

Glasgow Coma Scale (Continued)

VARIABLE	PATIENT RESPONSE	SCORE
Verbal response	Oriented	5
	Confused	4
	Inappropriate	3
	Incomprehensible	2
	None	1
Motor response	Obeys verbal commands	6
	Localizes (to pain)	5
	Withdraws (to pain, flexion)	4
	Flexion (to pain, decorticate)	3
	Extension (to pain, decerebrate)	2
	None	1

10. Can GCS be used to classify brain injury?

Yes. GCS is used to classify brain injury as follows:

Mild brain injury = GCS 13–15

Moderate brain injury = GCS 9–12

Severe brain injury and coma = GCS 8 or less

The widespread use of the GCS has made possible the comparison of homogeneous groups of head-injured patients, thus enabling further research into the evaluation and prediction of outcome of this group.

11. Describe the Abbreviated Injury Severity (AIS) scoring system.

The AIS is an anatomic scoring system used to calculate the ISS. It was first developed in 1971 and, since then, has been revised several times. The AIS identifies six body regions and uses a 6-point ordinal scale to classify severity. The **six body regions** are head and neck, face, thorax, abdomen and pelvic contents, extremities, and external. The **6-point ordinal scale** identifies the severity of each respective injury:

1 = minor
2 = moderate
3 = severe but not life threatening

4 = severe and life threatening
5 = critical, survival uncertain
6 = unsurvivable

12. What is the major limitation of the AIS? What system was designed to compensate for this limitation?

AIS only classifies individual injuries and thus does not accurately reflect the severity of multiple system injury. The ISS was developed to account for multiple system injury using the AIS. Each injury is assigned an AIS score and is then grouped into one of the six body regions. The three body regions with the highest scores (excluding a score of 6) are then squared and summed to get the ISS. A score of 6 is not squared as just described but rather is automatically calculated as ISS 75, an unsurvivable injury.

13. What are two major limitations of ISS?

ISS is a poor indicator of injury severity and probability of survival when multiple injuries occur in one body region *or* when severe isolated head injury is present. In both scenarios, the ISS will be falsely low. This underappreciation of injury severity occurs because the ISS calculations include only the *highest* AIS in each of three body regions (see question 14 for an example). For example, if a patient has multiple intra-abdominal injuries but no other system injury, only the highest abdominal injury can be used to calculate the ISS. Thus, the ISS does not reflect the severity of the patient's injury condition. In the case of a patient with isolated head injury, the maximum AIS is 5 (ISS of 25) despite potentially lethal cranial injury. Furthermore, injuries of similar AIS scores do not predict the same mortality. For example, a splenic rupture has the same score as an open comminuted humerus fracture.

14. Give an example of the AIS and ISS for a multiply injured patient.

REGION	INJURY DESCRIPTION	AIS	AIS SQUARED	THREE HIGHEST AIS
1. Head and neck	Subdural hematoma, small, < 30 ml	4	16	16
2. Face	Le Fort II fracture	2	4	
3. Chest	Unilateral hemothorax	3	9	9
4. Abdomen	Lacerated colon, partial thickness	2	4	
	Lacerated duodenum, full thickness	4	16	25
	Splenic laceration, moderate	3	9	
	Major mesenteric laceration	3	9	
	Massive avulsion of the pancreas	5	25	
5. Extremity	Femur fracture	3	9	
6. External	Lower extremity contusions	1	9	
			Total	50

As you can see from the above example, the three highest AIS scores for three body regions are selected and tabulated to yield an ISS of 50. This is a very high score and reflects major injury. However, despite the multiple serious abdomen injuries, only the single worst injury can be used in the calculation, illustrating one of the limitations of ISS in accurately reflecting injury severity.

15. What was the ISS for President Kennedy? How about for President Reagan after falling from a horse and sustaining a delayed subdural hematoma? Or the actor Christopher Reeve who sustained a spinal cord injury?

President Kennedy sustained two penetrating injuries, one to the head and one to the neck. The AIS for penetrating cranial injury is 5, so the ISS for a single penetrating head injury alone would be just 25. A penetrating neck wound without further details has an AIS of 1, thus yielding a total ISS of 26. While this ISS indicates a serious injury, it does not describe the true severity or potential lethality of the injury. Additionally, the lack of detailed autopsy data and description of anatomic injury limits accurate scoring. President Reagan's head injury is another example of how ISS underappreciates the potential severity of an injury. The severity of a subdural hematoma is determined by the clot size in milliliters. Often this size detail is not documented. The AIS for a small (< 50 ml of blood) subdural hematoma is 4, which translates to an ISS of 16. A large (> 50 ml) subdural hematoma yields an AIS of 5 (ISS 25), assuming no other injuries. Christopher Reeve sustained a complete, high cervical cord injury. ISS is determined by the level of the cervical injury. Complete cervical spinal cord injury at C3 or below is an AIS of 6 and ISS of 75, a "nonsurvivable injury." The following table summarizes the above conditions.

Samples of Isolated Head and Spine Injury Scores

INJURY DESCRIPTION	AIS	ISS
Penetrating head injury	5	25
Subdural hematoma < 50 ml	4	16
Subdural hematoma > 50 ml	5	25
Crush skull and brain	6	75
Complete cervical spinal cord injury C4 and below (with or without dislocation, fracture)	5	25
Complete cervical spinal cord injury C3 and above (with or without dislocation or fracture)	6	75

16. Why are autopsy data so important in trauma scoring?

The lack of a full surgical autopsy for trauma victims is a major cause of incomplete mortality data and, therefore, incomplete injury severity scores. The incomplete data are used to calculate the probability of survival, leading to results that are illogical. In most cases, particularly blunt injury from a motor vehicle crash, it is impossible to accurately calculate the ISS without an autopsy. The trauma surgeon should ensure an autopsy is ordered for all trauma deaths. This is especially critical for those cases where the details of anatomic injury are not known. Trauma death due to blunt injury is the most common emergency department situation for which needed autopsies are not requested. Autopsy data can have a dramatic impact on the ISS and accuracy of predictions of probability of survival. It is for these reasons that the availability of complete mortality data is so important. The future of trauma research and the quality improvement review process rely on these data to direct and optimize care.

17. What is the physician's role in trauma data collection and injury scoring systems?

Accurate injury scoring depends on detailed descriptions of a patient's clinical condition and anatomic injury data. By diligent attention to thorough documentation, physicians can play a significant role in the quality of data collected and used in these scoring systems. Consider, for example, the AIS for a liver laceration. If the physician's injury description is minimal, such as "liver laceration" without further detail, the AIS is 2 (ISS 4). However, the same liver injury described in more detail by the physician might include "moderate liver laceration > 3 cm deep and > 20% blood loss." This description would result in a higher AIS of 4 (ISS 16). Therefore, detailed documentation is necessary to accurately score the severity of injury. If data collection is poor, scientific endeavors to evaluate trauma care are hampered.

18. What is the Major Trauma Outcome Study (MTOS)?

MTOS is a large trauma database established to evaluate many aspects of trauma care nationwide. Numerous trauma centers from across North America contributed information on thousands of trauma cases to a central registry over a period beginning in 1982 and lasting through 1989. The primary goals of the registry were to establish outcome values for quality of care and to enable institutions to objectively evaluate and compare patient outcome data. The large size of the MTOS database made possible the evaluation of combined scoring systems known as TRISS. MTOS contributed greatly to the knowledge currently used to evaluate care.

19. What scoring system is used to predict probability of survival?

TRISS methodology. Commonly referred to simply as TRISS, this method draws relationships among the ISS, RTS, age, and mechanism of injury (blunt or penetrating). The combination of ISS and TS or TRS yields more accurate prediction of probability of survival based on outcome data from the MTOS. The information can be represented on a graph, as shown at the top of the next page. Nonsurvivors below the diagonal line on this graph represent "unexpected deaths." Such cases would prompt peer review by a multidisciplinary quality improvement committee to identify opportunities to improve care. Those deaths above the line represent unexpected survivors or "great saves."

CONTROVERSY

20. What is ICISS?

In recent years some trauma specialists have become more critical about the predictive value of ISS and TRISS. One of the major disadvantages of these systems is the GCS. The GCS is a major component of the RTS, yet it cannot be performed well on many of the sickest patients. This limitation has prompted certain researchers to pursue other tools for predicting survival. Rutledge and colleagues used ICD-9-CM codes to describe severity of anatomic injury. Their data show better predictive value for outcome than the ISS. This model is called ICISS, reflecting the combination of ICD-9-CM codes and Injury Severity Analysis. Critics of the study report limited use of only the most lethal diagnoses, small study sample size, and insufficient information for individual institutions to apply the model. Since the initial paper, Rutledge and colleagues recently reported on findings that extend beyond evaluating survival predictions by comparing the ICISS scoring system's ability to predict hospital charges and length of stay. They cite the cost of collecting ISS and TRISS data combined with the poor predictive quality as reasons for using the new ICISS scoring system described in their studies. ICISS is currently being tested in numerous states nationwide.

Trauma Scoring Systems

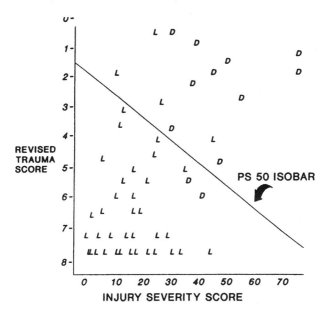

From Feliciano DV, Moore Ee, Mattox KL (eds): Trauma, 3rd ed. Norwalk, CT, Appleton & Lange, 1996, with permission.

BIBLIOGRAPHY

1. American College of Surgeons Committee on Trauma: Resources for Optimal Care of the Injured Patient: 1993. Chicago, American College of Surgeons, 1993.
2. Association for the Advancement of Automotive Medicine: The Abbreviated Injury Scale—1990 Revision. Des Plaines, IL, AAAM, 1985.
3. Baker SP, O'Neill B: The Injury Severity Score: An update. J Trauma 16:822, 1986.
4. Baker SP, O'Neill B, Haddon W Jr, Long WB: The Injury Severity Score: A method for describing patients with multiple injuries and evaluating emergency care. J Trauma 14:187, 1974.
5. Boyd CR, Tolson MA, Copes WS:Evaluating trauma care: The TRISS method. J Trauma 27:370–378, 1987.
6. Champion HR, Sacco WJ, Carnazzo AJ, Copes W, Fouty WJ: Trauma score. Crit Care Med 9:672–676, 1981.
7. Champion HR, Sacco WJ, Copes WS, et al: A revision of the Trauma Score. J Trauma 29:623–629, 1989.
8. Champion HR, Sacco WJ, Hannan DS, et al: Assessment of injury severity: The triage index. Crit Care Med 8:201–208, 1980.
9. Champion HR, Sacco WJ, Lepper RL, et al: An anatomic index of injury severity. J Trauma 20:197–202, 1980.
10. Copes WS, Champion HR, Saco WJ, et al: The Injury Severity Score revisited. J Trauma 28:69–77, 1988.
11. Gormican SP: CRAMS scale: Field triage of trauma victims. Ann Emerg Med 11:132–135, 1982.
12. Jennett B, Teasdale G, Braakman R, et al; Predicting outcome in individual patients after severe head injury. Lancet 1:1031–1034, 1976.
13. Knaus WA, Draper EA, Wagner DP, Zimmerman JE: APACHE II: A severity of disease classification system. Crit Care Med 13:818–829, 1985.

14. Knaus WA, Zimmerman JE, Wagner DP, et al: APACHE—Acute physiology and chronic health evaluation: A physiologically based classification system. Crit Care Med 9:591–597, 1981.
15. Rutledge R, Fakhry S, Baker C, Oller D: Injury severity grading in trauma patients: A simplified technique based upon ICD-9 coding. J Trauma 35:497–506, 1993.
16. Rutledge R, Osler T, Emery S, Kromhout-Schiro S: The end of ISS and TRISS: An ICD-9–based prediction tool, "ICISS," outperforms both ISS and TRISS as predictors of trauma patient survival, hospital charges, and length of stay. Presented at the 57th annual meeting of the American Association
for the Surgery of Trauma, Waikoloa, HI, September 24–27, 1997.
17. Teasdale G, Jennett B: Assessment of coma and impaired consciousness. A practical scale. Lancet 2:
81–84, 1974.
18. Tepas JJ 3rd, Mollitt DL, Talbert JL, Bryant M: The Pediatric Trauma Score as a predictor of injury severity in the injured child. J Pediatr Surg 22:14–18, 1987.

3. AIRWAY MANAGEMENT IN TRAUMA

Sujal Mandavia, M.D., and Diku Mandavia, M.D.

1. What are some general indications for intubation in the trauma patient?
Remember that the status of trauma patients is dynamic and that anticipation of any indication occurring in the near future should prompt airway management:
- Severely depressed level of consciousness, as in a severely head-injured patient (Glasgow Coma Score ≤9), demands airway management because airway reflexes often are lacking in these patients, making aspiration a potential problem.
- Protection of the airway may be effected to protect from aspiration, as in a patient with no gag reflex, or in the setting of impending obstruction, as in a patient with an expanding neck hematoma or with an inhalation injury. In these patients, delayed airway management may not be successful as the airway becomes more edematous and distorted.
- Therapeutic mild hyperventilation, as in the severely head-injured patient with elevated intracranial pressure, is an indication for airway management.
- Augmentation of ventilation, oxygenation, or both may be needed, as in the patient with flail chest and pulmonary contusion whose oxygenation or ventilation is failing.
- Facilitation of adjunctive diagnostic tests may be warranted for many trauma patients with potentially life-threatening injuries who are so agitated and combative that important imaging (e.g., scans for cervical spine clearance, computed tomography) cannot be obtained until the patient is sedated, paralyzed, and intubated.

2. What equipment is necessary for airway management in the trauma patient?
The following minimal equipment should be ready when any critical trauma patient is evaluated:
- Nonrebreathing masks connected to high-flow oxygen
- Bag-valve-mask ventilation with oxygen setup
- Pharyngeal airways, oral and nasal
- Laryngoscopes, multiple sizes with curved and straight blades
- Endotracheal tubes and stylets, multiple sizes
- Magill forceps to deal with foreign objects in the airway
- Yankauer suction
- End-tidal CO_2 detector or esophageal detector device for confirmation of tube placement
- Cricothyroidotomy equipment, including a scalpel, tracheostomy tube or small endotracheal tube (e.g., size 6), and tracheal hooks
- Drugs to facilitate intubation including sedative and paralytic agents

3. How is the pediatric airway different than the adult airway?
The pediatric airway is different from the adult airway in 10 important ways:
1. The head is proportionally larger, resulting in a natural "sniffing" position; a towel below the head to align the airway axes is therefore unnecessary.
2. The infant is an obligate nasal breather.
3. The mouth aperture is smaller, with a proportionately larger tongue and lymphoid tissue, making visualization more difficult.
4. The larynx is smaller and more anterior, obscuring visualization.
5. The cricothyroid membrane is much smaller so that only *needle* cricothyroidotomy can be performed in a small child.
6. The epiglottis is longer and floppier, often necessitating a straight blade to lift it out of view.

7. The cricoid is the narrowest part of the airway in children younger than 10 years, and cuffed tubes are unnecessary in most cases.

8. The mainstem bronchi bifurcation is symmetric, and right and left mainstem intubations are equally common.

9. Because of the small airway dimensions, mainstem intubation or extubation is more likely with minimal head motion.

10. Laryngeal manipulation in children often leads to significant bradycardia due to vagal stimulation. Atropine should be used as a premedication in children 6 years or younger to prevent this bradycardia.

4. What size endotracheal tube is needed in an adult or in a 6-year-old child?

A 7.5-mm tube suffices for most adult emergencies, with a 7.0-mm tube used for smaller adults and an 8.0-mm tube for larger patients. For children, the formula for endotracheal tube size is (age/4) + 4. A 6-year-old child would need a 5.5-mm tube. A rough guide for children is to choose an endotracheal tube that is the size of the patient's little finger. Always have one size smaller and larger tubes available and ready when intubating the patient.

5. What is rapid sequence intubation (RSI), and why is it performed?

RSI is the sequential administration of a sedative or anesthetic along with a neuromuscular blocking agent to facilitate endotracheal intubation while minimizing risk of aspiration. This combination of sedation and brief paralysis provides the optimal environment for emergency airway management from a variety of causes. RSI has several advantages:

Adequate sedation
Full muscle relaxation to facilitate vocal cord visualization atraumatically
Decreased risk of pulmonary aspiration
Minimal deleterious hemodynamic and intracranial pressure changes
High degree of success in placing an endotracheal tube

6. What are the proper steps in performing rapid sequence intubation (RSI)?

The steps can be summarized by the "6 Ps" as outlined below:

Prepare: Ensure all equipment is ready, including different sizes of blades and tubes and equipment to perform an emergency cricothyroidotomy. Preparation also involves evaluation of the airway anatomy before paralyzation. This helps to predict a difficult intubation and may change the plans for paralysis.

Preoxygenate: Five minutes of preoxygenation with 100% O_2 by a nonrebreathing mask is ideal to ventilate nitrogen from the lungs. If the entire lung volume is oxygen, up to 5 minutes of apnea can be experienced without hypoxia. In more emergent intubations, three full bag-valve-mask ventilations before intubation can also accomplish this. Assisted ventilation is needed to provide oxygenation and ventilation in the apneic patient.

Pretreat: Certain drugs should be given before the paralyzation. A priming dose of pancuronium (0.02 mg/kg) is given intravenously to help decrease fasciculations and other complications when using succinylcholine. Intravenous lidocaine (1.5 mg/kg) helps to decrease intracranial pressure associated with succinylcholine and laryngeal manipulation. An amnestic or sedative agent is necessary if the patient is awake, and a variety of medications are used, including midazolam, thiopental, fentanyl, or etomidate. The Sellick maneuver should be applied just before the paralytic agent is given to prevent passive regurgitation from the esophagus.

Paralyze: Paralysis is most often accomplished with the use of succinylcholine (1.5 mg/kg) because it acts rapidly (about 45 seconds) and has a short duration of action, which is usually less than 10 minutes. Nondepolarizing drugs that can be used are vecuronium, atracurium, and rocuronium.

Pass the tube: With an assistant providing in-line stabilization to prevent cervical spine movement, the endotracheal tube is passed through the vocal cords. Throughout intubation, pulse oximetry is closely watched. If hypoxia develops, further attempts are halted, and the patient is managed by bag-valve-mask ventilation until the hypoxia resolves. Throughout this period, the physician should always be ready to intervene with a surgical airway if subsequent oral attempts are unsuccessful or the patient cannot be managed with bag-valve-mask ventilation.

Postintubation assessment: This step is essential because an unrecognized esophageal intubation is universally fatal. Auscultate over the epigastrium to detect esophageal intubation, and then listen over the anterior chest and axilla to confirm intratracheal tube placement. End-tidal CO_2 detection is considered standard but may be falsely negative in extremely low-flow states such as cardiac arrest, and an esophageal detector is better in this circumstance. An arterial blood gas determination to assess oxygenation and ventilation and a chest radiograph for endotracheal tube placement should be obtained after every intubation.

7. What are the contraindications to RSI?

RSI should be avoided in patients with significantly distorted anatomy that would make oral intubation difficult. In this group of patients, "awake" intubation (with the use of a sedative) or fiberoptic intubation is preferred. This contraindication stresses the need for proper airway evaluation before performing RSI. Never take a patient's airway away with paralysis unless you know you can give it back to him or her.

8. What is succinylcholine?

Succinylcholine is a depolarizing, neuromuscular-blocking agent that is commonly used for RSI. It causes paralysis within 45 seconds, and the effects last less than 10 minutes. No other neuromuscular-blocking agent acts so quickly and lasts for so short a period. Its brief duration of action facilitates serial neurologic examinations in the CNS-injured patient.

9. What are the complications of and contraindications for succinylcholine?

Complications:
  Rise in serum potassium level (about 0.5 mEq/L)
  Increased intracranial pressure
  Increased intragastric pressure
  Increased intraocular pressure
  Rhabdomyolysis (rare)
  Malignant hyperthermia
  Fracture displacement from muscle contractions
Contraindications:
  Bag-valve-mask ventilation impossible because of airway distortion
  Known or suspected hyperkalemia
  Burn or crush injury more than 48 hours after injury
  Chronic denervating diseases
  Penetrating eye injuries
  Renal failure (relative contraindication) because of possibility of preexisting hyperkalemia

Despite these complications and contraindications, succinylcholine remains the neuromuscular blocking agent of choice in most emergency intubations. Pretreatment with a minidose (10% of paralyzing dose) of a nondepolarizing paralytic agent (e.g., pancuronium, vecuronium) can help alleviate complications such as fasciculations or muscle contractions.

10. What adjunctive medications help decrease intracranial pressure during intubation?

The following medications are useful in helping blunt the intracranial pressure rise with intubation: lidocaine, thiopental (or other barbiturates), etomidate, fentanyl, and propofol.

11. What steps are necessary for confirmation of endotracheal tube placement?

1. Direct visualization during intubation
2. Auscultation at the axilla and epigastrium

   3. End-tidal CO_2 detection or esophageal detector device
   4. Chest radiograph to determine depth of intubation *but not* esophageal intubation

12. What are initial ventilator settings after intubation?
The following adult settings are standard:
   Ventilator mode: assist-control
   Respiratory rate: 12 to 14/min or higher if hyperventilation is indicated
   Tidal volume: 7 to 10 mL/kg
   FiO_2: 100% to start; adjust as necessary with serial arterial blood gas determinations

13. What anatomic features predict difficult oral intubation?
   Short neck
   Prominent upper incisors
   Receding mandible
   Limited jaw opening ($<$4 cm or about 3 finger widths)
   Macroglossia
   Thyroid-mental distance of less than 4 cm (i.e., 3 finger widths)

14. What injuries predict difficult oral intubations?
Several injuries distort airway anatomy or cause significant airway hemorrhage, making oral intubation difficult:
   Blunt laryngotracheal injuries
   Penetrating neck injuries, especially with expanding hematomas
   Severe midface fractures, especially Le Fort III fractures, causing bleeding and collapse
      of airway support
   Mandible fractures causing problems similar to those of facial fractures
   Acute inhalation injuries causing rapid and significant airway edema

15. If oral intubation is unsuccessful, what options are available?
Blind nasal intubation is rarely used in modern airway management because the success rate is not high and the technique requires a spontaneously breathing patient.

Fiberoptic intubation is an excellent technique, especially in those with distorted airway anatomy. Unfortunately, it requires special expertise, and the equipment may not be readily available.

Retrograde wire intubation is an option in the patient who remains oxygenated with bag-valve-ventilation. The technique involves the placement of a guide wire through the cricothyroid membrane. The wire is advanced cephalad to the oropharynx and is used to guide an endotracheal tube into the trachea.

Digital intubation can be used in patients with little or no muscle tone. In this technique, the endotracheal tube is placed by tactile guidance through the vocal cords.

Jet ventilation involves the placement of a large-bore needle through the cricothyroid membrane and connection to a high-pressure oxygen source. Oxygenation is improved, but ventilation often remains poor, limiting the duration of its use.

Cricothyroidotomy is most often the procedure of choice after unsuccessful oral intubation. The surgical technique is relatively straightforward and requires equipment available in any emergency department.

Tracheostomy is the surgical airway of choice when cricothyroidotomy is contraindicated. This technique requires special training and takes significantly more time than cricothyroidotomy, even in experienced hands.

Laryngeal mask airway can be used to temporize the airway until further help arrives or another technique is used. It consists of a pharyngeal tube with a distal balloon that fits over the laryngeal inlet. It is inserted blindly with a very high success rate. Although the laryngeal mask does not protect against aspiration, it can provide temporary oxygenation and ventilation.

16. What are the indications for a surgical airway?

The single most important indication is the inability to orally intubate a patient because of conditions such as severe maxillofacial trauma, massive airway hemorrhage, anatomic variants, and oropharyngeal obstruction.

17. What are the contraindications to cricothyroidotomy?

There are no absolute contraindications to cricothyroidotomy. Relative contraindications include penetrating neck injuries, laryngotracheal injuries, and a bleeding diathesis. Needle cricothyroidotomy is recommended in children younger than 10 years.

18. Which surgical airway—cricothyroidotomy or tracheostomy—is preferred in emergency airway management?

Cricothyroidotomy is preferred for most cases for several reasons:
- Much faster than tracheostomy, therefore minimizing potential hypoxic insult
- Technically easier to perform
- Safer operation with fewer complications, especially when performed under emergency circumstances

Tracheostomy is reserved for patients with laryngotracheal injuries and pediatric patients in which needle cricothyroidotomy is unsuccessful.

19. What are the landmarks for a cricothyroidotomy? Describe the basic procedure.

The thyroid cartilage, or "Adam's apple," is usually easily identified by visualization or palpation. Just inferior to this site lies the cricoid cartilage, which is usually palpable:

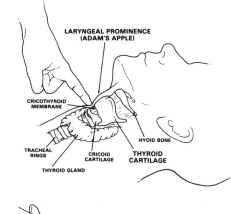

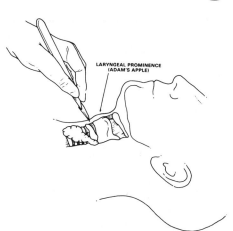

Between these cartilages lays the cricothyroid membrane, where a vertical skin incision is made.

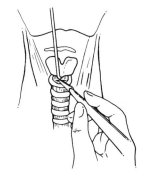

The cricothyroid membrane is identified, and a horizontal incision is made.

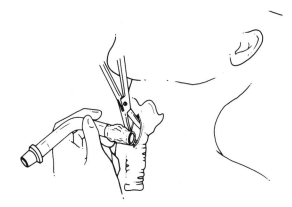

A small endotracheal tube (5.0 mm) or tracheostomy tube (Shiley no. 4) is then placed into the trachea.

(All figure parts from Roberts JR, Hedges JR: Clinical Procedures in Emergency Medicine. Philadelphia, WB Saunders, 1991, with permission.)

Confirmation of endotracheal placement is then performed in the usual manner.

20. What is the preferred technique for airway management in the patient with a cervical spine fracture?

Because it was previously thought that orotracheal intubation caused excessive motion of the cervical spine, nasotracheal intubation and surgical airways were the preferred techniques. However, it has since been shown that proper in-line stabilization of the neck adequately immobilizes the cervical spine during direct laryngoscopy, and orotracheal intubation with in-line stabilization is now the procedure of choice.

21. A patient suddenly decompensates shortly after intubation. What are the possible causes?

- Hypoxia: esophageal intubation, inadequate preoxygenation, prolonged intubation attempts, or right or left mainstem intubation
- Decreased venous return secondary to excessive bagging
- Tension pneumothorax
- Medication side effect
- Air embolism
- Vasovagal response (rare)

22. What are the differences between pediatric and adult prehospital airway management?

In addition to the intrinsic anatomic differences, prehospital pediatric airway management is fundamentally different from that for adults. (They are not just small adults!) A large, randomized trial showed no benefit from prehospital endotracheal intubation (ETI) compared with adequate bag-valve-mask (BVM) ventilation. Because pediatric ETI is difficult under the most controlled circumstances and BVM ventilation is associated with fewer complications, it is reasonable to train paramedics only in the art of BVM for pediatric patients. Reports on the benefit of prehospital ETI in adults are mixed, but the literature does show a trend toward improved outcomes, suggesting that intubation is helpful if it does not prolong transport time.

23. What are common airway devices used in the prehospital phase?

Depending on your locale and the sophistication of your emergency medical system, you may encounter any of the below devices:
- Endotracheal tube
- Esophageal obturator airway (EOA)
- Combitube
- Laryngeal mask airway (LMA)

24. What is an esophageal obturator airway (EOA)?

An EOA is a face mask attached to a 37-cm-long plastic tube with perforations at the level of the pharynx and a cuff at the distal end. The cuffed end is blindly passed into the esophagus and inflated to prevent air entry into the stomach and regurgitation of gastric contents into the airway. It should be used only in patients without a gag reflex. When properly placed, the patient can be ventilated through the mask and the perforations until a definitive airway can be established. This modality has fallen out of favor because of its high incidence of major complications.

25. What is a combitube?

A combitube is a double-lumen airway that is inserted blindly through the mouth. It should be used only in a patient with no gag reflex. Unlike the EOA, this tube can be passed into the esophagus or the trachea. In most cases, the distal end is placed in the esophagus. The clinician then assesses the location of the tube and can selectively ventilate the lumen that provides inflation of the lungs. The combitube has essentially replaced the EOA.

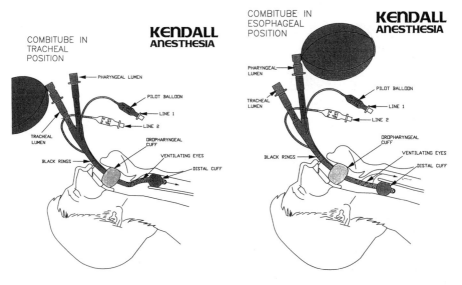

Combitube: trachael and esophageal positions. (Courtesy of Kendall Anesthesia, Mansfield, MA.)

26. What is a laryngeal mask airway (LMA)?

An LMA is a conventional endotracheal tube in which the distal end has been modified by the placement of a miniature inflatable mask designed to fit over the laryngeal inlet. The LMA can be lifesaving for patients who are difficult to intubate or ventilate, and it bridges the gap in airway management between bag-valve-mask ventilation and tracheal intubation. This device is inserted blindly into the pharynx so that the distal end, once inflated, forms a low-pressure seal around the laryngeal inlet. It is minimally stimulating to the airway, avoiding the undesirable effects of laryngoscopy. Medical and paramedical personnel have demonstrated the ability to place the LMA with a high rate of success and a low rate of complications. Most importantly, the LMA has an excellent clinical track record in "cannot ventilate, cannot intubate" situations. The LMA is widely recognized as a major advancement in airway management and has been incorporated into the American Society of Anesthesiologists' difficult airway algorithm.

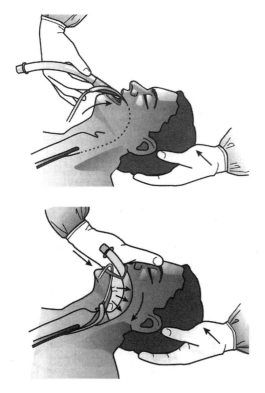

(Courtesy of LMA North America Inc., San Diego, CA.)

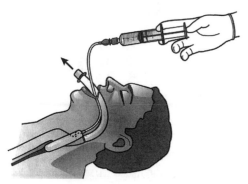

27. Can pupillary reflexes be evaluated in the head-injured patient after paralysis for intubation?

Yes! All currently used depolarizing and nondepolarizing agents preserve pupillary reflexes, enabling continued examination during paralysis.

28. What are the differences in airway management in the pregnant trauma patient?

Pregnancy, especially in the third term, produces physiologic changes that can alter emergency airway management. Pregnancy is associated with a much higher risk of aspiration because of the gravid uterus, delayed gastric emptying, and decreased lower esophageal sphincter function. Lung functional residual capacity (FRC) is decreased in pregnancy, leading to a shorter apnea time without hypoxia. Because of retained fluid, airway edema may be present or easily induced by laryngeal manipulation, and the use of a laryngoscope is often more difficult because of the larger breast size. Chronic respiratory alkalosis is induced by the progesterone state and may be identified on the arterial blood gas determination.

29. What are the two main adverse physiologic responses to laryngeal manipulation and endotracheal intubation? How can they be prevented?

The *hemodynamic response* results from a sympathetic outflow during intubation leading to increased blood pressure and heart rate. It may cause significant morbidity or mortality in those with poor cardiac reserves, such as the elderly. If unchecked, it may lead to myocardial ischemia or to infarction, arrhythmia, or stroke. It may be prevented or blunted by pretreating the patient with agents such as narcotics (e.g., fentanyl), thiopental, or etomidate.

The *intracranial pressure response* occurs when laryngeal manipulation and intubation cause a significant rise in intracranial pressure (ICP), which can be deleterious in those with preexisting ICP, such as head-injured patients. The ICP response is blunted by barbiturates (e.g., thiopental), etomidate, fentanyl, lidocaine, or propofol.

BIBLIOGRAPHY

1. American Society of Anesthesiologists: Practice guidelines for management of the difficult airway. Anesthesiology 78:597, 1993.
2. Benumof JL: Laryngeal mask airway and the ASA difficult airway algorithm. Anesthesiology 84: 686–699, 1996.
3. Benumof JL: Management of the difficult adult airway. Anesthesiology 75:1087, 1991.
4. Criswell JC, Parr MJ, Nolan JP: Emergency airway management in patients with cervical spine injuries. Anaesthesia 49:900–903, 1994.
5. Dailey RH, Simon B, Young GP, et al: The Airway: Emergency Management. St Louis, Mosby–Year Book, 1992.
6. Eckstein M: Effect of prehospital advanced life support on outcomes of major trauma patients. J Trauma 48:643–648, 2000.
7. Gausche M, Lewis RJ, Stratton SJ: Effect of out-of-hospital pediatric endotracheal intubation on survival and neurological outcome: A controlled clinical trial. JAMA 283:783–790, 2000.
8. Roberts JR, Hedges JR: Clinical Procedures in Emergency Medicine. Philadelphia, WB Saunders, 1991.
9. Rosenblatt W: The intubating laryngeal mask: Use of a new ventilating-intubating device in the emergency department. Ann Emerg Med 33:234–238, 1999.
10. Rotondo MF, McGonigal MD, Schwab W, et al: Urgent paralysis and intubation of trauma patients: Is it safe? J Trauma 34:242, 1993.
11. Salvino CK, Dries D, Gamelli R, et al: Emergency cricothyroidotomy in trauma victims. J Trauma 34: 503, 1993.
12. Walls RM: Rapid sequence intubation in head trauma. Ann Emerg Med 22:1008, 1993.
13. Yardy N: A comparison of two airway aids for emergency use by unskilled personnel: The Combitube and laryngeal mask. Anaesthesia 54:181–183, 1999.

4. SHOCK AND RESUSCITATION

Frederic S. Bongard, M.D.

1. Define shock.

Shock is a condition in which the cardiovascular system is no longer able to meet the body's metabolic and oxygen needs. Note that this definition does *not* include blood pressure limits. Although many practitioners believe that shock exists when the systolic blood pressure falls below 80 mmHg, some patients will still be able to maintain relatively normal metabolic function below this level.

2. What are the physiologic groups into which shock is divided?

Shock states are usually described by their etiology and physiology and can be segregated into three categories: hypovolemic, distributive, and cardiac.

3. What is the most common etiology of shock among injured patients?

Hypovolemic shock due to hemorrhage is, by far, the most common cause of shock among trauma patients.

4. How is total body water distributed?

Total body water constitutes approximately 70% of an adult's weight and is divided into three compartments:
1. Intravascular (7% of total body weight)
2. Interstitial (21% of total body weight)
3. Intracellular (42% of total body weight)

The intravascular portion constitutes blood circulation and is that portion of body water that we usually think of when a patient is hypovolemic. The interstitial and intracellular compartments together comprise the extravascular space.

5. What factors influence the movement of fluid between the different body compartments?

The balance of fluid shifts between the intravascular and extravascular spaces is governed by Starling's law, which relates net flux to differences in hydrostatic and osmotic pressure.

$$Q^{\cdot} = K[(P_c - P_i) - \rho(\pi_c - \pi_i)]$$

where $Q^{\cdot}$ is fluid flux, $(P_c - P_i)$ is the hydrostatic pressure gradient, $(\pi_c - \pi_i)$ is the osmotic pressure gradient, K is the permeability coefficient, and ρ is the reflection coefficient.

Usually, intravascular hydrostatic pressure (approximately equal to mean blood pressure) is greater than interstitial hydrostatic pressure, and fluid tends to move from the intravascular space into the interstitial space. Interstitial osmotic pressure, however, is usually less than intravascular osmotic pressure, thus favoring the movement of fluid back into the capillaries. When hypovolemia occurs, intravascular pressure falls, decreasing the hydrostatic gradient. This facilitates the movement of water from the interstitial space into the intravascular space. This vascular refill phenomenon is limited by an increase in extravascular osmotic pressure as fluid leaves the interstitial space. The degree of translocation is limited to a total of about 1–2 liters.

6. Is a change in the hematocrit a useful measure of the amount of acute blood loss?

No. Hematocrit is a measure of that portion of total blood volume that is composed of red blood cells. Recall that hematocrit is expressed as a percentage. If no exogenous fluid is given (e.g., blood cell free resuscitation fluid), a decrease in hematocrit depends on the refill of the intravascular space from the interstitial space and not on the loss of red blood cells.

A simple way to convince yourself of this is to think back to college chemistry where you were presented with the problem of a beaker that contained a dye solution of known concentration. If a spigot was opened and part of the solution drained, the concentration of the remaining solution would be the same—only the volume would be different. If the beaker was then filled with water, which contains no dye, the volume of solution in the beaker would return to normal but the concentration of dye particles within the beaker would decrease.

When a trauma victim loses blood, the concentration of red blood cells in the intravascular space remains the same until refill from the interstitial space begins (about 20–30 minutes) or until blood free solution is given intravenously. If you were to remove 2 liters of blood from a patient's arm over 10 minutes, the hematocrit would be the same as before phlebotomy. At 1 hour, however, after refill had begun, the hematocrit would be substantially lower.

7. What are the clinical features of mild blood loss ($< 20\%$ blood volume)?

This degree of volume loss causes a redistribution of blood away from the organs that are the most tolerant of ischemia, such as skin, fat, skeletal muscle, and bone. Organs that are less tolerant of ischemia have preserved blood flow. Clinical features include a subjective sense of cold; postural changes in blood pressure; and pale, cool, and clammy skin. Neck veins are flattened. Urine output decreases and becomes more concentrated.

8. What are the clinical features of moderate blood volume deficit ($20–40\%$)?

Perfusion of all organs decreases, including those less able to tolerate ischemia. Patients complain of thirst, and blood pressure is lower than normal even in the supine position. Oliguria is a prominent feature.

9. What are the clinical features of severe blood volume deficit ($> 40\%$)?

Perfusion decreases to the heart and brain, resulting in critical ischemia. If still conscious, the patient is restless, agitated, and often obtunded. Blood pressure is very low, and the pulse may be "thready." Tachypnea is often present. If hypovolemia is not corrected, cardiac arrest usually results.

10. What is the first physiologic response to hypovolemia?

An increase in heart rate (tachycardia). Remember that cardiac output is the product of heart rate and stroke volume. Stroke volume is the product of end diastolic volume and ejection fraction. Hypovolemia causes a decrease in end diastolic volume and a resultant fall in stroke volume. Therefore, heart rate must increase to return cardiac output to normal.

11. Why do hypovolemic patients feel clammy?

Blood pressure is the product of cardiac output and systemic vascular resistance. Hypovolemia causes a decrease in venous return and an increase in heart rate. The tachycardia may not be able to keep cardiac output constant, however, resulting in a decrease in blood pressure. The response to the decline in blood pressure is an increase in systemic vascular resistance. Vasomotor tone is largely under the influence of the sympathetic nervous system. The generalized sympathetic outflow also causes sweating, which, when combined with the coolness produced by vasoconstriction, results in the classic clammy sensation.

12. What is oxygen content, and what effect does hemorrhage have on it?

The amount of oxygen contained in an aliquot (usually 100 ml) of blood is referred to as the oxygen content. The oxygen content of a deciliter of arterial blood is calculated using the following formula:

$$CaO_2 = 1.34 \cdot Hb \cdot SaO_2 + (0.0031 \cdot PaO_2)$$

where CaO_2 is the arterial oxygen content (in ml/dl), Hb is the hemoglobin concentration (in gm/dl), SaO_2 is the fractional hemoglobin oxygen saturation (e.g., .95 for 95%), and PaO_2 is the partial pressure of oxygen dissolved in the blood. When hemoglobin concentration falls, the oxygen content of the blood decreases even though the saturation and PaO_2 remain constant. The oxygen content of venous blood (CvO_2) is calculated using the same formula, except that venous values are substituted for saturation and partial pressure. The relatively small difference between venous and arterial hemoglobin concentration is clinically unimportant. Normal oxygen content is about 20 ml O_2 per dl.

13. What is oxygen delivery?

Oxygen content simply tells us how much oxygen is present in a given quantity of blood; it tells us nothing about how much oxygen is reaching the tissues. The missing piece is the flow of blood—obtained from the cardiac output. Hence, oxygen delivery is calculated as:

$$DO_2 = CaO2 \cdot CO \cdot 10$$

where DO_2 is the systemic oxygen delivery (in ml/min), CaO_2 is the arterial oxygen content (in ml/dl), and CO is the cardiac output (in L/min). The conversion factor (10) is required because CaO_2 is expressed in ml of oxygen per dl of blood, and cardiac output is measured in liters per minute. Because there are 10 deciliters in a liter, the conversion factor is obtained. Normal oxygen delivery is approximately 1 L O_2 per min.

14. Why does oxygen delivery decrease with hemorrhage?

Oxygen delivery goes down because both the cardiac output and the arterial oxygen content fall.

15. What is systemic oxygen consumption?

Oxygen consumption is a measure of how much oxygen the entire body is using and is calculated by rearranging Fick's equation for cardiac output.

$$VO_2 = (a - v)DO_2 \cdot CO \cdot 10$$

where VO_2 is systemic oxygen consumption (in ml/min), $(a - v)DO_2$ is the arterial minus venous oxygen content (in ml/dl), and CO is cardiac output (in L/min). Normal oxygen consumption is about 250 ml O_2 per min.

16. What happens to systemic oxygen consumption during hypovolemic shock?

This topic is debated among physiologists, but most believe that oxygen consumption remains essentially constant during hypovolemic shock up to a point. This is made possible by increasing extraction of oxygen from the blood that is delivered. At some critical point, increased extraction can no longer keep pace with metabolic demand, and oxygen consumption falls.

17. What is the oxygen extraction ratio?

The oxygen extraction ratio is a measure of the degree of oxygen extraction. Because normal oxygen extraction is about 250 ml/min, and normal oxygen delivery is 1000 ml/min, the extraction ratio is about 25%. Physiologists debate how much extraction can increase before oxygen consumption becomes dependent on oxygen delivery. Clearly, this depends on the patient's premorbid physiology and the degree and acuity of the insult.

18. What effect does hypovolemic shock have on arterial-venous oxygen content difference?

Arterial-venous oxygen content difference reflects how much oxygen is extracted systemically from an aliquot of blood. When hypovolemia and anemia produce a decrease in oxygen delivery, the only way that oxygen consumption can remain constant is to extract more oxygen from the blood that is delivered. This process yields venous blood that is relatively more desaturated than usual. As the venous oxygen content decreases, the arterial-venous oxygen content difference increases. The normal $(a - v)DO_2$ is 5 ml/dl $\pm$ 1 ml/dl. As oxygen delivery falls and extraction increases, $(a - v)DO_2$ increases and often reaches values in excess of 7 ml/dl.

19. What does the term *crystalloid* mean?

Intravenous fluids used for resuscitation can be divided in a number of ways. One of the most useful is to segregate them based on their osmotic activity. Those with little protein (or large molecule) content are referred to as crystalloids, while those containing proteins are called colloids (like albumin or fresh-frozen plasma).

20. How do crystalloids work when given for resuscitation?

Crystalloids, such as normal saline and lactated Ringer's solution, acutely expand the intravascular space and thereby restore circulating blood volume. Because they contain no protein or large molecules, the free water contained in a crystalloid follows diffusion gradients (as defined by Starling's law) and quickly equilibrates with the interstitial and intracellular spaces. Hence, the benefit of rapid volume expansion obtained with these solutions is relatively short lived (1–2 hours), and more volume is required until equilibrium is reached.

21. Are there any advantages to using colloid solutions instead of crystalloids for resuscitation?

The theoretic advantage of colloid solutions is that the water they contain does not diffuse away into the interstitial space. In fact, these large species actually cause fluid to move from the interstitial into the intravascular space. Hence, a relatively small amount of a colloid solution is able to produce a relatively large effect on intravascular volume. The disadvantage is that the volume translocated into the intravascular space ultimately must be replaced. Colloid solutions have one other advantage. On the battlefield, where a medic can carry only a small amount of resuscitation fluid, high-osmolarity solutions such as 3% saline ("hypertonic saline") may be lifesavers. Because only a small amount is required, the medic can carry enough solution to treat a larger number of wounded than he would be able to with other solutions such as lactated Ringer's. In an urban trauma center, however, colloid solutions offer no advantage over crystalloids and are about 100 times more expensive.

22. If a patient is bleeding, why not resuscitate initially with blood?

Besides the obvious limitations of cost, availability, and the risks of hepatitis, HIV, and transfusion reaction, blood is still not a good choice for initial resuscitation. Recall that acute hemorrhage results in a drop in the intravascular hydrostatic pressure. Compensation occurs through capillary refill when interstitial volume moves into the intravascular space. The intracellular space, because of its larger volume, refills the interstitial source. While this compensatory mechanism works well, the fluid debts must be repaid. It is for this reason that crystalloids are chosen as the initial resuscitation fluid—they provide volume to repay these debts. If blood were used initially, subsequent hypotonic fluid would still be required to refill the interstitial and intracellular spaces.

23. What is the preferred resuscitation fluid?

Most authorities prefer lactated Ringer's solutions for initial resuscitation. Normal saline is an acceptable alternative, but its use produces a metabolic acidosis. Recall that the composition of normal saline is 154 mEq of sodium and 154 mEq of chloride. Both are contained in excess of what is normally present in the blood. The chloride presents a particular problem because the kidneys initially excrete bicarbonate in exchange for the chloride. This bicarbonate excretion makes normal saline act like a physiologic acid. Indeed, patients resuscitated with normal saline are readily recognizable the next day because they have elevated sodium and a hyperchloremic metabolic acidosis. Over the course of several days, the kidneys retain bicarbonate and excrete the excess chloride. Lactated Ringer's solution contains 130 mEq of sodium and only 110 mEq of chloride, with the remainder of the anions made up of lactate. The lower chloride concentration does not cause an acidosis, because the lactate is converted to bicarbonate on the first pass through the liver. Unless the patient is in profound shock, giving lactated Ringer's is like giving about half an ampule of bicarbonate. Ringer's lactate also contains a small amount of calcium, which, theoretically, can complex with the preservative in transfused blood, allowing it to clot. This is more a theoretic than real consideration.

24. What measures are used to assess the adequacy of resuscitation?

No single indicator can completely assess the adequacy of resuscitation. Blood pressure and heart rate are suboptimal, because the patient's blood pressure *prior* to injury is usually not known, and persistent tachycardia may be due to agitation or pain from associated injuries. Urine output provides a useful measure, but it takes a relatively long time (about an hour) to determine whether urine output has returned to normal levels. Furthermore, osmotically active substances in the urine, such as sugars or contrast material, will force a diuresis not related to the adequacy of resuscitation. Mentation is an often overlooked but useful measure of resuscitation. When head injury and toxic substances (such as alcohol or drugs) are not present, a return to normal sensorium and the ability to answer questions appropriately indicate adequate cerebral (and probably visceral) perfusion.

25. What is base excess, and how is it useful during resuscitation?

Base excess is calculated by most blood gas laboratories using a nomogram that incorporates the hematocrit, pH, and $PaCO_2$. Normal base excess is 0 ± 2. Base excess provides information on the metabolic component of acidosis. When base excess is negative, base is lacking and a metabolic component is present. Conversely, when base excess is positive, a metabolic alkalosis is present. For example, let's say a patient has a pH of 7.28, a $PaCO_2$ of 40, and a base excess of -6 (a base deficit). The negative base excess indicates that at least part of this patient's acidosis is of metabolic origin. One can calculate how much base would be required to correct the deficit completely using the following formula:

$$\text{mEq base required} = \text{B.E.} \cdot 0.4 \cdot \text{body weight (kg)}$$

Hence, if the patient weighs 70 kg, 168 mEq of bicarbonate would be required to correct the deficit completely ($6 \cdot 0.4 \cdot 70$).

Another patient has a pH of 7.28, $PaCO_2$ of 49, and a base excess of -1.0. Although a slight metabolic acidosis is present, the majority of this patient's acidosis is due to the respiratory component.

Base excess calculations obtained from serial blood gas determinations are very helpful in tracking the adequacy of resuscitation. For example, if a patient's base excess changes from -12 to -8 with resuscitation, progress is being made, but a metabolic component is still present and further resuscitation is required.

26. A patient arrives in the emergency room in shock. After initial resuscitation is begun, a Foley catheter is placed and returns 250 cc of pale urine. Is this patient adequately resuscitated?

You can't tell. The amount of urine obtained after the initial placement of a Foley catheter only represents urine output before the catheter was placed; it tells you nothing about what the patient's kidneys are doing currently. It is possible that the bladder was full prior to the onset of shock, and that no urine has been made since. Always disregard the initial amount of urine obtained and start measuring the urine after that.

27. What size intravenous catheters should be placed for resuscitation?

The flow of fluid through a tube is predicted by Poisuelle's law. The resistance is inversely proportional to the fourth power of the radius and directly proportional to the length. This means that a catheter with a larger radius and shorter length would be most desirable. While this sounds easy, it is often difficult to place large-bore catheters in hypotensive and hypovolemic patients because their veins are collapsed, difficult to find, and hard to cannulate.

28. Where should resuscitation catheters be placed?

The reflex answer is "upper extremities." The reason for this choice of site is that penetrating abdominal wounds may disrupt the vena cava or the iliac veins, causing fluid infused through lower extremity sites to extravasate into the abdomen. While this does happen, it is an infrequent occurrence.

29. I can't get an IV in the arms. Can I use the subclavian veins?

The subclavian veins are extremely undesirable alternatives for venous access. Recall that when the subclavian veins are cannulated for hyperalimentation or for central venous pressure monitoring, the patient is placed in Trendelenburg's position and a pillow is placed between the scapulae. These maneuvers open the thoracic inlet and help fill the subclavian vein, making it easier to cannulate. The vein lies in direct apposition to the pleura, making cannulation of the pleural space (a pneumothorax) easy if the vein is collapsed. Trauma patients are ideal candidates for a pneumothorax because their veins are collapsed due to hypovolemia, and they cannot be positioned adequately due to cervical spine precautions. Percutaneous cannulation of the femoral veins or a cutdown of the greater saphenous vein at the ankle or of the cephalic vein at the elbow are much safer options for venous access.

30. Are central venous pressure catheters useful measures of volume status during resuscitation?

Yes and no. A central venous pressure (CVP) catheter can guide volume resuscitation, but it is seldom necessary and often risky to place during the early phases of resuscitation when the great veins are collapsed and the risk of a pneumothorax from placement is high. When a patient fails to respond to volume infusion as expected, a CVP monitor might be useful to exclude other possible causes of hypotension.

31. A patient is stabbed in the left fourth intercostal space. On arrival, his blood pressure is 80 mmHg with a heart rate of 150 beats per minute (bpm). Two large-bore upper extremity catheters are placed and 3 L of fluid is given over 15 minutes. Despite this aggressive resuscitation, his blood pressure increases to only 90 mmHg and his heart rate remains elevated. His trachea is in the midline, and breath sounds are present bilaterally. What is the most likely cause?

This is the classic presentation of pericardial tamponade. The other feature which is *usually* present is dilated neck veins. When the knife entered the patient's chest, it passed through the pericardium and injured either a coronary artery or one of the cardiac chambers. As the knife was withdrawn, the pericardium closed around the hole, trapping blood within the pericardial sac. Because the pericardium is inelastic, the accumulated blood increased pressure and rapidly exceeded the central venous pressure. Because the heart could not fill properly, the heart rate increased to help return cardiac output to normal. Despite this compensation, cardiac output, and hence blood pressure, fell quickly. Patients with pericardial tamponade may compensate somewhat by increasing peripheral vascular resistance, but they are almost always in extremis and in immediate danger of dying. This situation constitutes a true surgical emergency and mandates immediate therapy, usually in the form of thoracotomy and control of the bleeding site.

32. How is the diagnosis of pericardial tamponade made?

Pericardial tamponade should be suspected based on mechanism (it almost always follows a thoracic or high-abdominal stab wound) and on physical examination. The patient is hypotensive, tachycardic, and diaphoretic. Neck veins are usually distended but may be collapsed if hypovolemia is present due to concomitant bleeding from another injury. Occasionally, patients present with compensated pericardial tamponade due to injuries of the right atrium or right ventricle. Because the pressure within these chambers is relatively low, high pressures within the pericardial sac cannot be achieved, and venous return, although impeded, continues to some extent. If fluid resuscitation fails to restore the blood pressure to the expected level, and physical examination is consistent with the diagnosis (e.g., distended neck veins), pericardial tamponade can be diagnosed with transthoracic ultrasound (if rapidly available) or with CVP monitoring. The risk of subclavian catheterization in this situation is relatively low because the veins are distended.

ACVP of more than 15 mmHg in the face of decreased blood pressure is virtually diagnostic, provided that congestive heart failure is not present.

33. Following a stab wound to the left chest, a patient presents with hypotension, tachycardia, tachypnea, and distended neck veins. He is severely dyspneic, and his trachea is deviated to the right. What is the diagnosis?

This patient has a tension pneumothorax, an immediately life-threatening condition in which air at supra-atmospheric pressure levels accumulates in one hemithorax. The increased pressure impedes venous return and decreases cardiac output. The pathophysiology is the same as that which occurs with pericardial tamponade except that the increased pressure is in the pleural space, rather than the pericardium. The elevated intrapleural pressure displaces the mediastinum to the opposite side (explaining the tracheal deviation) and embarrasses respiration as well as circulation. This patient's clinical presentation is classic. Auscultation of the affected chest would reveal absent breath sounds, while percussion would find hyperresonance. These patients represent hyperacute emergencies. If tension pneumothorax is suspected, time should not be wasted obtaining a chest x-ray to confirm the diagnosis. Rather, a large-bore intravenous catheter should be inserted into the chest (either second parasternal intercostal space or fourth intercostal space opposite the nipple) to decompress the tension rapidly. A tube thoracostomy can be inserted subsequently.

34. What is the difference between anaphylactic shock and an anaphylactoid reaction?

A naphylactic shock and anaphylactoid reactions are both due to the sudden release of preformed inflammatory mediators from mast cells and basophils. Symptoms may occur as rapidly as 1 minute after exposure. Anaphylactic shock is a true anamnestic response in which membrane-bound immunoglobulin E (IgE) causes mast cells and basophils to release histamine and platelet activating factor into the circulation. Anaphylactoid reactions occur when the offending agent causes direct release of the substances without mediation by IgE. The clinical presentations are virtually indistinguishable.

35. What is neurogenic shock?

Neurogenic shock is produced by loss of peripheral vasomotor tone as a result of spinal cord injury, regional anesthesia, or administration of neurogenic blocking agents. Blood pools in the peripheral circulation, thereby decreasing venous return and cardiac output. If cardiac sympathetic outflow is affected, bradycardia, rather than tachycardia, results. Signs and symptoms of spinal shock are usually present.

36. A patient sustains a penetrating injury of the neck and presents with flaccid paralysis and hypotension. Initial resuscitation should be directed toward treating what type of shock?

Always assume that a patient has hypovolemic shock until proven otherwise. Although this is a classic history and clinical presentation for neurogenic shock, associated injuries (such as external blood loss or an undiscovered abdominal wound) frequently cause hypovolemia. Therefore, remember that all hypotensive trauma patients are in hypovolemic shock until proven otherwise.

37. Following a chain saw injury to the leg with massive blood loss, a 70-kg patient presents with a systolic blood pressure of 80 mmHg. How much dopamine should be used initially?

None. Do not fall into the trap of using vasopressors for resuscitation. This patient has a volume (blood) deficit and needs crystalloid and blood. The use of pressors for resuscitation is almost always contraindicated and can result in dire complications such as renal failure. Always assume that a hypotensive trauma patient is in hypovolemic shock until proven otherwise.

38. What are the signs and symptoms of class I hemorrhage?

The American College of Surgeons Committee on Trauma, in their Advanced Trauma Life Support Course syllabus defines four classes of hemorrhage. While these are useful categories for thinking about the severity of shock, remember that treatment should be directed more by the response to therapy than by relying on any classification scheme or algorithm.

Class I hemorrhage constitutes a loss of up to 15% of circulating blood volume (about 750ml). The pulse rate is below 100 bpm, and the resting supine blood pressure is normal. Pulse pressure is also usually normal. The respiratory rate and urine output are also normal. The patient may appear anxious. Estimated blood loss should be replaced with crystalloid in the usual 3:1 ratio.

39. What are the signs and symptoms of class II hemorrhage?

Blood volume loss of between 15% and 30% (750–1500 ml) constitutes class II hemorrhage. The pulse rate is above 100, although the blood pressure is still normal. Pulse pressure is decreased. Urine output may also be decreased to 20–30 ml/hr. Patients are anxious and may be somewhat tachypneic. Crystalloids should be used to replace the estimated blood loss.

40. What are the signs and symptoms of class III hemorrhage?

A blood loss of between 30% and 40% (1500–2000 ml) constitutes class III hemorrhage. Blood pressure is decreased as are pulse pressure and urine output (5–15 ml/hr). Patients exhibit marked tachycardia (> 120 beats/min), tachypnea (30–40 breaths/min), and confusion. Blood, in addition to crystalloid, is required to replace the volume deficit.

41. What are the signs and symptoms of class IV hemorrhage?

Severe blood loss greater than 40% of the blood volume (in excess of 2000 ml) constitutes class IV hemorrhage. The pulse rate is greater than 140 bpm. The blood pressure is decreased, and the pulse pressure is widened. The respiratory rate is very high (> 35 breaths/min) and the urine output is negligible. Patients are confused and lethargic. Blood and crystalloids are required to replace the volume deficit.

42. What is the initial management of hemorrhagic shock?

The mnemonic is ABCDE:

Airway: A patent airway must be established to ensure adequate oxygenation and gas exchange. Although many trauma patients require endotracheal intubation, other means, such as the chin lift or the jaw thrust, can be used to keep an airway patent temporarily.

Breathing: An ambu (assisted manual breathing unit) bag or a ventilator may be required in a patient who is not breathing spontaneously after injury or who has required pharmacologic paralysis for intubation.

Circulation: The placement of large-bore intravenous access catheters ensures ready access to the circulation. Resuscitation should begin with crystalloid solution and uncrossmatched O-negative blood used in addition for larger volume deficits.

Disability: A rapid neurologic examination should be performed to determine the extent of injury.

Exposure: After life-threatening injuries have been addressed, the patient should be undressed completely, and a thorough "secondary survey" should be performed to identify all injuries. After the patient is undressed, nasogastric and urinary catheters should be placed to aid in abdominal decompression. The Foley catheter aids in evaluating the adequacy of resuscitation.

43. What is a M.A.S.T. suit?

The M.A.S.T. (military antishock trousers) suit, also called a PASG (pneumatic antishock garment), is a device that is placed around the patient's legs and abdomen to increase blood pressure. The exact mechanism of action of the M.A.S.T. suit has been debated for years and may be related either to an increase in systemic vascular resistance or to the production of an "autotransfusion." The devices are seldom used in rural trauma practice because the short transport times from the field to the hospital preclude placement of the garment. If you encounter one, remember that it must be deflated sequentially, starting with the abdominal compartment first. Partially deflate each section before removing it. If the garment is fully inflated, sudden release may cause an unrecoverable drop in the patient's blood pressure. Transient decreases are best treated with volume replacement.

44. What is an appropriate fluid challenge for initial resuscitation?
The usual dose is 1–2 L for an adult and 20 ml/kg for a pediatric patient. Response is judged by increase in blood pressure and urine output and decreased heart rate. Improvement in sensorium (in awake nonintoxicated patients) is another useful index.

45. What is the desirable urine output following resuscitation?
Although the volume will vary with the size of the patient, 50 ml/hr in an adult and 1 ml/kg/hr in the pediatric patient are desirable goals. For children younger than 1 year, 2 ml/kg/hr is desirable.

46. Are there any special requirements for fluid infusion and blood transfusion?
All fluids should be warmed to prevent hypothermia. Macropore (160 micron) blood filters should be used to remove microscopic clot. Micropore filters have not been shown to be of value.

47. Should calcium be given to trauma patients who require blood transfusions?
No. Most patients who require blood transfusions do not need calcium supplementation. Excessive supplementation may be harmful.

48. What is ATLS?
The letters ATLS stand for the Advanced Trauma Life Support course designed and sponsored by the American College of Surgeons. Anyone interested in emergency care or trauma surgery should take this 2-day course. Information can be obtained either by writing to the American College of Surgeons (55 East Erie Street, Chicago, IL 60611) or by visiting the Web site at http://www.facs.org.

49. What is AAST?
The letters AAST stand for the American Association for the Surgery of Trauma. It is an international organization dedicated to the care of injured patients and to research related to the field. The organization maintains an excellent Web site at http://www.aast.org.

50. Can radiology offer any treatment modalities in the treatment of shock?
Yes. Embolization of pelvic, hepatic, and other sources of blood loss by interventional radiologists have been very successful. It controls hemorrhage, while fluid resuscitation overcomes the shock.

BIBLIOGRAPHY

1. American College of Surgeons: Advanced Trauma Life Support Course for Physicians, 5th ed. Chicago, American College of Surgeons, 1993.
2. Bongard FS: Shock and resuscitation. In Bongard FS, Sue DY (eds): Current Critical Care: Diagnosis and Treatment. Norwalk, CT, Appleton & Lange, 1994.
3. Wilmore, Cheung, Harkin, et al: ACS Surgery: Principles and Practice. New York, 2002.

5. MECHANISMS OF WOUNDING BALLISTICS

Juan A. Asensio, M.D., and Patrizio Petrone, M.D.

1. What is ballistics?

Ballistics is the study of the dynamics of a missile (i.e., bullet) traveling through the barrel of a firearm, its subsequent trajectory through the air, and its final complicated motion after striking a target. Wound ballistics is the study of missile motion and damage produced when the final target is animal tissue.

2. Why must surgeons have a working knowledge of ballistics?

Knowledge of the principles of wound ballistics is crucial to the evaluation of gunshot wounds and their treatment. The surgeon who understands ballistics can more easily anticipate the potential injuries, identify which organs have been injured, and make decisions regarding whether an exploration is appropriate, what cavities should be explored, and in what order. The surgeon must also know how to evaluate the most potentially life-threatening injuries to a patient.

3. How are missiles fired?

When a cartridge consisting of primer, propellant (i.e., gun powder), and bullet is loaded into the chamber of a weapon, the initial step has been taken to fire the missile. The hammer on the weapon strikes the primer, resulting in sparks that ignite the propellant in the chamber. As the propellant particles ignite in the chamber, they are volatilized and converted into gas. The expanding volume of gas increases the energy of the propellant (i.e., kinetic energy pressure) in the chamber and subsequently overcomes the inertia of the missile, accelerating the missile through the barrel of the gun until it exits.

4. What are the three principles of wound ballistics?

1. Dissipation of kinetic energy
2. Damage from secondary missiles
3. Damage from cavitation

5. What are dissipation of kinetic energy and energy exchange?

To understand how missiles produce wounding, several physical principles must be understood. All missiles leave a weapon with a certain amount of kinetic energy that has been imparted to them as they are fired. Kinetic energy is defined as mass times velocity squared ($Ke = \frac{1}{2}MV^2$). Because energy is constant, meaning it is neither created nor lost, it must be exchanged. As a missile leaves the muzzle of a gun, it exits with a certain amount of kinetic energy. Some of the kinetic energy is lost to friction during its travel through air. The remaining kinetic energy is exchanged on impact with living tissue. The amount of damage to the tissue is determined by the energy exchange that occurs between the missile and the organs that it strikes. Tissue damage is proportionate to the kinetic energy of the missile on entrance into the living tissue minus the kinetic energy with which it exits.

6. How is this energy exchange responsible for wounding?

The energy exchange between the missile and living tissue displaces tissue away from the point of impact. A major determinant of the amount of energy exchanged is the number of living tissue particles involved. The greater the number of living tissue particles displaced or hit, the more they are set in motion away from the path of the missile and the greater the energy that is lost by such missile. It follows that organs of greater density (i.e., more tissue particles per volume of tissue) have more of their particles impacted and therefore sustain greater injury corresponding to the greater dissipation of kinetic energy. For example, when a missile impacts air-containing tissues such as the lung, fewer tissue particles are impacted and less tissue damage is sustained than in fluid-containing organs such as muscle, solid organs, and blood vessels. Denser structures such as bone receive the greatest transfer of energy and damage.

7. How do secondary missiles create wounding?
As a missile impacts dense objects, such as bone from buttons or metal in buckles worn by the patient, the missile may fragment to create multiple secondary missiles. Secondary missiles can become more destructive than primary missiles and often follow unpredictable courses. Bony fragments or spicules can also cause considerable damage to soft tissue.

8. How does the phenomenon of cavitation cause tissue damage?
A cavity is created by the missile as it strikes living tissue and displaces tissue particles. A missile that has low energy produces a cavity of slightly larger size than its diameter, whereas a missile of high kinetic energy pushes a large volume of tissue away from its track, generating a bigger cavity and causing more extensive tissue damage. This cavity is also enlarged by the amount of expanding gases. This allows energy to be transmitted into larger areas. In the case of high-velocity missiles, the cavity continues to enlarge even after the missile has passed. As a cavity is formed by the missile, tissue damage occurs by stretching, compressing, and shearing tissue. Organs that are more elastic can better withstand these forces and sustain less damage than organs that are relatively inelastic.

9. Do all missiles strike with their pointed ends?
No. Missiles usually produce a larger frontal profile. The larger the frontal profile, the larger the number of tissue particles that are struck and the larger the energy exchange that causes tissue wounding. The frontal area of a bullet may be increased in three ways:
1. Profile modification
2. The missile's tumble and yaw patterns
3. Fragmentation

10. How does profile modification affect wounding?
Increasing the frontal area of the missile by modifying its nose creates a larger surface with which the missile can impact the target. This alteration can be done by creating a small cavity within the nose of the missile. As heated gases accumulate within this cavity, the energy level within the cavity increases and allows the missile to expand or flatten on contact. A full or a partial jacket placed around the missile can "mushroom out" or expand on contact. Similarly, a plastic covering can be attached to the tip of a missile, covering its hollow point and allowing the heated gases within the hollow point to increase in temperature, which shatters the missile into smaller secondary missiles possessing greater energy and produces greater tissue destruction.

11. How do tumble and yaw affect the wounding produced by missile?
Tumbling is the action of forward rotation around the center of mass of the missile. Tumbling is best described by imagining a missile doing cartwheels. *Yaw* represents the deviation of the missile in its longitudinal axis from the straight line of flight. Yaw can best be described by imagining the missile dipping its nose and then raising it again along its entire trajectory. These mechanisms may cause the missile to impact not with its entire length instead of the nose. This larger area of impact produces more rapid dissipation of kinetic energy, a greater volume of cavitation, and greater tissue wounding.

12. How does fragmentation affect tissue wounding?
As a missile splits into several fragments, the total frontal area presented to the tissue increases, maximizing the opportunity for energy dissipation. As these fragments travel over wider areas, the possibility of energy dissipation on organs and other adjacent tissues increases.
Soft missiles that have built-in grooves fragment easily and cause greater damage; jack-

eted missiles with grooves on the outside of the jacket achieve the same effect. Shotgun shells and fragmentation grenades represent the ultimate fragmentation weapons, causing very extensive tissue damage.

13. What makes shotgun injuries so unique?

A shotgun fires a projectile, or *shell,* that consists of a charge and a plastic cup or wad, which contains multiple, small, round balls made of lead or steel called *shot.* The wad is designed to split away quickly after leaving the barrel of the shotgun and scatter the shot. These multiple missiles impact a fairly large area of tissue, providing a greater opportunity for energy dissipation and wounding.

Shot varies in size depending on its purpose. A cartridge with many small pellets, called *birdshot,* creates a broad scatter pattern of injury. However, at a distance, each individual pellet impacts with lower energy because of losses from air friction. A cartridge with a few heavy pellets, called *buckshot,* tends to deliver much higher energy than birdshot, creating highly lethal injury patterns.

14. Are shotguns effective weapons?

They can be, depending on the range from which they are fired. The kinetic energy of shot dissipates rapidly when traveling through air. The closer the target, the greater the tissue damage that can be imparted by the shot.

The standard classification system used for shotgun wounds is helpful in determining the surgical management of these injuries, but clinical judgment is of the utmost importance. This classification is listed below:

Type I: Injuries occur at long range, generally more than 7 yards. Wounds are usually scattered, and the shot has less ability to penetrate tissue. Many of these injuries can be observed. If surgical management is required, it is generally limited to soft tissue débridement.

Type II: Injuries are sustained at intermediate ranges of 3 to 7 yards. In general, many deep structures sustain significant damage, and in most cases, these injuries warrant surgical intervention.

Type III: Injuries occur at close ranges of less than 3 yards. These injuries are often immediately lethal. If the patient survives, there will be extensive tissue damage that warrants operative intervention. Often, wadding, fragments of the patient's clothing, foreign material, and necrotic tissue are found within the tissues, requiring extensive tissue débridement.

15. Should all missiles be removed?

No. Missiles that are easily accessible should be removed using meticulous surgical technique so as not to damage the missile. Digital extraction is the preferred method to extract a missile. Attempting to remove the missile with hemostats or other surgical instruments usually creates grooves in the metal of the missile, thereby modifying its structure. No change to the missile should be made by the surgeon that would create difficulty in matching the missile with the offending weapon. Missiles that are inaccessible and require extensive dissection to be removed should be left alone. Remember that all removed missiles must be turned over to the authorities as forensic evidence.

16. What are the indications for missile removal?

Missiles should be removed if they are found within a cardiac chamber, within the lumen of a blood vessel, or within an intra-articular surface. Missiles that are near major blood vessels and that may come in direct contact with the vessel wall as the vessel transmits its pulsatile flow should be considered for removal; these missiles have been known to erode into the vessel lumen, causing pseudoaneurysms and missile emboli.

17. What is a missile embolus?

A missile embolus is a missile that has penetrated a vascular conduit and has traveled within this conduit to an area remote from the site of entrance. Missile emboli have been reported in the arterial and venous circulations, and they can travel great distances, even traversing the heart. Missile emboli should be removed to prevent organ damage and infarction.

18. Do missiles carry microorganisms?

Yes. Although some assume that all missiles are sterile because of the heat generated by combustion and friction, this is not always true. Bacteria can be carried on the surface of missiles. After the missile implants in an area of devitalized tissue surrounded by hematoma, it can be a source of bacterial contamination. When missiles traverse hollow viscera, particularly the colon, and are implanted in areas of hematoma or devitalized tissue, abscesses can and do form.

19. What kind of organisms have been cultured from missiles and missile abscesses?

Staphylococcus aureus is known to survive on the surface of missiles and has been cultured from missile tracks. In patients sustaining missile injuries of the large bowel, *Escherichia coli* and *Enterobacter cloacae* have been cultured from missile abscesses. *Blastomyces dermatitidis* has been rarely cultured.

20. How should missile tracks be managed?

Missile tracks are managed based on the extent of tissue damage. Low-velocity missiles generally do not cause much tissue destruction, but higher-velocity missiles create much devitalized tissue. Any significant amount of devitalized tissue must be removed. The area must be carefully débrided, hemostasis should be maintained, all foreign particles must be removed, and the area must be copiously irrigated. Failure to do so will result in infection.

21. What is the difference between low-velocity and high-velocity missiles?

Low-velocity missiles are defined as those traveling less than 1200 feet per second. High-velocity missiles travel more than 2000 feet per second. Most hand guns are considered low velocity. Because a missile's kinetic energy is proportional to mass and the square of velocity, high-velocity missiles cause the greatest tissue destruction. Military assault rifles have the ability to create the most tissue destruction because their missiles have significant mass and are ejected at velocities of approximately 3000 feet per second.

22. What are the important ballistic properties of commonly used handguns?

Missiles of these handguns are shown in Figure, and the muzzle velocities of the missiles are listed in the Table:

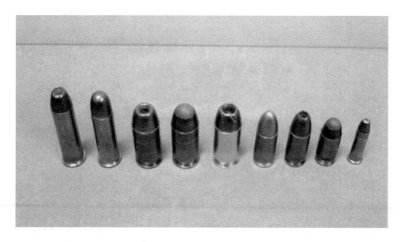

Handgun missiles are depicted from left to right: 38 Special, 357 Magnum, 45-caliber soft hollow point, 45-caliber soft hollow point grooved, 9 mm, 9 mm soft hollow point, 380 plastic covered copper-jacketed hollow point, 22 caliber

Handgun Caliber	Muzzle Velocity (ft/sec)
22	865
25	820
32	970
380	955
38	870
38 (Special)	1085
38 (Supervelocity)	1450
45	860
357 Magnum	1295
44 Magnum	1520

23. What are the important ballistic properties of the most commonly used military assault rifles?

Most military assault rifles (see Figure) use two types of ammunition: 5.56-mm missiles for the American-made M-16 in any of its models or 7.62-mm missiles for the Russian AK-47 and any of its models made in China, Korea, Finland, Romania, and The Czech Republic. The most common ballistic properties of these military assault rifles are listed in the Table:

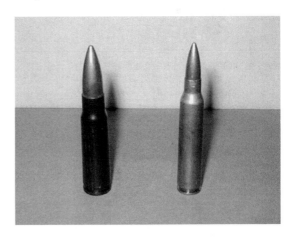

The military assault rifle missiles are 7.62 mm from an AK-47 (*left*) and 5.56 mm from an M-16 (*right*).

Assault Rifle	Muzzle Velocity (ft/sec)
M-16	3240
AK-47	2850

24. What about nonlethal weapons and their missiles?

In the interest of subduing civilians involved in domestic riots and for riot control, less destructive missiles with allegedly less wounding potential have been created. They include rubber and plastic missiles and bean bags. These "nonlethal" weapons are quite capable of inflicting severe injuries and causing death. Neither rubber nor plastic missiles are radiopaque. Bean-bag rounds are projectiles enclosed in 2-inch, heavy, clothlike cordura nylon bags filled with pellets. They are packaged into shotgun shells and can travel 280 ft/sec. Once liberated, the bags unroll after being fired from a 12-gauge shotgun. They are claimed to be nonpenetrating missiles and are designed to deliver a blow that causes minimal trauma, but they can cause significant muscle spasm that can briefly render an individual incapacitated. There have been case reports of bean bags causing thoracic penetration requiring thoracotomy and of abdominal penetration requiring laparotomy.

25. What are antipersonnel devices?

Antipersonnel devices are military weapons that include hand grenades, land mines, personally triggered mines such as the Claymore mine used in Vietnam, and any other explosive devices with great wounding and killing capabilities. White phosphorus grenades can cause extensive tissue destruction and burns simultaneously from the phosphorus. Fléchettes are small arrows packed in a shell fired from an artillery piece that explodes in midair, impaling soldiers with the steel darts. They were first used during the Vietnam conflict and were made by Russians and Americans.

BIBLIOGRAPHY

1. Charles A, Asensio JA, Forno W, et al: Penetraing "bean bag" injury: Intrathoracic complication of a non-lethal weapon. J Trauma 53(5):997–1000, 2002.
2. McSwain NE Jr: Ballistics. In Ivatury RR, Cayten CG (eds): Textbook of Penetrating Trauma. Media, PA, Williams & Wilkins, 1996, pp 105–128.
3. Olivas T, Jones B, Canulla M: Abdominal wall penetration by a police "bean bag." Am Surg 67:407–409, 2001.
4. Swan KG, Swan RC: Gunshot Wounds: Pathophysiology and Management, 2nd ed. Chicago, Year Book Medical Publishers, 1989.
5. Swan KG, Swan RC: Principles of ballistics applicable to the treatment to gunshot wounds. Surg Clin North Am 71:221–239, 1991.

6. HEMODYNAMIC MONITORING OF SHOCK AND CIRCULATORY DYSFUNCTION

William C. Shoemaker, M.D.

1. What is shock, and how is it diagnosed?

Shock is the clinical manifestation of circulatory dysfunction and failure. It is diagnosed by hypotension, oliguria, and collapse. It is usually due to hypovolemia and low flow but also may be due to high but maldistributed (uneven) flow from trauma, sepsis, cirrhosis, and other forms of stress. The common denominator is that blood flow is inadequate to supply tissue perfusion and oxygenation particularly when body metabolism is increased. This leads to global tissue hypoxia, organ failures, and death.

2. How is shock recognized at the earliest time?

Shock is first recognized by subjective, nonspecific signs and symptoms such as cold clammy skin, pallor, weak thready pulse, unstable vital signs, cyanosis mottled skin, restlessness, central nervous system (CNS) depression or agitation, and altered level of consciousness. There are secondary effects of acute circulatory failure; they are not the principle pathophysiologic problem.

3. How is cardiac function clinically evaluated?

Cardiac function is commonly evaluated by the Starling myocardial performance curve, in which some function of the heart, such as cardiac output, cardiac index, stroke volume, stroke work, or cardiac work, is plotted against the corresponding preload or inflow pressure (central venous pressure [CVP] or pulmonary artery [PA] occlusion or wedge pressure). This is usually simplified in an X-Y plot of these two variables by a line representing the lower limit of normal cardiac index (2.5 L/min/m^2 measured by thermodilution and a line representing the upper limit of normal for preload of PA wedge pressure (20 mmHg): these two lines divide the field into quadrants that define four clinical subgroups according to whether they have high or low flow as well as high or low inflow pressures. A patient's observed value is then evaluated according to these criteria, and therapy for each quadrant is suggested.

4. When do low-flow states commonly occur?

Low-flow states commonly occur when hypotension, oliguria, and tachycardia are initially restored without adequately correcting the underlying hypovolemic low-flow state: other situations include inadequate tissue perfusion from cardiodepressant effects of anesthetics, oxygen debt from delays in keeping up with blood losses, and the increased metabolism of postoperative states, immunochemical responses, sepsis, febrile states, and organ failure.

5. What is the conventional therapy for low-flow states?

The current conventional therapeutic paradigm for hemorrhage, trauma, postoperative states, septicemia, septic shock, and other acute circulatory states is to give promptly and vigorously sufficient fluid therapy to correct vital signs as well as other clinical manifestations of shock, including arterial blood gases, hematocrit, and urine output.

6. What are the common circulatory problems that result in low-flow states?

Low-flow states may occur when the blood pressure of the initial shock syndrome is restored without adequately correcting the underlying hypovolemia and low flow. This may occur when crystalloids increase blood pressure with incomplete or temporary restoration of the intravascular space and blood flow; this problem is particularly evident in elderly hypertensive patients who are often very responsive to salt.

7. What are the consequences of massive fluid replacement in terms of the distribution of body water?

In the critically ill patient, 80% of the crystalloids leave the intravascular space before the end of the infusion; 30 to 40 minutes later, most of the infused fluid has diffused (i.e. equilibrated) into the interstitial space. With large crystalloid infusions, the patient may have peripheral edema from overexpansion of the interstitial space, but with persistent hypovolemia.

Overexpansion of the peripheral and pulmonary interstitium may increase CVP and pulmonary artery occlusion pressures (PAOP), and this may be misinterpreted as adequately reflecting blood volume. The restoration of blood pressure is not well correlated with restoration of blood flow and tissue oxygenation; the latter are needed to reestablish the circulatory function that is necessary to maintain tissue oxygenation and body metabolism.

8. What are the clinical consequences of unrecognized low-flow states?

Specific circulatory problems associated with inadequate resuscitation include inadequate tissue perfusion and tissue oxygenation, oxygen debt, and organ failures such as adult respiratory distress syndrome (ARDS), acute renal failure, sepsis in the uncontaminated patient, hepatic failure, and disseminated intravascular coagulation (DIC). These are often the end-organ failures of prior tissue hypoxia from low—(or uneven) flow states.

9. What is mean arterial pressure and how is it measured?

Mean arterial pressure (MAP) is defined as the sum of the diastolic pressure plus one third the pulse pressure. It may also be calculated as one third of the sum of the systolic pressure plus two times the diastolic pressure. It is more frequently measured directly as a dampened "electrical mean" of the systolic and diastolic pressures in various electronic recording systems. Manometric measurements of blood pressure may be obtained with the sphygmomanometer cuff using the Korotkoff blood pressure sounds to identify the systolic and diastolic pressures.

10. What is the normal blood pressure?

The normal arterial blood pressure is approximately 120/80 mmHg for healthy young adults. The pressure may gradually increase with age, but the systolic pressure should not be more than 100 mmHg plus the patient's age. Systolic pressures greater than 160 mmHg and diastolic pressures greater than 90 mmHg suggest hypertension. Young adults, especially teenage girls, may normally have pressures as low as 90/60 mmHg. Therefore, it is important to know the patient's preillness baseline pressures.

Pressures should be measured in both arms early in the patient's hospital course, since unilateral arteriosclerotic or traumatic vascular lesions may result in 10–20 mmHg differences between the left and right side. Normally femoral arterial pressures are 5–10 mmHg higher than brachial pressures. After trauma to the femoral or iliac arteries on one side, there may be appreciable differences in the cuff pressures of the two legs.

11. What is the significance of abnormal blood pressure?

Arterial pressure may reflect overall circulatory status or more particularly the cardiac status, but it lacks diagnostic specificity. Pressure falls after hypovolemia from hemorrhage or other fluid losses, acute injury, sepsis, acute myocardial infarction, and acute cardiac failure particularly in patients with chronic congestive heart failure, anaphylactic reactions, neurogenic shock, dehydration, and vasovagal attacks. Blood pressure is useful for screening and for rapid assessment of trends in emergency conditions but is of limited physiologic and diagnostic significance.

Decreased pressure may reflect either circulatory decompensation or failure of therapy. Increased pressure may reflect acute hypertensive crisis, improved circulatory status, adrenomedullary stress response, anxiety, or excessive vasopressor therapy. Pressure and heart rate are useful as screening measures, but their changes are nonspecific and poorly reflect deficits of blood flow and blood volume because of compensatory adrenomedullary stress responses. Thus, arterial pressure does not directly reflect either blood flow or blood volume, but rather the failure of neural and neurohormonal circulatory compensations. The interactions of blood pressure, flow, and volume are extremely complex; however, the major overall aspects of circulatory dysfunction are generally reflected by serial blood pressure measurements.

12. What are the important time relationships in the evolution of traumatic shock syndromes?

Arterial pressure decreases during shock and trauma states, but these responses may be delayed because of the adrenal stress response that maintains pressure in the face of falling blood flow. In general, arterial pressures fall after compensatory mechanisms are exhausted, which may be some time after the precipitating hypovolemic event. Severely reduced cardiac output often occurs for periods of 40 minutes to 2 hours before significant reductions in arterial pressure.

On the other hand, arterial pressure may be rapidly restored by saline solutions before cardiac output and oxygen transport are corrected. This is often the case in elderly and hypertensive patients who develop hypertension after going off their low-salt diets.

13. What is pulse pressure, and what is the significance of its abnormal values?

The pulse pressure is the difference between the systolic and diastolic pressures. Decreased pulse pressures may precede decreases in diastolic pressures in hypovolemic patients; this is a suggestive, but not reliable, sign of shock.

14. How is heart rate measured, and what is its significance?

Heart rates are usually determined by manual palpation of the radial artery just above the wrist timed for at least 30 seconds. Heart rates may be measured automatically from EKG wave or the arterial pulse wave.

Heart rates above 100 beats per minute are regarded as tachycardia. When premature ventricular contractions or other rhythm abnormalities are present, the true heart rate may be determined by auscultation at the apex: the difference between the apical and radial rates represents the number of dropped beats.

15. How is blood flow measured in high-risk clinical circumstances?

Cardiac output or cardiac index, which is cardiac output per square meter of body surface area, is measured by the direct Fick method (indirect calorimetry), by indicator dilution or thermodilution methods, or by noninvasive impedance cardiography.

16. What is the direct Fick method, and how is the measurement made?

The physilogist's gold standard for cardiac output measurements has been the direct Fick method, which measures oxygen consumption (Vo_2) directly by a Douglas bag or measures the inspired and expired oxygen concentration and the tidal volume; the cardiac output is calculated from the measured Vo_2 divided by the arterial-venous O_2 content difference. The Vo_2 is measured noninvasively, but the cardiac output measurement requires calculations with invasive arterial and mixed venous (pulmonary artery or right ventricular) hemoglobin concentrations and saturations, and oxygen contents.

In general, the direct Fick method is applicable when the patient is in steady state conditions, when the FiO_2 is less than 0.6, and when the system is well calibrated and free of air leaks. It is not applicable in unstable, severely ill shock and trauma patients, particularly in early states where nonsteady states are common.

17. What is the difference between Vo_2 measurements by the direct Fick method and those calculated by thermodilution technique?

The direct Fick method measures oxygen consumption of all tissues from the outside, of the capillary-alveolar membrane including the lung parenchyma. The indirect Fick method, which measures cardiac output by thermodilution with arterial and mixed venous blood gases, measures oxygen consumption of all tissues inside the capillary-alveolar membrane, which excludes the lung parenchyma. When careful concomitant indirect Fick measurements using PA catheters were made, the calculated Vo_2 closely followed the direct Fick Vo_2 measurements made by inspired and expired O_2 concentrations with tidal volumes. Confirmation of the validity of these two approaches under ideal circumstances has been reported.

18. What are the hemodynamic and oxygen transport measurements obtained with PA catheters?

Hemodynamic variables can be repeatedly measured with a systemic arterial catheter and a PA catheter with measurements of arterial and venous pressures of the systemic and pulmonary circulations, cardiac output, arterial and mixed venous gases, and hemoglobin or hematocrit. Several hemodynamic and oxygen transport variables are claculated:

Cardiac index (CI)
Systemic vascular resistance index (SVRI)
Pulmonary vascular resistance index (PVRI)
Left and right ventricular stroke work (LVSWI, RVSWI)
Left and right cardiac work (LCWI, RCWI)
Arterial and mixed venous Po_2, (Pao_2 and $P\overline{v}o_2$)
Arterial and mixed venous hemoglobin saturation (Sao_2 and $S\overline{v}o_2$)
Oxygen delivery (Do_2)
Oxygen consumption (Vo_2)
O_2 extraction

All flow and volume measurements should be indexed to body surface area (BSA) or body weight to standardize values from patients of various sizes and body habitus.

19. Does systemic vascular resistance (SVR) reflect the average metarterial vessel tone?

SVR is measured as the ratio of blood pressure (MAP) to flow (cardiac index). This is an application of Ohm's law, which states resistance equals voltage divided by amperage ($R = i/e$). However, this concept is based on the direct current analogue, which is clearly inappropriate for the periodic changes of pressure and flow that occur in the cardiac cycle. Moreover, the arterial circuits in humans and animals are "parallel" not "in series." This means that if the resistance of ten or more circuits increases but one circuit's resistance decreases, the calculated resistance of the whole will decrease. Finally, there are no significant differences in the early period of postoperative and posttraumatic shock between survivors and nonsurvivors. Thus, SVR is an incorrect use of Ohm's law and may give misleading interpretations that lead to inappropriate therapy.

20. How is tissue perfusion measured?

Conventionally, tissue perfusion has been inferred from the subjective signs and symptoms of shock, but not specifically measured. However, invasive monitoring has been used to quantify the measurements of tissue perfusion and tissue oxygenation by the temporal patterns of Do_2 and Vo_2. Also, noninvasive transcutaneous O_2 and Co_2 tensions have been used to measure perfusion and oxygenation of skin of the trunk or shoulder as a surrogate of Vo_2

21. How is oxygen transport measured in critically ill patients in ICU conditions?

Overall measurement of the peripheral circulation and tissue perfusion may be quantitatively evaluated by oxygen delivery (Do_2), which is the product of cardiac output and arterial content. Similarly, overall body metabolism may be evaluated by oxygen consumption (Vo_2), which is the product of cardiac output and the arteriovenous content difference [$C(a-v)o_2$]. The oxygen contents of arterial and mixed venous blood are the products of hemoglobin concentration, the percent hemoglobin saturation, and a constant (1.36). This constant represents the volume of oxygen carried by each gram of saturated hemoglobin plus a small amount of oxygen dissolved in plasma ($0.0031 \times Pao_2$ mmHg).

22. **What is the significance of oxygen transport in the evaluation of circulatory function?**
    The bulk movement of oxygen is a useful measure of tissue perfusion because:
    - Oxygen is easily measured in arterial and mixed venous blood.
    - It has the largest arteriovenous gradient.
    - It is related to overall tissue perfusion and outcome.
    - Since it cannot be stored, the oxygen taken up by the cells is a measure of the overall rate of body metabolism.

    Oxygen delivery represents the supply side reflecting the overall function of the circulation, that is, the amount of oxygen delivered to the tissues per minute. As such, DO_2 reflects the circulatory function to peripheral tissues; increases over the normal baseline range represent compensations. That is, spontaneous increases in DO_2 in the face of exercise, trauma, stress, infection, and other forms of stress represent compensatory responses to inadequate tissue oxygenation and may reflect the reserved capacity of the circulation. The amount of increase in CI and DO_2 in response to a standard fluid volume load is also an indirect measure of circulation's capacity to compensate.

    The temporal pattern of DO_2 changes is more informative than a single set of measurements; the sequential pattern of changes in DO_2 provides a history of physiologic events that lead to shock, resuscitation, and the subsequent events.

23. **How is aerobic body metabolism measured?**
    The rate of body metabolism is measured by oxygen consumption (VO_2), which represents the total of all oxidative metabolic reactions and reflects the overall status of body metabolism. It represents the actual amount of oxygen consumed, not the real need, which may be more than the amounts that are burned, especially in trauma, postoperative states, sepsis, and burns.

24. **What factors limit body metabolism?**
    The VO_2 may be limited by progressively decreasing DO_2, which is the "supply side" of the equation. When VO_2 is limited by DO_2, the VO_2 is said to be "supply-dependent." That is, supply-dependent VO_2 is seen when sudden DO_2 increases produce significant increases in VO_2, DO_2-VO_2 relationships have been demonstrated in experimental laboratory conditions, but the patterns are not as obvious in clinical conditions where many other associated problems may obscure them. In practical terms, supply-dependent VO_2 is indicated by increased $VO_2 > 15$ ml/min.m^2 when DO_2 increases > 80 ml/min.m^2 after rapid administration of a standard volume of fluids, such as 100 ml of 25% albumen, 500 ml of 5% albumen. 6% hetastarch, and 1000–2000 ml of crystalloids.

25. **What are the aims of hemodynamic monitoring?**
    - To allow prompt recognition of circulatory problems at the earliest possible time
    - To diagnose or describe the physiologic alterations involved
    - To institute and evaluate early corrective therapy
    - To develop and use criteria to titrate therapy to its most effective end point

26. **What biochemical measurements of shock or tissue hypoxia are clinically available?**
    The venous pH, base deficit, anion gap, blood lactate, lactate/pyruvate ratio, and gastric mucosal pH (pHi) are blood gas or tissue fluid measurements that reflect tissue acidosis. These measure complex interrelationships that involve acidosis and indirectly reflect tissue hypoxia from anaerobic tissue metabolism.

27. **What are the advantages of the invasive pulmonary arterial (Swan-Ganz) catheter?**
    Circulatory measurements by invasive PA balloon-tipped thermodilution catheter – or Swan-Ganz catheter – are the gold standard for clinical evaluation of circulatory function. Although this technology is expensive, time consuming, and personnel intensive, it is currently

the most circulatory monitoring that can be used logistically at the bedside of the critically ill, unstable patient.

28. How reliable are individual thermodilution measurements?

The difference between repeated pairs of thermodilution measurements made at random times throughout the respiratory cycle average 7.4% $\pm$ 0.5 (SD). There is an average of 15% decrease with expiration and 12% to 15% increase with inspiration for the thermodilution method.

29. Can noninvasive hemodynamic monitoring systems provide comparable information to that of invasive PA catheter monitoring?

Multiple noninvasive monitoring includes bioimpedance cardiac output for condusive function, pulse oximetry to reflect changes in pulmonary function and transcutaneous O_2 and CO_2 to reflect changes in tissue perfusion. These noninvasive systems are feasible and useful surrogates for invasive PA catheter monitoring. They can be used in the Emergency Department, ambulance, and pre-hospital areas. They provide continuous displays, evaluate effects of therapy and predict outcome.

BIBLIOGRAPHY

1. Bishop MH, Shoemaker WC, Kram HB, et al: Prospective randomized trial of survivor values of cardiac index, oxygen delivery, and oxygen consumption as resuscitation endpoints in severe trauma. J Trauma 38:780–787, 1995.
2. Boyd O, Bennett D: Enhancement of perioperative tissue perfusion as a therapeutic strategy for major surgery. New Horiz 4:453–465, 1996.
3. Boyd O, Grounds M, Bennett D: Preoperative increase of oxygen delivery reduces mortality in high risk surgical patients. JAMA 270:2699–2704, 1993.
4. Forrester JS, Diamond G, Chatterje J, et al: Medical therapy of acute myocardial infarction by application of hemodynamic subsets. N Engl J Med 295:1356–1364, 1976.
5. Kern J, Shoemaker WC: Meta-analysis of hemodynamic optimization in high risk patients. Crit Care Med, In press.
6. Shoemaker WC, Appel PL, Kram HB, et al: Prospective trial of supranormal values of survivors as therapeutic goals in high risk surgical patients. Chest 94:1176–1186, 1988.
7. Shoemaker WC, Appel PL, Kram HB: Role of oxygen debt in the development of organ failure, sepsis, and death in high risk surgical patients. Chest 102:208–215, 1992.
8. Shoemaker WC, Wo CCJ, Bishop MH, et al: Noninvasive monitoring of high risk surgical patients. Arch Surg 131:732–737, 1996.
9. Shoemaker WC, Wo CCJ, Demetriades D, et al: Early physiologic patterns in acute illness and accidents. New Horiz 4:395–412, 1996.
10. Shoemaker WC, Wo CCJ, Chan L, et al: Outcome prediction of emergency patients by noninvasive hemodynamic monitoring. Chest 120:528–537, 2001.
11. Shoemaker WC, Bayard DS, Wo CCJ, Botnan A, Jelliffe RW: Hemodynamic evolution and outcome prediction of noninvasively monitored patients by a stochastic control program. Crit Care Med, In Press.

7. RESPIRATORY INSUFFICIENCY AND MECHANICAL VENTILATION

Jesús I. Ramírez, M.D., and Howard Belzberg, M.D.

1. What are the five general medical indications for mechanical ventilation?
- Acute respiratory failure
- Depressed level of consciousness
- Neuromuscular impairment
- Impending upper airway obstruction
- Acute exacerbation of obstructive airway disease

2. When do these indications commonly apply in trauma patients? List specific diagnoses.
- Acute respiratory failure in trauma is often seen in cases of acute respiratory distress syndrome (ARDS), pulmonary contusion, or pneumonia. It may also occur with cardiovascular failure of any cause.
- A depressed level of consciousness may occur with intoxication, head injury, or shock.
- Neuromuscular impairment may occur with flail chest, diaphragmatic rupture, abdominal compartment syndrome, or spinal cord injury above C5–C7, the origin of the phrenic nerves.
- Impending upper airway obstruction may result from an expanding neck hematoma, facial trauma, facial burns, or thermal inhalation injury.
- Acute exacerbation of obstructive airway disease my occur, although it does not usually result from trauma.

3. In the mechanically ventilated patient, what two basic ventilator adjustments can be made to alleviate hypercapnia?
Increase the respiratory rate (RR) or increase the tidal volume (V_T); either adjustment increases the amount of air moving through the respiratory system, thereby "blowing off" CO_2. The effects of altering RR or V_T may be seen in the formula for minute ventilation (V_E), which measures the volume of air moving through the respiratory system in 1 minute: $V_E = V_T \times RR$.

4. What two basic ventilator adjustments can be made to alleviate hypoxemia?
Increase the fraction of inspired oxygen (FiO_2) or the positive end-expiratory pressure (PEEP).

5. Why does increasing ventilation result in CO_2 being blown off but not significantly improve blood oxygenation?
Carbon dioxide is more soluble in water than oxygen; it therefore diffuses more readily across biologic membranes. It equilibrates almost instantaneously across the capillary-alveolar interface and is rapidly removed from the alveoli by air moving through the system, allowing further CO_2 diffusion. Oxygenation is limited by the rate of oxygen diffusion through the interface.

6. How does PEEP improve oxygenation?
- By "recruiting" alveoli, positive pressure keeps alveoli from collapsing at the end of expiration. The increased number of patent alveoli provides increased surface area for gas exchange.
- By increasing mean airway pressure.

7. What do PaO_2 (pO_2) and SaO_2 (O_2Sat) measure? Which is a better measure of blood oxygen content?
PaO_2 measures the oxygen *dissolved* in arterial blood. SaO_2 measures the oxygen *bound to*

hemoglobin in arterial blood. The total amount of oxygen carried by the blood is determined by these two variables. Because most of the oxygen in blood is bound to hemoglobin, SaO_2 is a more accurate measure of oxygen content. The PaO_2 can change considerably without significantly altering blood oxygen content. This minimal contribution of PaO_2 is reflected in the correction factor of 0.003 found in the equation for arterial oxygen concentration (CaO_2): $CaO_2 = (1.34 \times Hgb \times SaO_2) + (0.003 \times PaO_2)$.

8. What is the minimum level of blood oxygen desired to maintain adequate tissue oxygenation?

A minimum arterial oxygen saturation of 90% should maintain oxygenation near the maximum level. Increasing oxygen saturation above 90% has little effect on oxygen delivery because of the nonlinear nature of the oxyhemoglobin dissociation curve. Hemoglobin delivers most of its bound oxygen as it goes from a saturation of 90% to 50%, as reflected in the increased slope of the curve between these two points (see Figure).

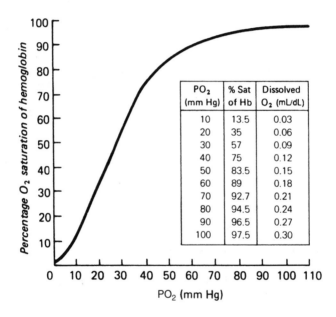

PO_2 (mm Hg)	% Sat of Hb	Dissolved O_2 (mL/dL)
10	13.5	0.03
20	35	0.06
30	57	0.09
40	75	0.12
50	83.5	0.15
60	89	0.18
70	92.7	0.21
80	94.5	0.24
90	96.5	0.27
100	97.5	0.30

9. Why is it sometimes beneficial to limit inspired oxygen in trauma patients?

Oxygen is toxic. Oxygen itself is only a weak oxidizing agent, but neutrophils and macrophages use it to generate reactive oxygen species. This is part of the normal response to infectious organisms. However, these cells are systemically activated during the inflammatory response to trauma, leading to systemic release of free radicals and tissue injury.

10. Which organ is most commonly affected by oxidative stress?

The lungs, resulting in acute lung injury (ALI). In its most severe form, it results in ARDS.

11. What are the diagnostic criteria for ARDS?

All of the following must be present for the diagnosis of ARDS, as defined in 1994 by the American-European Consensus Conference on ARDS:
- Inflammatory state
- Acute onset

- Ratio of PaO_2 to FiO_2 less than 200 mmHg
- Bilateral infiltrates on the chest radiograph
- No evidence of pulmonary edema (as defined by pulmonary artery wedge pressure $\leq$ 18 mmHg)

12. What is the optimal ventilatory strategy for patients with ARDS?

Low tidal volume (<6 mL/kg) combined with high PEEP (2 cm H_2O greater than P_{FLEX}). This strategy has been shown to decrease 28-day mortality by 25% to 50%. It is the only strategy proved to improve survival of ARDS patients. Despite substantial interest and research in high-frequency ventilation and prone ventilation (i.e., ventilating patients in the prone position), these strategies have not been shown to affect survival. However, all three strategies have improved oxygenation in ARDS patients.

13. What is P_{FLEX}?

P_{FLEX} is the level of pressure at the lower inflection point on the static respiratory pressure–volume curve (see Figure). It is the point where the slope of the curve (which represents compliance) exceeds a value of 1 and rapidly increases; if inflating a balloon rather than the lungs, this would be the point at which the balloon suddenly "gave" and started to rapidly expand. Many investigators argue that this is the pressure where optimal alveolar recruitment is attained.

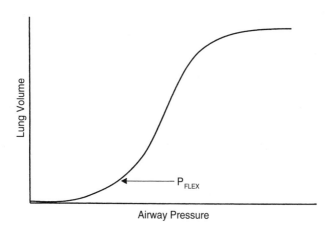

14. Why is the combination of low-volume ventilation and PEEP set at P_{FLEX} thought to be beneficial in treating ARDS?

It decreases overdistention and cyclic reopening of alveoli during mechanical breaths. In ARDS, these two factors are thought to create sheer stress that perpetuates injury to the alveolar-capillary interface.

15. Name six toxic effects of mechanical ventilation.

1. Oxygen toxicity
2. Volutrauma
3. Barotrauma
4. Hemodynamic changes
5. Auto-PEEP
6. Toxicities associated with concomitant therapies

16. Describe the pathophysiology for each of the toxic effects?

1. Oxygen toxicity: tissue is injured by reactive oxygen species (see Questions 9 and 10).

2. Volutrauma: sheer stress damages the alveolar-capillary interface, altering its permeability.

3. Barotrauma: positive pressure in the airway ruptures alveoli, small airways, or blebs.

4. Hemodynamic changes: positive-pressure ventilation increases intrathoracic pressure, decreasing thoracic venous inflow (return) during diastole and increasing thoracic arterial outflow during systole.

5. Auto-PEEP: air "trapping" in alveoli occurs as a result of incomplete exhalation; patients who are ventilated with an increased inspiration to expiration (I:E) ratio or excessive tidal volume are at higher risk for this effect, as are those who have distal airway collapse or increased airway resistance.

6. Concomitant therapies: treatments used to support mechanical ventilation, such as paralysis, sedation, or tracheal suctioning, may lead to a variety of problems by altering the body's normal autoregulation.

17. What are the clinical manifestations of each of the toxic effects?

1. Oxygen toxicity: acute lung injury, ARDS, or multiple organ dysfunction syndrome may result.

2. Volutrauma: progressive respiratory failure can occur.

3. Barotrauma: pneumothorax, pneumomediastinum, subcutaneous emphysema, or pulmonary interstitial emphysema may result.

4. Hemodynamic changes: decreased cardiac output occurs when the ventricular filling is already compromised (as in hypovolemia); increased cardiac output occurs when filling is adequate.

5. Auto-PEEP: increased dead space, increased airway pressure, decreased cardiac output, or barotrauma may occur.

6. Concomitant therapies: paralysis and sedation may result in pressure sores, muscle atrophy, or peripheral polyneuropathy; the effects may be prolonged well beyond the patient's acute illness and need for mechanical ventilation. Tracheal suctioning may contaminate the airway and facilitate development of respiratory infections.

18. Name seven serious complications of laryngeal intubation independent of those directly related to mechanical ventilation.

1. Pulmonary infection
2. Vocal cord injury
3. Posterior glottic stenosis
4. Subglottic stenosis
5. Tracheal stenosis
6. Tracheomalacia
7. Tracheoesophageal fistula

19. Describe the pathophysiology of each of the serious complications of laryngeal intubation.

1. Pulmonary infection: stenting of the epiglottis by an orotracheal tube facilitates aspiration and impairs coughing. Obstruction of the trachea by the tube impairs mucociliary clearance of secretions.

2. Vocal cord injury: granulation tissue may form as a reaction to the tube, the cords may be directly injured during intubation, or the recurrent laryngeal nerves may be compressed during intubation

3. Posterior glottic stenosis: abrasions to the posterior glottis heal with granulation tissue or scar, narrowing the airway. Such abrasions may occur during intubation or from the endotracheal tube itself.

4. Subglottic stenosis: mucosal compression by the endotracheal tube leads to submucosal edema and subsequent fibrosis, narrowing the airway. Healing of a tracheostomy stoma may also lead to stenosis.

5, 6, and 7. Tracheal injury: mucosal compression by the tracheal tube cuff leads to ischemia. Depending on the degree of injury and healing process, it may produce flaccidity of the tracheal wall (i.e., tracheomalacia), scarring and narrowing of the lumen (i.e., stenosis), or posterior tracheal erosion into the esophagus (i.e., fistula). With tracheomalacia, the flaccid tracheal wall may collapse, obstructing the airway.

20. What are the diagnostic criteria for ventilator-associated pneumonia (VAP)?
The diagnostic criteria for VAP include an infiltrate seen on the chest radiograph and the presence of two of the following variables: leukocytosis, fever, or purulent tracheal secretions. According to the American College of Chest Physicians (ACCP), these criteria should be used for screening. Because these findings are nonspecific, the ACCP also recommends establishing the diagnosis by culturing specimens obtained through invasive testing, such as bronchioalveolar lavage or protected-specimen brush sampling.

21. Is it preferable to treat VAP when the diagnosis is suspected, or is it preferable to wait until the diagnosis and pathogens are established by culture?
Early, empiric treatment has been shown to significantly improve survival. However, broad-spectrum empiric treatment also increases unnecessary antibiotic use and may lead to selection of resistant organisms. The preferred clinical strategy is to simultaneously obtain cultures and start broad-spectrum treatment as soon as the diagnosis of VAP is suspected and then tailor treatment to specific pathogens as culture results become available.

22. How is early-onset VAP defined? What pathogens are associated with early-onset VAP?
Early-onset VAP occurs during the first 4 days of mechanical ventilation. The most common pathogens are endogenous upper airway flora: *Streptococcus pneumoniae, Haemophilus influenzae,* and *Moraxella catarrhalis.*

23. What pathogens are associated with late-onset VAP?
Late-onset VAP occurs after 5 or more days of mechanical ventilation. It is commonly caused by pathogens not often seen outside the hospital: *Pseudomonas aeruginosa,* methicillin-resistant *Staphylococcus aureus, Acinetobacter* species, and *Enterobacter* species. Resistance is more common among these organisms than among those associated with early-onset VAP.

24. Why is prompt extubation of mechanically ventilated patients important?
Prompt extubation avoids complications, the risk of which increases with the duration of ventilation.

25. Describe four popular strategies for weaning patients from mechanical ventilation.
1. Progressively lower the number of ventilator-assisted breaths
2. Progressively lower the level of pressure support with each breath
3. Perform "wind sprints," allowing spontaneous breathing for progressively longer periods
4. Perform a single daily trial of spontaneous breathing

26. Which of the strategies for weaning patients from mechanical ventilation is most effective?
A once-daily trial of spontaneous breathing has been shown to result in extubation more promptly than strategies that gradually decrease ventilator support, and the term *weaning* is therefore a misnomer.

27. What parameters may be measured at bedside during spontaneous breathing to assess the likelihood of successful extubation?
- Adequate oxygenation with FiO_2 of 50% (or less) and PEEP of 5 cm H_2O (or less)
- Spontaneous respiratory rate less than 25

- Spontaneous tidal volume greater than 5 mL/kg
- Spontaneous minute volume less than 10 L/min
- Negative inspiratory force greater than –20 cm H_2O
- Respiratory rate–tidal volume ratio less than 100 breaths/min/L

28. Which of the previous parameters has the highest predictive value for successful extubation?

A respiratory rate–tidal volume ratio less than 100 breaths/min/L has the highest predictive value for successful extubation.

BIBLIOGRAPHY

1. The ARDS Network: Ventilation with lower tidal volumes as compared with traditional tidal volumes for acute lung injury and the acute respiratory distress syndrome. N Engl J Med 342:1301–1308, 2000.
2. Esteban A, Frutos F, Tobin MJ, et al: A comparison of four methods of weaning patients from mechanical ventilation. N Engl J Med 332:345–350, 1995.
3. Gardner GM: Posterior glottic stenosis and bilateral vocal fold immobility: diagnosis and treatment. Otorynolaryngol Clin North Am 33:855–878, 2000.
4. Gattinoni L, Tognoni G, Pesenti A, et al: Effect of prone positioning on the survival of patients with acute respiratory failure. N Engl J Med 345:568–573, 2001.
5. Grossman RF, Fein A: Evidence-based assessment of diagnostic tests for ventilator-associated pneumonia: executive summary. Chest 117:177S–181S, 2000.
6. Krishnan JA, Brower RG: High-frequency ventilation for acute lung injury and ARDS. Chest 118: 795–807, 2000.
7. Lesperance MM, Zalzal GH: Assessment and management of laryngotracheal stenosis. Pediatr Clin North Am 43:1413–1427, 1996.
8. Mecca RS, Vaz Fragoso AC. The lungs and their function. In Civetta JM, Taylor RW, Kirby, RR (eds): Critical Care. Philadelphia, Lippincott Williams & Wilkins, 1997, pp 189–208.
9. Passos Amato MB, Valente Barbas CS, Machado Medeiros D, et al: Effect of a protective-ventilation strategy on mortality in the acute respiratory distress syndrome. N Engl J Med 338:347–354, 1998.
10. Yang KL, Tobin MJ: A prospective study on indexes predicting the outcome of trials of weaning from mechanical ventilation. N Engl J Med 324:1445–1450, 1991.

II. Head and Neck Trauma

8. BRAIN INJURY

Marvin Bergsneider, M.D., and Daniel F. Kelly, M.D.

1. Does traumatic brain injury pose a serious health care problem in this country?

In the United States, trauma is the leading cause of death in individuals younger than 45 years of age, and brain injury results in more trauma deaths than injuries to any other body region. One half of the 150,000 injury-related deaths that occur annually in the U.S. involve a head injury that is primarily responsible for the patient's demise. Overall, 500,000 head injuries requiring hospital admission occur annually in the U.S.

2. What is the meaning and significance of *secondary brain injury*?

Primary injury occurs at the moment of impact and may lead to irreversible cell damage from mechanical disruption. **Secondary injury** is any physiologic event occurring within minutes, hours, or days after the initial injury that leads to further damage of nervous tissue, contributing to permanent neurologic dysfunction. Hypotension, hypoxia, intracranial hypertension, and seizures are probably the most serious and frequently seen secondary injuries after head injury. The probability of a meaningful recovery of function after head injury is greatly increased if secondary injuries are prevented or minimized.

3. What does the Glasgow Coma Scale assess, and why is it important?

The Glasgow Coma Scale (GCS) is a widely used method of defining a patient's level of consciousness following a traumatic brain injury. A score, ranging from 3 to 15, is obtained by adding the patient's best motor, verbal, and eye-opening responses.

Glasgow Coma Scale

EYE OPENING	VERBAL RESPONSE	MOTOR RESPONSE
1. None	1. None	1. None
2. To painful stimulus	2. Incomprehensible sounds	2. Abnormal extensor posturing
3. To verbal stimulus	3. Inappropriate words	3. Abnormal flexor posturing
4. Spontaneous	4. Confused	4. Withdrawal to pain
	5. Fully oriented	5. Localization to pain
		6. Following commands

The advantage of this scaling system is its objectivity, reproducibility, and simplicity. The GCS has strong prognostic value in head-injured patients regarding eventual neurologic recovery. Head injury severity is generally categorized into three levels based on the GCS after initial resuscitation:

Mild: GCS 13–15
Moderate: GCS 9–12
Severe: GCS 3–8
In general, any patient with a GCS of 8 or less is considered to be in a coma.

4. Describe the essentials of the neurologic and general examinations in the acutely head-injured patient.

As always, address the ABCs first: **A**irway, **B**reathing, and **C**irculation. The neurologic examination is necessarily abbreviated and should focus on the level of consciousness (GCS), pupillary light reflexes, and lower brain stem reflexes for patients in deep coma. The head should also be palpated to detect bony step-offs, and all scalp lacerations should be probed gently to assess for depressed fractures and foreign bodies. Signs of basal skull fracture should also be sought, including hemotympanum, cerebrospinal fluid (CSF) otorrhea or rhinorrhea, and retromastoid (Battle's sign) or periorbital ecchymosis ("raccoon eyes") and tenderness. This initial assessment, along with inspection of the neck and thoracolumbar spine, should take no longer than 5–10 minutes.

5. Explain the significance of a dilated pupil following traumatic brain injury.

A dilated pupil often signifies compression of the third cranial nerve as it courses from the midbrain to the orbit. Most commonly, this pupillary change after trauma is due to the uncus (medial temporal lobe) being pushed over the tentorial edge by an expanding hematoma. As the uncus herniates further, compression of the ipsilateral cerebral peduncle and the reticular activating system results in a contralateral hemiparesis and a deteriorating level of consciousness, respectively (see figure). Thus, a dilated pupil following trauma may be indicative of an expanding intracranial hematoma, brain stem compression, and elevated intracranial pressure (ICP). In most cases, the hematoma is on the same side as the dilated pupil. This finding should prompt empiric treatment to reduce ICP in a comatose patient and should heighten the urgency to obtain a computed tomogram (CT) of the head. A third nerve palsy, however, can also be caused by direct trauma to the orbit.

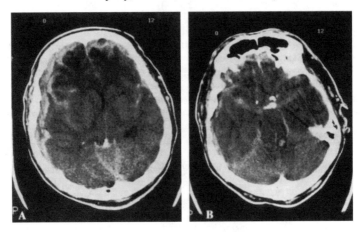

Noncontrast axial head CT showing *A*, acute right-greater-than-left subdural hematomas with midline shift and subarachnoid hemorrhage, and *B*, midbrain compression secondary to right-sided uncal herniation. A contusion of the midbrain is also seen. The patient sustained this contrecoup injury by falling off a roof onto the back of his head sustaining an occipital skull fracture. He eventually expired. Note that the subdural hematoma on the right extends over the entire frontoparietal area.

6. What are the three main types of brain herniation?

The most common types of herniation are uncal, subfalcian, and tonsillar herniation. **Uncal herniation** results from the herniation of the medial part of the temporal lobe (the uncus) across the tentorial edge (see figure in question 5), thereby compressing the third nerve and the cerebral peduncle. The triad of a deteriorating GCS, pupillary dilatation, and a contralateral hemiparesis strongly suggests an uncal herniation. **Subfalcian herniation** occurs when the singulate gyrus of one frontal lobe herniates below the falx cerebri. **Tonsillar herniation** refers to the cerebellar tonsils through the foramen magnum.

7. Do patients with uncal herniation always present with an ipsilateral pupil dilatation and a contralateral hemiparesis?

No. Kernohan's notch phenomenon occurs when the motor deficit is ipsilateral to the side of the lesion due to a mass causing brain stem shift with resultant compression of the contralateral cerebral peduncle against the opposite tentorial edge. Thus, signs of herniation can be falsely localizing.

8. How do the neurologic findings differ among patients with epidural, subdural, or intra-cerebral hematomas?

There are no characteristic neurologic findings that reliably distinguish epidural, subdural, or intracerebral hematomas from one another.

9. Why is an imaging study needed to evaluate head-injured patients?

The neurologic examination is frequently unreliable in predicting intracranial pathology, and signs of herniation may be falsely localizing. A CT scan of the brain is always indicated in the acutely head-injured patient. An axial CT without contrast rapidly and unequivocally defines in-tracranial lesions and determines whether urgent neurosurgical intervention is required. Obtaining both brain and bone "windows" will help determine the significance of focal neurologic findings and whether a skull fracture is present. Magnetic resonance imaging (MRI) is not practical in the acute setting and is poor at demonstrating acute hemorrhage.

10. Is a head CT required for every head-injured patient?

A CT is indicated in all head-injured patients with a depressed level of consciousness (GCS < 15), including those who are heavily inebriated. A timely CT is also indicated in all patients with a GCS of 15 who sustained a loss of consciousness, are amnestic to the injury, have a focal neurologic deficit, or have signs of a basilar or calvarial skull fracture.

11. What is cerebral perfusion pressure, and what importance does it have in the manage-ment of traumatic brain injury?

Conceptually, cerebral perfusion pressure (CPP) is the difference between the internal carotid artery blood pressure (input) and the cerebral venous pressure (output). Because cerebral venous pressure and ICP typically are very similar in magnitude, CPP is estimated clinically by the mean arterial pressure (MAP) minus ICP. In normal subjects, MAP ranges from 80–100 mmHg, and ICP is 5–10 mmHg; thus, CPP ranges from 70–95 mmHg. In an analogous fashion to Ohm's law, cerebral blood flow is proportional to the CPP divided by the cerebrovascular resistance. One major goal in treating severe head injury patients is to maintain CPP $\geq$ 70 mmHg.

12. Why is the maintenance of an adequate blood pressure important following a severe head injury?

Pressure autoregulation is the mechanism by which a constant cerebral blood flow is maintained despite wide fluctuations in systemic MAP or CPP. Autoregulation is achieved by cerebral arteriolar vasodilatation in response to a decrease in blood pressure and, conversely, by vasoconstriction in response to an increase in MAP. Pressure autoregulation normally has a lower CPP limit of 40–50 mmHg and an upper limit of 140 mmHg. After head injury, pressure autoregulation is often impaired, and most severe head injury patients require a CPP of at least 60–70 mmHg to maintain autoregulation and reduce the risk of cerebral ischemia.

13. Why and how is hyperventilation used in treating elevated ICP?

Hyperventilation-induced hypocarbia results in cerebral vasoconstriction that lowers cerebral blood volume, thereby decreasing ICP. Despite the effectiveness of hypocarbia in reducing ICP, it must be used with caution in severe head injury patients because excessive hyperventilation ($PaCO_2$ 25–30 mmHg) can cause cerebral ischemia. It is recommended that $PaCO_2$ be maintained in the range of 30–35 mmHg when treating head-injured patients in whom there is a suspicion of elevated intracranial hypertension.

14. What initial measures should be taken to treat intracranial hypertension?

Initial treatment should begin prior to obtaining a CT in individuals who are in a coma (GCS ≤ 8), who have a precipitous decline in level of consciousness, or who develop pupillary asymmetry or hemiparesis, because of the likelihood that a traumatic mass lesion is responsible for their deterioration. Such interventions include:

- **Intubation:** This controls the airway, prevents hypoxia, and allows controlled ventilation.
- **Mild hyperventilation:** Maintain $PaCO_2$ at 30–35 mmHg with adequate tidal volume.
- **Sedation:** This assists ventilation; typically morphine or fentanyl is used.
- **Neuromuscular blockade:** This is required for intubation and prevents increase of ICP in agitated or abnormal posturing patients. Vecuronium or pancuronium is preferred.
- **Mannitol bolus** (1.0 gm/kg IV bolus): This lowers ICP by osmotic means and increases CPP. Mannitol should not be given to hypotensive patients.
- **Prophylactic phenytoin** (18 mg/kg IV loading dose): Seizures can cause precipitous increases in ICP with resultant herniation.
- **Volume resuscitation and prevention of hypotension:** This is critical to prevent cerebral ischemia. Aggressive fluid replacement (typically normal saline) and inotropic support may be necessary.

15. What factors should be considered before a craniotomy is performed to evacuate a traumatic intracranial hematoma?

The most critical factors are the patient's neurologic status and CT findings. Surgical intervention is indicated in all deteriorating patients harboring an expanding intracranial hematoma causing significant mass effect and brain shift. In general, all acute epidural, subdural, or intracerebral hematomas with significant mass effect and evidence of raised ICP warrant urgent evacuation. Acute intracranial hematomas cannot be adequately removed through burr holes because of their solid consistency; instead, a craniotomy is required for evacuation.

16. Describe the etiology and radiographic appearance of epidural hematomas.

Epidural hematomas typically result from an injury directly over the site of the hematoma (coup injury) and frequently involve a skull fracture that results in tearing of a meningeal artery (most commonly the middle meningeal artery). Because the outer layer of the dura mater is actually the cranial periosteum, arterial pressure is required to lift the periosteum from the bone. The periosteum is very adhesive at the cranial suture lines, and, therefore, these landmarks often limit the extent of epidural hematomas. Tenting of the dura results in a biconcave (lens) shape of epidural hematomas (see figure).

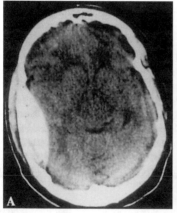 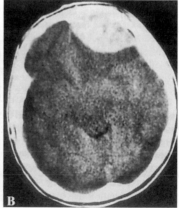

Noncontrast axial head CTs showing acute epidural hematomas in two different patients: *A*, right middle fossa (temporal) hematoma, and *B*, left frontal fossa hematoma. Both hematomas are limited in their extension by the coronal suture.

17. Describe the etiology and radiographic appearance of acute subdural hematomas.

Subdural hematomas often occur opposite the site of mechanical impact (contrecoup injury). In most cases, bridging veins between the brain and dura are torn as the brain rebounds away from the contralateral calvarium, resulting in hematoma formation in the subdural space. The subdural space is a potential space that allows the relatively unimpeded expansion of the hematoma. As such, the subdural hematoma often extends over the entire cerebral hemisphere in a crescent shape (see figure in question 5). Severe underlying parenchymal injury is much more common with acute subdural hematomas than with epidural hematomas.

18. Do all depressed skull fractures warrant surgical treatment?

The indications for surgical elevation of a depressed skull fracture are generally:
- A contaminated wound
- An underlying hematoma that necessitates evacuation irrespective of the skull fracture
- A significant cosmetic deformity
- Involvement of a paranasal sinus

Uncomplicated, open depressed skull fractures can be treated in the emergency department with wound irrigation and closure.

19. What is the significance of CSF rhinorrhea or otorrhea following a head injury and how should it be treated?

A CSF leak nearly always signifies a skull base fracture and carries the risk of the development of meningitis. The most common fracture sites are the floor of the frontal fossa and the petrous bone. Conservative therapy of maintaining head elevation at or above 30° for 72 hours is effective in most cases. Prophylactic antibiotics should not be administered because there is no proven benefit in preventing meningitis, and, if meningitis occurs, this treatment may promote the growth of resistant strains. For CSF leaks resistant to conservative therapy, the placement of an external lumbar CSF drain is usually effective.

20. Describe the essential monitoring parameters in severe head injury patients (GCS ≤ 8).

Monitoring equipment for the severe head injury patient should include an ICP monitor, central venous line, and arterial pressure line. The monitors provide continuous data from which to assess and correct ICP, volume status, and blood pressure, respectively.

21. Which patients should receive an ICP monitor?

Nearly every patient with an initial postresuscitation GCS of 8 or less warrants monitoring. In most cases, a ventriculostomy is preferred because it allows both for the monitoring of ICP and for the ability to drain CSF. Other types of ICP transducers that monitor brain parenchymal pressure are available, as well. An ICP monitor is sometimes referred to as a "bolt," a term that is no longer applicable and is misleading.

22. What ICP constitutes intracranial hypertension requiring treatment?

The normal ICP for a healthy adult is 5–10 mmHg. An ICP of over 20 mmHg sustained for more than 5 minutes typically warrants treatment.

23. Describe the standard measures for treatment of increased ICP.

Routine preemptive measures include maintenance of normothermia, head elevation to 30° with neutral alignment, and mild hyperventilation to a $PaCO_2$ of 30–35 mmHg. Because of the risk of acute increases in ICP with seizure activity, anticonvulsants (phenytoin) should also be administered for at least the first week postinjury. When acute and sustained rises in ICP occur, additional therapies to control ICP are used, often simultaneously. These include ventricular drainage, narcotic sedation (morphine or fentanyl), and neuromuscular blockade (vecuronium or pancuronium), followed by bolus mannitol (0.5–1.0 gm/kg). In patients with persistent or worsening intracranial hypertension, the possibility of a new or a reaccumulating intracranial hematoma should be investigated by head CT and, if present, should be urgently evacuated.

24. What is CPP therapy of elevated ICP, and how is it accomplished?

CPP therapy is based on the theory that severely head-injured patients are not able to regulate cerebral blood flow normally, even in the presence of normal blood pressures. By increasing the systemic blood pressure with the aim of achieving a CPP > 70 mmHg, it is predicted that reflexive vasoconstriction will result in a decrease in ICP, yet cerebral blood flow will remain optimized. The first step in CPP therapy is vascular volume expansion with the goal of a central venous pressure of 5–10 mmHg. If perfusion pressure remains insufficient after volume therapy and treatment to reduce ICP, the use of induced hypertension (by inotropic or α-constrictor agents) is usually indicated. The efficacy of CPP therapy has not been demonstrated in a randomized study, although the concept of volume resuscitation, prevention of systemic hypotension (systolic blood pressure < 90 mmHg), and maintenance of CPP $\geq$ 70 mmHg remain accepted goals of head injury treatment.

25. What are the indications for high-dose barbiturate therapy in severe head injury patients?

In patients refractory to the standard measures outlined above to treat high ICP, barbiturates can be used in some individuals. Theoretically, high-dose barbiturates reduce cerebral metabolism with a decrease in cerebral blood flow, blood volume, and ICP. The response rate (i.e., control of ICP) has ranged from 30–80% in different series. For therapy to be effective, it should be instituted before irreversible brain stem injury has occurred. Indications to begin high-dose pentobarbital include persistence of ICP over 30 mmHg with CPP less than 70 mmHg and ICP over 40 mmHg despite a CPP of 70 mmHg. These patients must be monitored vigilantly because of the increased risk of hemodynamic and pulmonary complications.

26. What role do steroids have in treating head injury patients?

None. The inability of high-dose corticosteroid therapy to control ICP or improve outcome in patients with head injury has been shown in numerous clinical trials. Additionally, associated complications, including blunt immune response, masking of infection, gastrointestinal hemorrhage, poor wound healing, and elevation in serum glucose levels, make high-dose glucocorticoids unsuitable for head-injured patients.

27. Are posttraumatic seizures common? Do anticonvulsants reduce the risk?

Early posttraumatic seizures, occurring in the first week after injury, are seen in approximately 25% of patients with traumatic intracranial hematomas and contusions. Use of phenytoin during the first week after head injury reduces the risk of posttraumatic seizures by 70–75% during this period. Use of phenytoin with maintenance of high therapeutic serum levels is thus recommended during the acute injury period. Prophylactic anticonvulsant therapy does not appear to reduce the risk of the development of posttraumatic epilepsy, however; therefore, this therapy is usually discontinued after 1 week postinjury.

28. Why is hyponatremia such a problem after head injury?

Hyponatremia lowers the seizure threshold and can exacerbate cerebral edema. Low serum sodium (< 135 mmol/L) occurs in almost 10% of moderately or severely injured patients. Hyponatremia in head-injured patients is caused by either cerebral salt wasting or the syndrome of inappropriate anitdiuretic hormone (SIADH); both are characterized by low serum sodium and serum osmolality and by inappropriately high urine sodium and urine osmolality, in a setting of normal renal, adrenal, and thyroid function. The major distinction is that patients with SIADH are generally responsive to fluid restriction, while those with cerebral salt wasting respond to volume addition and sodium administration. Hypertonic saline or IV urea therapy are effective for treating significant hyponatremia of < 130 mmol/L.

29. What are the most important determinants of neurologic recovery after head injury?

The most important predictors of poor outcome include older age, low GCS, abnormal motor response (decorticate or decerebrate posturing), pupillary dilatation, hypotension, hypoxia, and sustained intracranial hypertension. CT predictors of poor outcome include acute subdural and intracerebral hematomas, multiple contusions and subarachnoid hemorrhage, presence of compressed mesencephalic cisterns, and midline shift of over 3 mm (see the table and figure below). Importantly, these variables have an additive effect on morbidity and mortality; when multiple factors are present, such as older age, low GCS, pupil dilation, and midline shift on CT, the chances for a good recovery are markedly diminished.

Major Predictors of Poor Outcome after Closed Head Injury

CLINICAL FINDINGS	CT FINDINGS
Older age	Mass lesions (subdural, intracerebral hematoma,
Lower GCS	multiple contusions)
Abnormal motor response	Compressed or absent mesencephalic cisterns
Abnormal pupillary response	Midline shift > 3 mm
Sustained ICP > 20 mmHg	Subarachnoid hemorrhage
Hypotension SBP < 90 mmHg	
Hypoxia PaO_2 < 60 mmHg	
Systemic complications	

These clinical and CT findings constitute the strongest prognostic indicators in head-injured patients.

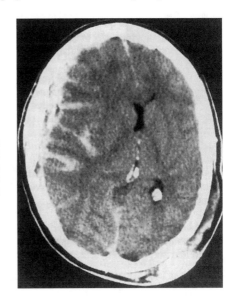

This noncontrast axial head CT shows an extensive right-sided acute subdural hematoma, subarachnoid hemorrhage, and early cerebral contusions with a large right-to-left midline shift. These findings, despite the patient's relatively young age of 32, are predictive of a poor neurologic outcome.

30. How many patients actually make a functional neurologic recovery after sustaining a severe head injury?

In the most recent reports, a favorable outcome, defined as good recovery or moderate disability by the Glasgow Outcome Scale, was achieved in approximately 50% of patients, with a mortality rate of approximately 25%. Despite intensive intervention, long-term disability occurs in a large portion of the survivors of severe head injury. Significant neuropsychologic sequelae and physical disabilities are also common in patients sustaining milder injuries.

31. Why is it important to obtain a cervical spine x-ray in head-injured patients, and what are the key points about performing this study?

Five to ten percent of head injury victims sustain a cervical spine injury. The lateral cervical spine x-ray must visualize the cervicothoracic junction. If the C7–T1 junction is not seen on the lateral view despite arm traction or swimmer's view, then a CT through the C7–T1 level should be obtained.

32. What are the short- and long-term sequelae of head injury?

In the early weeks after discharge, complaints of persistent headache, confusion, or gait disturbance should prompt a repeat CT to evaluate for the development of posttraumatic hydrocephalus. Long-term follow-up is dictated largely by the degree of neurologic and physical disability. For patients discharged fully conscious and independent, the most common complaints are neuropsychological in nature, with memory and behavioral disturbances occurring most frequently. Referral to a neuropsychologist for evaluation is often indicated. Patients with significant neurocognitive impairment are best managed at a comprehensive rehabilitation unit for several weeks or months. *Recovery of function from the time of discharge to 6 months postinjury can be dramatic, even in severely impaired or vegetative individuals.* Improvement generally begins to plateau at 6 months postinjury and is typically maximal by 1 year.

33. What patients are at risk for developing a chronic subdural hematoma?

Chronic subdural hematomas typically occur in individuals older than age 40. A history of head trauma is obtained in only one half to three quarters of patients. Chronic alcoholism is also a common associated factor. Preexisting brain atrophy is seen in many individuals. Other factors include ventricular shunts, seizure disorders, and anticoagulant (Coumadin) therapy.

34. Name the typical manifestations of a chronic subdural hematoma.

Chronic subdural hematoma may mimic a number of other neurologic conditions including dementia, stroke, transient ischemic attacks, encephalitis, and other mass lesions. The patient or patient's family often does not remember a traumatic event or has only a vague recollection of a seemingly trivial head injury. *An initial misdiagnosis of dementia is particularly common in the elderly patient presenting with an insidious global decline in mental function, without focal neurologic findings.* An erroneous admission diagnosis occurs in up to 40% of cases. The most common complaint is headache, seen in up to 80% of individuals. Other symptoms include lethargy, memory impairment, confusion, weakness, nausea, vomiting, and seizures. Motor deficits and gait disturbance are common.

35. How is a chronic subdural hematoma diagnosed?

CT and MRI are the primary imaging modalities for diagnosis. On CT, these lesions are typically iso- or hypodense to brain and may extend over a large portion of the cerebral convexity (see figure, top of facing page).

36. How does treatment of a chronic subdural hematoma differ from treatment of an acute subdural hematoma?

Patients with chronic subdural hematomas are effectively and safely treated with twist drill craniostomy at the patient's bedside or by burr holes and drainage in the operating room. A craniotomy is rarely needed. In contrast, patients with an acute subdural hematoma require a craniotomy for evacuation because the hematoma is clotted and cannot be drained via burr holes.

BIBLIOGRAPHY

1. Alberico AM, Ward JD, Choi SC, et al: Outcome after severe head injury, relationship to mass lesions, diffuse injury, and ICP course in pediatric and adult patients. J Neurosurg 67:648–656, 1987.
2. Cooper PR (ed): Head Injury, 3rd ed. Baltimore, Williams & Wilkins, 1993.
3. Marshall LF, Gautille T, Klauber MR, et al: The outcome of severe closed head injury. J Neurosurg 75(Suppl):S28–36, 1991.
4. Bouma GJ, Muizelaar JP, Choi SC, et al: Cerebral circulation and metabolism after severe traumatic brain injury: The elusive role of ischemia. J Neurosurg 75:685–693, 1991.

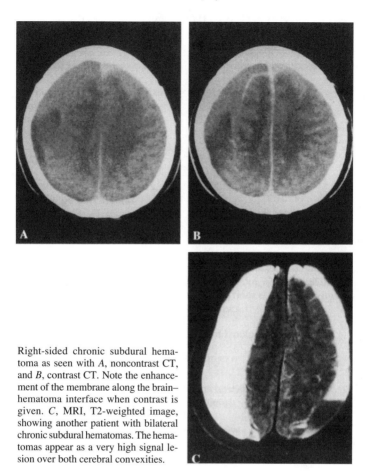

Right-sided chronic subdural hematoma as seen with *A*, noncontrast CT, and *B*, contrast CT. Note the enhancement of the membrane along the brain–hematoma interface when contrast is given. *C*, MRI, T2-weighted image, showing another patient with bilateral chronic subdural hematomas. The hematomas appear as a very high signal lesion over both cerebral convexities.

5. Bouma GJ, Muizelaar JP, Bandoh K, et al: Blood pressure and intracranial pressure-volume dynamics in severe head injury: Relationship with cerebral blood flow. J Neurosurg 77:15–19, 1992.
6. Kelly DF, Nikas DL, Becker DP: Diagnosis and treatment of moderate and severe head injuries in adults. In Youmans J (ed): Neurological Surgery, 4th ed. Philadelphia, W.B. Saunders, 1995, pp 1618–1718.
7. Marmarou A, Anderson RL, Ward JD, et al: Impact of ICP instability and hypotension on outcome in patients with severe head trauma. J Neurosurg 75:S59–S66, 1991.
8. Muizelaar JP, Marmouov A, Ward JD, et al: Adverse effects of prolonged hyperventilation in patients with severe head injury: A randomized clinical trial. J Neurosurg 75:731–739, 1991.
9. Narayan RK, Wilberger JE, Povlishock JT (eds): Neurotrauma. New York, McGraw-Hill, 1996.
10. Paulson OB, Strandgaard S, Edvinsson L: Cerebral autoregulation. Cerebrovasc Brain Metab Rev 2:161–192, 1990.
11. Rosner MJ, Rosner SD, Johnson AH: Cerebral perfusion pressure: Management protocol and clinical results. J Neurosurg 83:949–962, 1995.
12. Rosner MJ: Pathophysiology and management of increased intracranial pressure. In Andrews BT (ed): Neurosurgical Intensive Care. New York, McGraw-Hill, 1993, pp 57–112.
13. Teasdale G, Jennett B: Assessment of coma and impaired consciousness. A practical scale. Lancet 2:81–84, 1974.

9. MAXILLOFACIAL TRAUMA

Dennis-Duke R. Yamashita, D.D.S., and James P. McAndrews, D.D.S.

1. What are the indications for performing orbital floor exploration in the treatment of a zygomatic complex fracture?
- Enophthalmos greater than 3 mm
- Limitation of extraocular function
- A large orbital floor defect with herniation of soft tissue into the maxillary sinus as evaluated on the computed tomography (CT) scan

2. In the evaluation of orbital trauma, what would be the significance of subconjunctival ecchymosis that has no lateral limit?
The bleeding suggests a fractured orbital bony structure such as the lateral orbital wall, orbital floor, or the zygomaticofrontal suture.

3. What is an orbital blow-out fracture?
In the classic orbital blow-out fracture, the integrity of one or more of the walls of the orbital cavity is lost without fracture of the surrounding orbital rim. The trauma results from an almost instantaneous increase in intraorbital pressure. The orbital floor is most often involved, with concomitant injury of the medial wall occurring in about 50% of the cases.

4. What are the clinical signs of an orbital blow-out fracture?
Enophthalmos
Diplopia (i.e., difference in visual axis)
Extraocular muscle limitation (i.e., entrapment)
Infraorbital nerve paresthesia, if fracture traverses infraorbital canal
Subconjunctival hemorrhage (i.e., violation of periosteum)
Periorbital ecchymosis and swelling
Pain around the eye and in the area of the maxillary sinus

5. Which is the most common orbital wall to be involved in an orbital blow-out fracture?
The inferior wall, although not the thinnest, is the most frequently fractured wall of the orbit, particularly in the area medial to the infraorbital groove. The lateral wall is the thickest, strongest, and least frequently fractured wall of the orbit.

6. Which bones make up the structure of the orbit?
The orbit is composed of the frontal, zygoma, maxilla, lacrimal, ethmoid, sphenoid, and palatine bones (i.e., orbital process). The orbital process of the palatine bone is most often forgotten.

7. What is the average depth from the orbital rim to the optic canal?
Two measurements are important in the exploration and reconstruction of the orbit:
Infraorbital rim to optic canal: 42 mm
Superior orbital notch to optic canal: 45 mm

8. How is traumatic telecanthus described? What are the normal intercanthal, interpupillary, and lateral canthal measurements?
Traumatic telecanthus is an increase in the distance between the medial canthi of the eyes due to fracture of the bones to which the medial canthal ligaments are attached. The normal related measurements are approximately as follows:

Intercanthal distance: 30 mm
Interpupillary distance: 60 mm
Lateral canthal distance: 90 mm
(*Hint:* Remember the 30, 60, 90 right triangle.)

9. Which signs and symptoms characterize the superior orbital fissure syndrome?

The contents of the superior orbital fissure are compressed by trauma or neoplasms, resulting in this particular syndrome. Symptoms are related to the anatomic structures within the fissure:

Lacrimal nerve	Oculomotor nerve
Frontal nerve	Nasociliary nerve
Trochlear nerve	Abducens nerve

The syndrome has associated signs and symptoms:

Ophthalmoplegia	Fixed dilated pupil
Ptosis	Sensory deficits to the forehead
Proptosis	Loss of corneal reflex

10. Provide a list of implant materials that are used to restore the continuity of the orbital floor.

Autogenous bone
Cartilage and homologous grafts
Alloplastic materials:
  Teflon
  Silicone sheeting
  Methylmethacrylate
  Calcium phosphate (hydroxyapatite)
  Nylon
  Metal alloys
  Marlex
  Medpor (porous polyethylene) the most often used alloplastic material
  Bioresorbable agents (i.e., Gelfilm, Vicryl, PDS, and Lactosorb)
The most often used alloplastic material is Medpor.

11. What is the anatomic attachment of the medial canthal ligament? The lateral canthal ligament?

The medial canthal ligament (tendon) has two heads: the thin, deep head inserts on the posterior lacrimal crest, and its thick, superficial head inserts into the anterior lacrimal crest.

The lateral canthal tendon (lateral palpebral ligament) inserts at Whitnall's tubercle. The tubercle is on the lateral orbital wall approximately 2 mm inferior to the zygomaticofrontal suture.

12. What is an ocular forced duction test, and how is it performed?

The forced duction test is used to determine if there is muscle weakness or a physical impediment to ocular motility. The corneoscleral junction is grasped in the area of the muscle tendon in question, and the globe is gently rotated. Inability to rotate indicates muscle or fascial entrapment. The test should also be performed after orbital floor or wall repair to determine impingement of graft material on orbital soft tissue with resultant reduced motility.

13. What are the Jones 1 and Jones 2 tests (primary and secondary dye tests), and what is each one's significance?

Jones 1 test: 2% fluorescein dye is injected into the conjunctival sac. The nose is examined after 5 minutes to see if the dye emerges through the normal ductal flow.

Jones 2 test: 2% fluorescein dye is injected into the inferior puncta to see if any obstruction to flow is encountered. If the dye finds its way to the superior puncta, there is an obstruction of the drainage in the area below the lacrimal sac. If the dye appears in the nose, after a failure in the Jones 1 test, there is an obstruction of the drainage below the sac, which is usually reparable by means of dacryocystorhinostomy.

14. What is the clinical difference between the superior orbital fissure syndrome and the orbital apex syndrome?

The orbital apex syndrome includes all the clinical signs and symptoms of the superior orbital fissure syndrome plus optic nerve involvement (primarily visual).

15. What is the Knight and North classification of orbitozygomatic fractures?

In 1961, Knight and North described the classification of six groups of orbitozygomatic fractures based on the direction of displacement as seen on a Water's radiographic view.

Group I: Undisplaced fracture with no clinical or radiographic evidence of displacement.

Group II: Arch fractures. A pure fracture of the zygomatic arch is caused by a direct lateral blow to the arch. Classically, three fracture lines form a V-shaped deformity as seen on a submental vertex radiograph.

Group III: Unrotated body fractures are caused by a direct blow to the zygomatic prominence that drives the zygoma posteriorly and medially, resulting in a flattening of the cheek.

Group IV: Medially rotated body fractures are caused by a blow from above the horizontal axis of the zygoma that drives the bone medially, inferiorly, and posteriorly with rotation. Radiographs show the bone displaced inferiorly at the infraorbital rim and outward at the malar buttress or inward at the frontozygomatic suture.

Group V: Laterally rotated body fractures are caused by a blow originating below the horizontal axis of the zygoma, resulting in displacement medially and posteriorly with lateral rotation. Radiographs demonstrate the upward displacement at the infraorbital rim and lateral displacement at the frontozygomatic suture.

Group VI: Complex fractures, such as comminuted fractures of the body of the zygoma (see Figure).

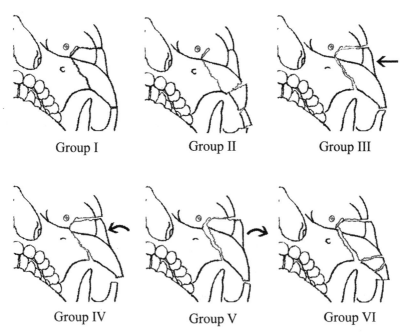

Group I   Group II   Group III

Group IV   Group V   Group VI

16. List the signs and symptoms that accompany zygomatic bone fractures.

Periorbital ecchymosis and edema	Trismus
Abnormal nerve sensibility	Epistaxis
Flattening of the malar prominence	Crepitation from air emphysema
Flattening of the zygomatic arch	Unequal pupillary level

Ecchymosis of the maxillary buccal sulcus
Subconjunctival ecchymosis
Deformity of the orbital margin

Diplopia
Enophthalmos

17. What sort of fracture of the malar complex would produce limited mandibular movements? Which anatomic structures are involved?

Limitation of mouth opening frequently accompanies zygomatic injuries (33%), and the incidence is increased with isolated fractures of the zygomatic arch (45%). Although controversial, the reason most cited for postfracture lack of mobility is impingement of the coronoid process of the mandible by the displaced zygomatic arch fragments. A more likely cause is muscle spasms of the temporalis muscle from impingement of the displaced fragments.

18. How are isolated subcondylar fractures treated in a growing child versus an adult?

In general, children are treated nonsurgically to avoid potential disruption of the growth center (see Table). A short period of intermaxillary fixation and applied, immediate immobilization for pain relief, followed by physical therapy, reduces the chance of bony ankylosis with resultant mandibular deformity. Many clinicians feel that the potential for remodeling of the condylar remnants or the formation of a new condylar head is quite likely in the growing child.

Treatment of Condyle Fractures

SEVERITY OF FRACTURE	ADULT	CHILD
Nondisplaced to moderately displaced		
Centric occlusion with no pain	Soft diet and observation	Soft diet and observation
Malocclusion with no pain	Arch bars and guidance elastics	Arch bars and guidance elastics
Pain with or without malocclusion	Intermaxillary fixation for 2–4 weeks and guidance elastics as necessary	Intermaxillary fixation for 1–3 weeks and guidance elastics as necessary
Severely displaced	Open reduction with osteosynthesis is the best option	Same as nondisplaced

19. Bony ankylosis of the temporomandibular joint (TMJ) after trauma is caused by which mechanism?

The two classically recognized causes of this tissue destruction are TMJ trauma (i.e., nonsurgical and iatrogenic) and osteomyelitis (i.e., otitis media and mastoiditis). Multiple factors predispose the TMJ to ankylosis:

- The displacement of the articular disk allows direct bony contact between the condyle and glenoid fossa.
- The hematoma and bony splinters in the joint area provide an osteoinductive environment.
- Immobility of the joint after trauma from splinting, from intermaxillary fixation, or in a comatose states optimizes abnormal bony healing.

20. In the clinical evaluation of the trauma patient, which nerve supplies sensory innervation to the skin over the mandibular angle?

The great auricular nerve, a branch of the cervical plexus (C2, C3) provides this innervation.

21. Which facial fractures can cause an open-bite deformity with a skeletal class III mandibular position? With a skeletal class II mandibular position?

Bilaterally displaced subcondylar or angle fractures of the mandible may cause the open-bite deformity with a skeletal class II mandibular position (i.e., relative retrusion of the mandible). The displaced Le Fort fractures can cause a skeletal class III appearance (i.e., relative protrusion of the mandible) and an open-bite deformity.

22. How are mandibular fractures managed in the edentulous patient?

Surgical splints (or modified dentures) that are fixed to the maxilla and mandible can be used for closed reduction of an edentulous mandibular fracture. If physiologic mobility of the mandible is required, rigid skeletal fixation using plates and screws or extraoral devices may be used.

23. Which mandibular fractures are not considered compound fractures?

By definition, any fracture in which there is communication with an external wound involving the skin, mucosa, or periodontal membrane (key) is a compound fracture. These fractures include coronoid process fractures, subcondylar fractures, and fractures in all edentulous areas of the mandible where the mucosa remains intact.

24. What is the most common site for a mandibular fracture?

In descending order of occurrence, the most common sites are the body, condyle, angle, symphysis, ramus, and coronoid process.

25. In the treatment of highly comminuted fractures of the mandible, such as gunshot wounds, what factors affect treatment?

It is often impossible to create stable units by the placement of internal plates, screws, and wires. The greatest concerns follow:
- Judicious débridement of necrotic and contaminated tissues with appropriate manipulation and lavage
- Immediate use of parenteral antibiotics
- Hemostasis and elimination of dead space, using proper drainage techniques
- Preservation of the blood supply to the comminuted segments because open surgical techniques increase the potential for osteonecrosis
- Maintaining the stability of osseous segments

26. How are mandibular third molars managed when they are involved in angle fractures of the mandible?

The third molars are maintained if they are in sound condition and are not mobile or if they are fully impacted within the bone and are not mobile nor fractured. In general, diseased or partially erupted third molars are removed.

27. Which facial bones are the most commonly fractured bones?

The nasal bones are most commonly fractured because of their prominent position.

28. Epiphora is caused by the disruption of flow through which structure?

Naso-orbital trauma has the potential to fragment and fracture the nasolacrimal duct, through which tears flow. The nasolacrimal duct, the connection between the lacrimal sac and the nasal cavity, lies within the bony nasolacrimal canal.

29. What is the significance of "raccoon eyes"?

Raccoon eyes are bilateral periorbital ecchymoses that commonly occur as a result of fracture to the base of the anterior cranial fossa.

30. What is the significance of Battle's sign?

Battle's sign is ecchymosis behind the ear that indicates a basilar skull fracture of the middle cranial fossa.

31. Which is the greatest determining factor in destructive force of a bullet: its mass or its velocity?

The answer is evident in the equation for kinetic energy (KE) and its relationship to mass (m) and velocity (v) of the bullet:

$$KE = \frac{½ \, m \, v^2}{2}$$

32. What is the protocol for the management of high-energy ballistic injuries to the maxillo-facial region?
- Immediate primary repair of existing tissue
- Serial, conservative débridement of the wound
- Early, definitive reconstruction

33. With regard to velocity, how are the ballistic injuries classified?
>   Low velocity (<2000 ft/sec)
>   High velocity (>2000 ft/sec)
>   Ultrahigh velocity (>4500 ft/sec)

34. How are shotgun injuries classified?
The closer the victim is to the shotgun, the less the pellets scatter. The greater mass and energy create devastating wounds similar to rifle wounds.
>   Type I: more than 25 cm of scatter (>7 yards)
>   Type II: 10 to 25 cm of scatter (3–7 yards)
>   Type III: less than 10 cm of scatter (<3 yards), with a 38% mortality rate for abdominal injury and higher rate for craniomaxillofacial injury

35. What are the contraindications to tracheal intubation in the patient who has sustained head and neck trauma?
- Suspected or confirmed cervical spine injuries. Establishment of a protected airway requires cricothyrotomy in an emergency situation or controlled, fiberoptic-aided intubation or tracheotomy.
- Suspected fractures of the anterior cranial fossa with cerebrospinal fluid (CSF) rhinorrhea. The nasal route is relatively contraindicated because of contamination of the meninges or violation of the cranium by the endotracheal tube (or nasogastric tube).
- Retropharyngeal swelling seen on cervical spine films. Pharyngeal walls may be violated, with subsequent aspiration of materials.
- Fractured larynx. This may make endotracheal intubation impossible.

36. What causes a fixed, dilated pupil in a patient with head trauma?
Rapidly increasing supratentorial pressure, usually from a mass lesion or epidural bleeding, can compress the ipsilateral third cranial nerve from uncal or tentorial herniation. Contralateral spastic weakness of the arm and leg can be seen with uncal herniation.

37. What is the Le Fort classification of maxillary fractures?
Le Fort I maxillary fracture is a transverse fracture above the apices of the teeth, through the maxillary sinus, and across the nasal septum. It runs posteriorly across the pyramidal processes of the palatine bones and through the pterygoid processes of the sphenoid bones.
Le Fort II maxillary fracture is known as the pyramidal fracture. This fracture follows the same posterior course as the Le Fort I and continues anteriorly, coursing upward near the zygomaticomaxillary suture and the infraorbital foramen, through the inferior orbital rim onto the orbital floor, across the medial orbital wall to the frontal process and nasal bones (or the nasofrontal suture), and through the nasal septum.
Le Fort III maxillary fracture is known as a craniofacial dysjunction fracture. The fracture begins at the nasofrontal suture area and continues through the frontal process, following the medial orbital walls across to the frontozygomatic suture. The fracture continues through the zygomatic arches and continues through the pterygoid processes of the sphenoid bone (see Figure).

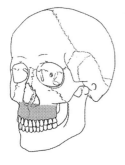
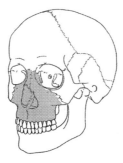
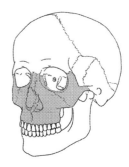

Le Fort I   Le Fort II   Le Fort III

38. What are the causes of traumatic binocular diplopia in midfacial injuries?
Binocular diplopia is primarily caused by restriction or entrapment of extraocular muscles, as seen in orbital floor, medial wall, and blow-out fractures. Diplopia may also be caused by medial or lateral suspensory ligament displacement caused by nasoethmoidal fractures or zygomaticomaxillary complex fractures.

39. Name the vertical buttress areas of the middle third of the facial skeleton. What is their significance?
The buttresses are the nasomaxillary, zygomaticomaxillary, and the pterygomaxillary. They are significant because the nasomaxillary and the zygomaticomaxillary areas are most often used for the placement of rigid fixation systems.

40. Where does the frontal sinus drain? Maxillary sinus? Ethmoid sinus?
- The frontal sinus drains through the nasofrontal duct to the middle meatus.
- The maxillary sinus drains into the middle meatus.
- The ethmoid sinus drains primarily into the superior meatus.

41. How much force would it take to fracture the frontal sinus area of the skull?
Approximately 800 to 1600 pounds of force is needed, which is two to three times greater than the force required to fracture the zygoma, maxilla, or mandible.

42. What is the Stanley classification of frontal sinus fractures?
    Anterior table fractures (type I)
      Isolated to anterior table
      Accompanied by supraorbital rim fractures
      Accompanied by nasoethmoidal complex fractures
    Anterior and posterior table fractures (type II)
      Linear fractures
      Transverse
      Vertical
    Comminuted fractures (type III)
      Isolated to both tables
      Accompanied by nasoethmoidal complex fractures

43. What are the complications associated with frontal sinus fractures?

Short-term complications	*Long-term complications*
Wound infection	Mucocele
CSF leak	Mucopyocele

Fluid accumulation under a coronal flap
Paresthesia of the supraorbital nerve
Meningitis
Acute sinusitis
Brain abscess
Frontal headache

Osteomyelitis of the frontal bone
Cosmetic defect
Brain abscess
Headache

44. How is a nondisplaced fracture of the anterior table managed?
Nondisplaced fractures require no treatment other than medical management consisting of antibiotic coverage and a systemic decongestant or nasal decongestant (or both). These medications are administered to keep the nasofrontal duct patent and to prevent infection.

45. To maintain viability to supporting structures of avulsed teeth, what is the maximum allowable amount of time that the teeth can remain out of the mouth before reimplantation?
Treatment objectives are replantation at the earliest possible time and minimization of damage to the dental ligament and pulp tissue. The speed with which replantation is accomplished is the most important factor: The critical time appears to be 20 to 30 minutes, after which the success rate drops significantly. Contact with the root surface should be avoided, and the tooth should not be allowed to dry out. Treatment, if there is a reasonable expectation of success, includes semirigid stabilization of the tooth for 7 to 10 days and reevaluation to determine the need for further treatment.

46. Why should you perform an intraoral examination on a patient with maxillofacial injuries?
Examination of the oral cavity can give the clinician important information. If there is a malocclusion, the maxilla or mandible may be fractured. Missing or fractured teeth as a result of trauma may have been aspirated or may be embedded in adjacent soft tissue injuries. Tongue lacerations can bleed profusely, and swelling in the floor of the mouth can obstruct the airway. Movement of segments of the dentition may indicate alveolar fractures that require stabilization.

BIBLIOGRAPHY

1. Alling CC, Osborn DB: Maxillofacial Trauma. Philadelphia, Lea & Febiger, 1988.
2. Assael LA: The treatment of comminuted fractures of the mandible. Atlas Oral Maxillofac Surg Clin North Am 5:159–162, 1997.
3. Bailey BJ, Johnson JT, Kabut RI, et al: Head and Neck Surgery–Otolaryngology. Philadelphia, JB Lippincott, 1993.
4. Clark N, Birely B, Manson PN, et. al.: High-energy ballistic and avulsive facial injuries: classification, patterns, and an algorithm for primary reconstruction. Plast Reconstr Surg 98:583–601, 1996.
5. Ellis E, Zide MF: Surgical Approaches to the Facial Skeleton. Baltimore, Williams & Wilkins, 1995.
6. Fonseca RJ (ed): Oral and Maxillofacial Surgery. Philadelphia, WB Sanders, 2000.
7. Foster CA, Sherman JE (eds): Surgery of Facial Bone Fractures. New York, Churchill Livingstone, 1987.
8. Greenberg MS: Handbook of Neurosurgery, 3rd ed. Lakeland, FL, Greenberg Graphic, 1994.
9. Ochs MW, Buckley MJ: Anatomy of the orbit. Oral Maxillofac Surg Clin North Am 5:419–429, 1993.
10. Pearl RM: Management of secondary orbital deformities. Oral Maxillofac Surg Clin North Am 5:507–521, 1993.
11. Perrott DH, Kaban LB: Acute management of orbitozygomatic fractures. Oral Maxillofac Surg Clin North Am 5:475–493, 1993.
12. Trope M: Protocol for treating the avulsed tooth. J Calif Dent Assoc 24:43–49, 1996.
13. Weber WD: Treatment of mandibular fractures. Atlas Oral Maxillofac Surg Clin North Am 5:77–125, 1997.

10. TRAUMATIC OPHTHALMOLOGIC INJURIES

Jonathan C. Song, M.D.

1. What kinds of injuries can be caused by blunt trauma to the eye?

Corneal abrasions

Hyphemas

Traumatic iritis

Traumatic mydriasis

Cataracts

Lens dislocation

Vitreous hemorrhage

Retinal holes or tears

Retinal detachment

Blow-out fracture of the orbit

2. When should a ruptured globe be suspected?

An open globe (ruptured globe) should be suspected with any history of a sharp object entering the globe or of significant blunt trauma. Clinical signs include irregular pupil (i.e., pointing to the direction of injury), soft-appearing globe from decreased intraocular pressure, and severe subconjunctival hemorrhage. Careful, gentle examination of the eye is mandatory to minimize additional pressure on the globe. As soon as a ruptured globe is diagnosed or suspected, a Fox shield should be placed over the eye, and an emergent ophthalmology referral should be made.

3. Which lid lacerations require more than simple skin closure?

Most periorbital lacerations can be repaired with simple skin closure. Lacerations involving the lid margin or gray line require additional techniques for approximation of the lid margin. A laceration involving the tear duct or lacrimal system may require placement of nasolacrimal tubes. Laceration involving the tarsal plate or levator muscle may require reattachment of the muscle before skin closure. These types of lid lacerations should be referred to an ophthalmologist or plastic surgeon for repair.

4. What are the common complaints of patients with corneal abrasions or corneal foreign bodies?

Patients usually present with red, teary eyes and complain of photophobia and pain. Topical anesthesia can be used to improve comfort to allow for examination but should never be dispensed to the patient. Frequent use of topical anesthetics can cause corneal melts. After the eye is anesthetized, it can be stained with fluorescein and illuminated by a Wood or ultraviolet lamp. Corneal epithelial defects take up fluorescein and stain yellow-orange. Careful inspection of the whole cornea must be made to rule out foreign bodies. Nonembedded foreign bodies can be removed with a wet cotton swab. An embedded foreign body may require removal with a 25- or 27-gauge needle or eye spud. Do not remove foreign bodies that involve full-thickness cornea; immediate referral to an ophthalmologist should be made in this case. A larger corneal abrasion (involving more than one fourth of the cornea) may require pressure patching to limit ocular motion and instillation of cycloplegic eyedrops to prevent ciliary body spasm for the patient's comfort. The need for tetanus prophylaxis should also be determined.

5. What is the management of an anterior hyphema?

After trauma, an anterior hyphema can be seen as a layering of red blood cells that pool at the bottom of the anterior chamber of the eye. It can also manifest as a diffuse haziness of the anterior chamber. The patient should be kept upright with minimal activity to prevent rebleeding. Complications include glaucoma and corneal blood staining. The patient should be referred to an ophthalmologist.

6. How do you treat a chemical burn to the eye?

Determine whether the chemical is alkali or acidic. Alkali chemicals can penetrate through the anterior segment of the eye, rapidly causing extensive damage. Initial use of Nitrazine paper helps determine the pH before and after irrigation. Copious irrigation is the key, using at least 2 L of normal saline and 15 to 20 minutes of irrigation. Adequate irrigation is achieved when the pH is corrected to neutral level (pH 7). The pH level should be checked 15 minutes after the last irrigation with Nitrazine paper.

7. What causes traumatic anisocoria (mydriasis)?

An efferent pupillary defect in which a pupil is dilated (usually irregular) and nonreactive to direct or consensual light is usually a result of sphincter tears in the iris from trauma. A careful eye examination is mandatory to rule out other ocular injuries. Uncal herniation from intracranial injuries should be considered if there is a decreased level of consciousness in the presence of a round, nonreactive, dilated pupil.

8. How do you treat subconjunctival hemorrhages?

Subconjunctival hemorrhages are usually benign and resolve spontaneously within 2 to 3 weeks without treatment. However, a careful eye examination must be performed to rule out other ocular injuries in the setting of ocular trauma.

9. What radiographic tests should be ordered if an intraocular foreign body is suspected?

History from the patient about the type of foreign body is important. Metallic objects can be visualized with orbital plain films. However, computed tomography (CT) scans of the orbit with axial and coronal cuts is needed for three-dimensional localization. Orbital ultrasound is useful for detection of nonmetallic objects. Magnetic resonance imaging (MRI) should not be initially ordered.

10. What are the signs and symptoms of a retinal detachment?

Classic symptoms include seeing floaters and flashes of light. Patient may also see curtain-like shadows in the peripheral vision. Central vision may be initially preserved if the detachment begins at the periphery. As the detachment progresses to involve the macula, the central vision diminishes.

11. What are the symptoms and signs of a blow-out fracture?

Patients with inferior orbital wall fractures (i.e., blow-out fractures) can present with pain, local tenderness, and binocular double vision. Critical signs include restricted eye movement (especially in upward gaze) from entrapment of the inferior rectus muscle, decreased sensation over the inferior orbital rim, palpable step-off along the orbital rim, and enophthalmos (i.e., sunken appearance of the eye), which may initially be masked by orbital edema.

12. How do you diagnose a retrobulbar hemorrhage?

A traumatic retrobulbar hemorrhage may occur after moderate to severe facial or head trauma. Proptosis with resistance is felt when pushing on the involved eye compared with the unaffected eye. Measurement of the intraocular pressure dictates the course of management. Lateral canthotomy and cantholysis should be reserved for cases with very high pressures in which there is an immediate risk to vision. CT scans of the orbits should be obtained to document blood in the retrobulbar space. However, management can be instituted before the scan if vision is threatened.

13. What are the most common cranial nerve palsies after trauma?

After trauma, III, IV, and VI nerve palsies can occur. Traumatic cranial nerve palsies usually improve with time, with full resolution by 6 months.

14. What ophthalmic trauma injuries require immediate ophthalmologic referral?

- Ruptured globes
- Chemical burns to the cornea
- Lens rupture or dislocation

- Retrobulbar hemorrhage with increased intraocular pressure
- Lacerations of the lid involving the lid margin, lacrimal system, or tarsal plate
- Signs or symptoms of retinal detachment

BIBLIOGRAPHY

1. Cullom RD, Chang B: The Wills Eye Manual: Office and Emergency Room Diagnosis and Treatment of Eye Disease, 3rd ed. Philadelphia, JB Lippincott, 1994.
2. Friedman NJ, Pineda R, Kaiser PK: The Massachusetts Eye and Ear Infirmary Illustrated Manual of Ophthalmology. Philadelphia, WB Saunders, 1998.
3. Joondeph BC: Blunt ocular trauma. Emerg Med Clin North Am 6:147–167, 1988.
4. Sternberg P, Aaberg TM: The persistent challenge of ocular trauma. Am J Ophthalmol 107:421–424, 1989.

11. EAR, NOSE, AND THROAT INJURY

Joel Sercarz, M.D.

1. What is the first step in the management of patients with injuries to the neck?

It is critical to secure the airway in patients with head and neck injuries. Frequently, patients with severe blunt injuries have both soft tissue and bony injuries that compromise the airway. Intubation may be attempted, but some injuries require a surgical airway because blood and soft tissue trauma obscures visualization of the larynx. Trauma surgeons should be familiar with the indications and techniques for both cricothyrotomy and tracheotomy.

Because of the risks of airway obstruction and aspiration, it is necessary to have a proactive approach to airway management in trauma patients.

2. Is cricothyrotomy possible in all age groups?

In children younger than 7, the cricothyroid membrane is very short in height and close to the vocal cords. There is a considerable risk of injury to the vocal cords and the immediate subglottis when cricothyrotomy is performed in this age group. In young children, cricothyrotomy or tracheotomy is preferable.

3. In severe penetrating injuries to the larynx, is intubation recommended?

When there is severe disruption of the larynx from trauma, intubation is not recommended. There is risk of worsening the injury to the mucosa or displacing the laryngeal cartilages. It is best to perform a tracheotomy to secure the airway, followed by a computed tomography (CT) scan of the larynx or an open exploration (laryngofissure) to determine the extent of the injuries.

4. What maneuvers can be used to improve airway obstruction caused by displacement of the tongue on the pharyngeal wall?

The jaw thrust is performed by lifting the mandible, grasping the ramus and angle, and displacing it anteriorly. This maneuver will help to temporarily stabilize the airway.

5. In penetrating neck trauma, what are the zones of the neck?

A zone 1 injury occurs at the base of the neck between the cricoid cartilage and the sternal notch. Zone 2 is between the cricoid and the angle of the mandible. Zone 3 is between the angle of the jaw and the skull base. The most common site for penetrating injuries is zone 2.

6. What are some of the findings that indicate the need for immediate exploration of zone 2 injuries to the neck?

There are several indications for immediate neck exploration for zone 2 injuries. These include a rapidly expanding hematoma or the presence of a large wound with obvious injury to the larynx, trachea, or esophagus. If the patient is hemodynamically unstable from blood loss, neck exploration should also be performed.

7. Should all zone 2 injuries to the neck be explored?

Most trauma specialists believe that not all injuries to zone 2 that penetrate the platysma need to be explored surgically. Selective exploration is performed based on clinical presentation and diagnostic studies.

In general, patients who are not explored should undergo angiography to rule out injuries to the neck arteries. The use of color flow Doppler imaging has proven to be sensitive for vascular injuries, suggesting that noninvasive imaging may reduce the need for angiography in the future.

8. Are all serious vascular injuries in the neck clinically apparent?

Some significant vascular injuries, especially in low-velocity wounds, are not clinically apparent and may cause delayed complications. Such arterial injuries include arteriovenous fistulas and false aneurysms.

9. How are zone 3 injuries to the neck evaluated?

In zone 3 injuries of the neck, there is the risk of vascular injuries at the skull base. In most cases, angiography is necessary to assess the great vessels at the skull base. A CT scan of the temporal bone, sinuses, or orbits may help define bony injuries in zone 3 trauma.

The need for other diagnostic studies is based on the trajectory and nature of the injury. In most cases, a CT scan of the neck and skull base are necessary to better define the injury.

10. How are patients with penetrating injuries to zone 1 injuries managed?

Zone 1 major vascular injuries can occur within the chest and may be difficult to identify clinically. Therefore, angiography is necessary in the evaluation of these injuries.

Further studies, such as contrast studies of the esophagus, CT scanning, and bronchoscopy are performed if clinically indicated.

11. How is a penetrating injury to the esophagus ruled out?

Esophageal injuries can be ruled out with contrast studies, endoscopy, or direct examination during neck exploration. If the injury is identified, primary repair is generally successful.

12. What is the consequence of a delay in the diagnosis of an esophageal injury?

Early diagnosis of esophageal injuries is critical to prevent neck abscess, mediastinitis, sepsis, and stricture.

13. When the facial nerve is lacerated by a knife wound, how is the injury managed?

If the facial nerve is lacerated on the face, this can be elicited easily on physical examination in an awake patient. If there is weakness of a significant branch of the facial nerve, such as the ramus mandibularis or frontal (zygomaticotemporal) branch, surgical exploration is performed to attempt a repair.

It is frequently difficult to identify the distal facial nerve branches. When these branches are found, the nerve is reapproximated and sutured with a fine nylon suture under the surgical microscope. If there is a gap in the nerve segments that prevents a tension-free repair, an interposition nerve graft is required.

14. When the facial nerve is paralyzed following a gunshot wound to the temporal bone, how is the patient evaluated and treated?

A gunshot wound that damages the facial nerve produces a much more serious injury than a knife wound. An injury to the facial nerve in the temporal bone should be explored via a mastoidectomy approach. If the injury occurs in a medial location, such as the geniculate ganglion in the middle ear, the approach must be extended to identify the nerve proximally, for example, in the internal auditory canal.

After a gunshot wound, there is usually a full-thickness loss of a segment of the nerve at the point of impact. If both the proximal and distal segments can be located, a cable nerve graft is sutured between the two segments. A sensory nerve from the neck is used as a donor, because it is accessible and has a convenient branching pattern. The sural nerve from the lower extremity is another potential nerve donor site.

15. What are the two types of temporal bone fractures, and what types of hearing loss do they cause?

There are two types of temporal bone fractures. These are longitudinal, which are roughly parallel to the petrous bone, and the transverse, which are perpendicular to the petrous.

Because the transverse temporal bone fracture typically traverses the cochlea, patients typically are deaf in the involved ear. Longitudinal fractures tend to produce hearing loss because of ossicular dislocation or external canal fracture but rarely lead to catastrophic hearing loss.

16. What are the indications to surgically explore a temporal bone fracture?

Temporal bone fractures are explored if there is complete facial nerve paralysis or persistent cerebrospinal fluid (CSF) leak. Exploration of a paralyzed facial nerve may allow removal of bony spicules in the fallopian canal or interposition grafts if there has been destruction of a facial nerve segment.

Most CSF leaks that follow temporal bone fractures resolve with observation alone.

17. How is the larynx evaluated for significant injury after neck trauma?

There are two critical tests in the evaluation of a potential laryngeal injury. First, the airway should be examined with a flexible laryngoscope. If there are significant mucosal lacerations, laryngeal exploration is necessary. A CT scan should also be obtained, if possible. This is the best way to evaluate the laryngeal framework. If a displaced fracture of the thyroid or cricoid cartilage is identified, further treatment will be necessary.

18. How are laryngeal fractures treated?

A displaced thyroid cartilage should be treated with neck exploration and anatomic reduction of the involved cartilages. If a displaced fracture of the thyroid cartilage is untreated, subtle voice changes may result because of a loss of symmetry of the vocal folds.

If there is significant mucosal injury, thyrotomy with open repair of the mucosal lacerations will generally prevent severe laryngeal scarring and stenosis.

The cricoid cartilage is the only complete ring in the airway, and it creates a potential site of narrowing within the area. Cricoid fractures, therefore, can produce subglottic stenosis, either because of membranous stenosis or because of displaced fracture of the cartilage framework.

19. What is laryngotracheal separation?

A separation of the trachea and larynx is a potentially fatal injury in which a transverse injury to the trachea produces a discontinuity to the airway. Such patients usually present with a massive neck injury and breathe through the laceration. Attempts at oral intubation may be fruitless or even harmful.

20. How is laryngotracheal separation treated?

Immediate tracheostomy is necessary to stabilize the airway in cases of laryngotracheal separation. Unfortunately, the trachea may retract into the chest, making lifesaving tracheostomy difficult.

21. What are the most common sites for mandibular fractures?

The three most common sites for mandibular fractures are the parasymphyseal fracture through the mental foramen, the angle of the mandible, and the subcondylar area inferior to the temporomandibular joint. Most commonly, two fractures occur simultaneously because mechanical forces produced at the point of the injury are transmitted to other areas of the jaw.

22. What is the primary goal in the treatment of mandibular fractures?

The most important goal in the treatment of mandibular fractures is reestablishment of anatomic occlusion of the teeth. Incorrect repair of mandible fractures frequently produces significant malocclusion.

23. Are any types of mandibular fractures emergencies?

If there are bilateral parasymphyseal mandible fractures, the tongue is free to be displaced posteriorly and obstruct the airway. This occurs because there is loss of anterior tongue support provided primarily by the genioglossus muscle and tendon. Such bilateral fractures require immediate fixation.

24. What are some of the complications of mandible fracture treatment?

Injuries to the marginal mandibular branch of the facial nerve, inferior alveolar nerve, and mental nerves are all too common. Malocclusion is also a common potential problem, especially with badly comminuted fractures.

25. What is maxillomandibular fixation?

Maxillomandibular fixation (MMF) involves securing the upper and lower teeth in their normal anatomic relationships, thereby producing normal occlusion. In some mandibular fractures, immobilization with MMF is helpful in the healing process, analogous to the use of a cast for the extremities.

26. Why is MMF necessary during the management of complex midfacial fractures?

MMF provides anatomic alignment of the teeth, which is necessary to produce normal occlusion. If maxillary fractures are repaired without attention to the occlusion, the mandibular and maxillary teeth will not oppose. This problem is much more difficult to treat after healing of the fractures.

27. What is a Le Fort fracture?

Severe maxillary fractures are known as Le Fort fractures. They are classified by level as Le Fort I, II, and III. These fractures are produced by anterior forces and follow the three weak areas of the midfacial skeleton. Each of these fractures produces mobility of the upper teeth and maxilla, a valuable clinical sign.

These fractures are extremely varied and often occur in association with frontal sinus, nasoethmoid, and mandible fractures. A Le Fort I fracture is a low transverse facture of the maxillary sinus. A Le Fort II fracture involves the floor of the orbit and lateral buttress of the midface. The Le Fort III fracture is through the frontozygomatic suture line at the lateral orbit and creates a complete separation of the maxilla from the frontal bone.

These fractures typically produce an elongation of the midface, malocclusion, and maxillary rotation. The fractures commonly occur in combination, with significant asymmetry of the fracture sites.

28. What is the radiographic hallmark of a Le Fort fracture?

All Le Fort fractures include fractures of the pterygoid plates, which allow mobility of the palate. There also are obvious injuries to the anterior maxilla and zygoma, although these findings vary substantially, depending on the level and severity of the fractures.

29. How are Le Fort fractures repaired?

In order to treat Le Fort fractures, wide exposure of the injured maxilla is necessary. Small titanium plates are then placed across the various fracture lines and secured with titanium screws.

Generally, both the medial and lateral buttresses of the maxilla are reconstituted. It is necessary to fixate the maxilla to stable bone. In the case of Le Fort III fractures, the maxilla and zygoma are fixated to the frontal bone of the skull, which typically is a stable point. In some cases with severe comminution, bone grafts are necessary for adequate repair of Le Fort fractures.

In the future, bioabsorbable plates will probably be used more frequently. These are currently available and have proven to be particularly helpful for the repair of pediatric facial fractures, where the ongoing presence of plates may be counterproductive to facial growth.

30. How is the midface exposed for fracture fixation?

The midface is exposed from below with the facial degloving approach, which involves an incision in the gingivobuccal sulcus superior to the maxillary teeth. Then, the soft tissue and mucosa are elevated off the maxilla. This allows direct repair of the lateral (or zygomaticomaxillary) and medial (or nasomaxillary) buttresses of the face.

31. What is the bicoronal approach, and what areas of the facial skeleton can it expose?

The bicoronal approach is a very versatile technique for severe fractures to the facial skeleton and frontal bone. An incision is placed posterior to the hair line in the forehead and is extended to the preauricular crease. A flap is then raised immediately superficial to the pericranium. This flap allows exposure of the frontal sinus, orbital roofs, frontozygomatic suture, and zygoma.

If the supraorbital nerves are elevated out of their foramina, it is possible to expose the entire nasal bone and nasoethmoid complex via the bicoronal incision.

32. What is a trimalar fracture?

When a lateral impact injures the facial bones, the malar eminence often absorbs the blow, producing a fracture of the zygoma upon its attachments to the maxilla and frontal bone. The zygomatic arch may also be fractured. The malar eminence is very important for facial cosmesis, and symmetry should be restored to this area during fracture repair.

33. How are trimalar fractures repaired?

As in Le Fort fractures, the maxilla is exposed and the anatomic position of the bone fragments is assured with titanium plate fixation. Usually the lateral brow incision is used to repair the frontozygomatic suture line, and the orbital rim is exposed to repair the fracture that is usually present through the infraorbital foramen.

34. What problems does a nasal fracture produce?

Nasal fractures cause displacement of the nasal bones and nasal septum. This causes both cosmetic and functional problems. If a hematoma forms adjacent to the septal cartilage, the septum can lose its blood supply and necrose, with collapse of nasal support.

35. When is a nasal fracture repaired?

A nasal fracture should be repaired within 7 days of the injury, while there is still some mobility of the bones. In most cases, closed reduction and casting of the nose is attempted in order to optimize the position of the nasal bones. Some specialists recommend open reduction with rhinoplasty techniques when closed reduction is not possible.

36. What is a nasoethmoid complex fracture?

In the nasoethmoid fracture, there is posterior displacement of the nasal and ethmoid bones. The fracture frequently produces traumatic telecanthus, in which the medial canthi of the eye is displaced laterally due to disruption of the medial canthal tendon. It also causes a posterior displacement to the upper nose that is a serious cosmetic problem.

This type of injury is usually due to severe blunt trauma, such as automobile or industrial accidents.

37. How is a nasoethmoid complex fracture treated?

Like many other fractures of the facial bones, nasoethmoid complex fractures are repaired by exposing the fractures and then placing titanium microplates to secure the bones in an anatomic position. If possible, the lamina papyracea is reconstituted, and the medial canthal ligament is securely attached to the bone by the repair, to correct the traumatic telecanthus.

BIBLIOGRAPHY

1. Asensio JA, Valenziano CP, Falcone RE, Grosh JD: Management of penetrating neck injuries. The controversy surrounding zone II injuries. Surg Clin North Am 71:267–296, 1991.

2. Gerst PH, Sharma SK, Sharma PK: Selective management of penetrating neck trauma. Am Surg 56:553–555, 1990.
3. Gruss JS, Mackinnon SE: Complex maxillary fractures: Role of buttress reconstruction and immediate bone grafts. Plast Reconstr Surg 78:9–22, 1986.
4. Schaefer SD, Close LG: Acute management of laryngeal trauma. Ann Otol Rhinol Laryngol 98:98–104, 1989.

12. PENETRATING NECK INJURIES

Juan A, Asensio, M.D., and Gustavo A. Roldán, M.D.

1. What makes the anatomy of the neck unique?

The neck harbors many vital structures confined within a very small space. The cardiovascular, respiratory, digestive, endocrine, and central nervous systems are represented. The neck structures are invested by fascial layers that provide for compartmentalization of all the structures within the neck. This arrangement limits external bleeding from vascular injuries, minimizing the chance for exsanguination.

2. How is the neck anatomically divided for the purpose of evaluating penetrating neck injuries?

The neck is divided into three zones:

Zone I extends from the clavicle to the cricoid cartilage

Zone II extends from the cricoid cartilage to the angle of the mandible

Zone III extends from the angle of the mandible to the base of the skull

Knowledge of cervical anatomy, coupled with an effort to conceptualize which structures lie within each zone, allows the trauma surgeon to institute a systematic diagnostic search for injuries.

3. What structures are contained within the carotid sheath?

The carotid sheath is formed by three components of the cervical fascia. It contains the carotid artery, the jugular vein, and the vagus nerve. It communicates with the mediastinum, and the nerves of Hering innervate the carotid bulb.

4. What are the historical and physical examination findings associated with injuries to the vascular structures of the neck?

A history of bleeding, which can be profuse at the scene of the traumatic incident; the presence of shock; neurologic deficits such as hemiparesis or hemiplegia and coma; and the presence of aphasia indicate the presence of a carotid artery injury. Jugular venous injuries may also present with profuse bleeding but do not produce neurologic changes.

Physical examination findings may include the presence of a pulsatile or expanding hematoma, the absence of pulses, the presence of bruits, and active external hemorrhage. Findings of neurologic deficits on physical examination are also important.

5. What are the historical and physical examination findings associated with pharyngoesophageal injuries?

A history of hematemesis, dysphagia, or odynophagia indicates the presence of pharyngoesophageal injuries. The incidence of dysphagia and odynophagia is quite low, estimated to occur in approximately 3% to 5% of patients. Tenderness over the neck, crepitus, subcutaneous emphysema, and the presence of air bubbling or escaping from the wound are important physical examination findings. The presence of blood in the pharynx may also indicate pharyngoesophageal injuries.

6. What are the historical and physical examination findings associated with laryngotracheal injuries?

A history of dyspnea, changes in the tone and quality of the voice, and inability to phonate accompanied by hemoptysis should alert trauma surgeons to the presence of a laryngotracheal injury. Physical examination findings include tenderness over the thyroid, cricoid cartilages, or tracheal rings. The presence of crepitus, subcutaneous emphysema, and air bubbling from the wound also indicate these types of injuries.

7. How are penetrating neck injury patients resuscitated?

All trauma patients should be resuscitated using the Advanced Trauma Life Support (ATLS) protocols. However, the airway of the patient with a penetrating neck injury should be secured early, because expanding hematomas may rapidly occlude the airway. Early intubation can prevent loss of the airway. The performance of a surgical cricothyroidotomy can be dangerous because of violation of fascial planes that are responsible for containing cervical hematomas.

Nasogastric tubes should not be placed during the resuscitation phase; they may cause patients to retch, releasing a tamponaded vascular injury that results in active external hemorrhage. Nasogastric tubes should be put in place in the operating room when the patient is under general anesthesia.

8. What is the best way to control active external bleeding from the neck during the initial evaluation and resuscitation of penetrating neck injuries?

Direct pressure should control all significant hemorrhage until definitive control can be obtained in the operating room. Blind clamping in the presence of active external hemorrhage may damage vital structures.

9. How are hemodynamically stable patients with penetrating neck injuries evaluated?

Hemodynamically stable patients who need immediate surgical intervention can be evaluated by investigating the three key anatomic components of the neck—the cardiovascular, respiratory, and digestive systems. The investigative armamentarium includes arteriography, color flow duplex scanning, laryngoscopy and bronchoscopy, esophagoscopy and esophagography, and computed tomography (CT) scans.

Arteriography remains the gold standard in evaluating vascular injuries; however, color duplex scanning is reliable and noninvasive. Laryngoscopy and bronchoscopy facilitate the exclusion of laryngeal and tracheal injuries. CT scanning can be a valuable adjunct to these techniques in assessing the structures of the laryngotracheal complex, evaluating missile trajectory and assessing the cervical spine. Esophageal injuries can be diagnosed with esophagography, which has a sensitivity of 70% to 80%. Rigid esophagoscopy has a higher sensitivity for diagnosing cervical esophageal injuries; however, it requires general anesthesia and poses a risk of esophageal rupture. Flexible endoscopy is not a useful tool in establishing the diagnosis of pharyngoesophageal injuries. Simple cross-table lateral and anteroposterior (AP) views of the neck are helpful diagnostic tools because they aid in missile location and trajectory determination in patients sustaining gunshot wounds to the neck.

10. What are the indications for formal neck exploration of penetrating neck wounds?

The indications for exploration of penetrating anterior neck wounds that have violated the platysma can be subdivided according to the organ systems represented in the neck. Vascular indications for exploration consist of a history of substantial blood loss, persistent and ongoing hemorrhage, and a pulsatile or expanding hematoma. Respiratory indications include hemoptysis, crepitation, and dysphonia. Digestive indications include hematemesis, dysphagia, and crepitation. Central nervous system indications for exploration include neurologic deficits such as aphasia and hemiparesis or hemiplegia.

11. Should all penetrating neck injuries be explored?

Mandatory exploration of all penetrating neck injuries yields an approximately 50% rate of negative explorations. Selective management of penetrating neck injuries is a management philosophy that seeks to evaluate the neck using a variety of diagnostic tools. Only patients who exhibit clinical signs or symptoms consistent with an injury should be explored. Patients who have positive findings in their diagnostic workup that demand operative interventions are explored. Physical examination is considered a valuable triage tool and, accompanied by many diagnostic modalities, is used to select patients who merit surgical intervention. This management approach increases the yield of positive explorations to approximately 70%.

12. What are transcervical gunshot wounds?

Transcervical gunshot wounds are defined as injuries that have crossed the midline of the neck. Their severity can be quite high because they may injure vascular structures in both sides of the neck. Although a significant number of these injuries require immediate surgical intervention, this is not the rule. For hemodynamically stable patients sustaining transcervical gunshot wounds, a thoughtful selective approach is usually quite successful, although all key anatomic structures must be thoroughly investigated.

13. What are the standard operating room approach, incisions, and maneuvers used in the management of penetrating neck injuries?

On the operating table, the patient is placed supine, with the head extended and rotated to the side opposite of the area to be explored, provided that the cervical spine has been radiographically cleared. The face, neck, supraclavicular, and chest areas are included in the operating fields because extension of the standard neck incision may become necessary. The contralateral groin or ankle areas are also prepared and draped separately should the need arise to harvest the saphenous vein for a bypass.

The neck is explored through the standard incision on the anterior border of the sternocleidomastoid muscle, starting from the angle of mandible to the sternoclavicular junction. This incision provides exposure of all structures within zone II of the neck. The neck incision may also be extended as a supraclavicular incision for the management of most zone I injuries, and it can be extended as a median sternotomy or combined with an anterolateral thoracotomy to create the "trap door" or "book" thoracotomy. Extension of the standard zone II neck incision toward the origin of the sternocleidomastoid muscle may be made to gain better exposure to zone III injuries.

14. What makes carotid artery injuries unique?

Carotid artery injuries are the most difficult and immediately life-threatening of all injuries to the neck. They are prone to active hemorrhage, which can occlude the airway, making surgical intervention challenging. Their potential for causing fatal neurologic problems demands excellent surgical judgment in their approach and management.

Between 11% and 13% of all penetrating neck injuries are carotid artery injuries. The common carotid artery is the most frequently injured carotid artery, followed by the external and internal carotid arteries. The most common presentations include shock, active bleeding, and an accompanying pulsatile or expanding hematoma. These injuries may include neurologic deficits.

15. What is the operative approach to the management of carotid artery injuries?

The most important goal of operative approach to penetrating carotid artery injuries is the control of hemorrhage. The operative approach should be based on the preoperative classification of the neurologic presentation of the patient. All patients should be thoroughly evaluated with regard to neurologic presentation, and they should be classified as follows:

A. Normal neurologic examination; no deficits

B. Mild neurologic deficits defined as weakness of an upper or lower extremity in the absence of other neurologic injuries

C. Severe neurologic deficits defined as aphasia or hemiplegia

D. Coma

E. Indeterminate neurologic status secondary to the presence of shock

Patients who fit into categories A, B, C, and E should undergo primary repair and revascularization. Ample evidence suggests that primary repair and revascularization results in better outcomes compared with ligation. Many neurologic deficits correct on revascularization. In patients presenting with coma and fixed neurologic deficits, ligation is the better approach. In those presenting with indeterminate neurologic status, primary repair and revascularization result in better outcomes. Frequently, a thorough neurologic examination cannot be performed in the presence of shock.

16. Should shunts be used during carotid artery injury repair?

Shunts should be used at the discretion of the surgeon. The surgical management of small carotid injuries that can be repaired rapidly may be safely accomplished without their use, generally these are caused by stab wounds . Shunts may be used in the management of complex carotid injuries, particularly those that may require the use of a bypass graft and in which there is diminished back flow from the distal stump. The use of shunts should also be considered in patients presenting with neurologic deficits and severe hypotension.

17. How many types of shunts are available?

There are four types of shunts in general use. The *Javid* shunt was the first shunt designed and requires special clamps to hold it in place. Similarly, the *Sundt* shunt requires clamps to secure it. The *Pruitt-Inahara* shunt is held in place by balloons that are inflated through separate ports. This shunt also has a separate irrigating port trough which heparinized saline may be infused. Perhaps easier to use are the straight *Argyle* shunts, which come in several sizes and can be held in place by clamps or sutures (see Figures).

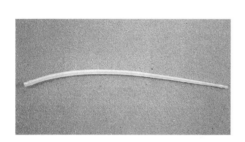

(Figure 1) Javid shunt

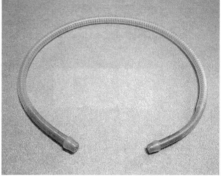

(Figure 2) Sundt shunt

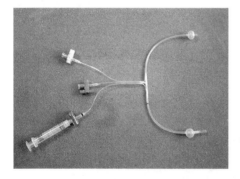

(Figure 3) Pruitt-Inahara shunt

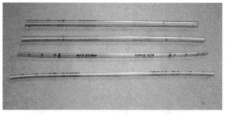

(Figure 4) Straight Argyle shunts

18. How could vertebral artery injuries be best described? Do they usually occur alone?

Vertebral artery injuries are uncommon and account for approximately 1% of all penetrating neck vascular injuries. They are increasingly being diagnosed because of the liberal use of angiography. Many of the clinical findings result from associated injuries. Associated vascular injuries occur with a frequency of 13% to 19%. Arteriovenous fistulas among the vertebral artery and its paired accompanying veins occur with a frequency of 11%, and the incidence of associated pharyngoesophageal injuries is 19%. These injuries usually are associated with other severe injuries.

19. Is any shunt superior to others?

No, the type of shunt employed is generally at the surgeon's discretion. The type of shunt use is not as important as the indications for their use.

20. How are vertebral artery injuries best managed?

If the patient presents with hemodynamic instability and profuse bleeding from a vertebral artery injury, he or she is best managed operatively. Knowledge of the anatomy of the vertebral artery is important in determining the operative approach, which can be difficult. The vertebral artery emerges from the subclavian artery and enters the intervertebral foramina at the level of the sixth cervical vertebra (C6). It then courses upward and exits at the level of the second cervical vertebra (C2) before entering the skull.

If the injury is located in the first part of the vertebral artery, between its origin and its entrance into the intervertebral foramina, the artery can be ligated. Ligation of the artery at its second part within the intervertebral canal requires unroofing the canal, which can be challenging. Ligation of its third portion as it emerges at the level of C2, as well as ligation within its fourth portion that is intracranial, necessitates combined approaches by the trauma and neurosurgical teams. Most vertebral artery injuries do not require this approach.

21. What are the alternate approaches to the management of vertebral artery injuries?

With the advance of interventional radiology, embolization has become the procedure of choice in many patients. Brisk bleeding usually requires proximal and distal embolization. The same can be said for the control of false aneurysms or arteriovenous fistulas. Thrombosed vertebral arteries do not require further treatment. Sometimes, small intimal injuries to the vertebral artery are detected and require no treatment. Angiographic evaluation at a later date usually reveals complete healing of the vessel.

22. Are pharyngoesophageal injuries frequent in cases of penetrating neck injuries?

Pharyngoesophageal injuries are relatively uncommon, occurring in 7% to 9% of all penetrating injuries to the neck. They represent the most commonly missed injuries in the neck. Exclusion of these injuries is the most frequently cited indication for neck exploration.

23. How do delays in diagnoses and repair of pharyngoesophageal injuries affect outcome?

Diagnostic delays and delays in definitive surgical intervention are cited as the most important factors in the rising morbidity and mortality of penetrating cervical esophageal injuries. Their morbidity and mortality rises if these injuries are not detected and definitively repaired within a 24-hour period.

24. How are pharyngoesophageal injuries surgically repaired?

Surgical exploration of the neck must be carried out in a meticulous fashion. All areas where crepitus is noted or surrounding hematomas must be carefully explored. Advancing a nasogastric tube to the level of the origin of the cervical esophagus and infusing saline on a dry operative field or air in a flooded operative field may detect cervical esophageal lacerations. Instillation of methylene blue may also outline these injuries. Cervical esophageal injuries may be hard to detect and have been missed during surgical exploration.

Because the esophagus does not have a serosal layer, repairs can be difficult. Primary repair using a two-layer closure is recommended. The mucosal layer is approximated with fine absorbable sutures, and the muscular layer of the esophagus can be approximated with fine nonabsorbable sutures. In all cases, a closed drainage system should be used in case a fistula develops. A cervical esophagostomy is rarely needed to deal with these injuries.

25. How are jugular vein injuries managed?

The clinical presentation of jugular vein injuries is similar to that of the arterial injuries in the neck. Jugular veins are the most frequently injured vascular structures in the neck. They tend to bleed profusely, requiring rapid proximal and distal control. The risk of air emboli should also be considered. Jugular veins may be ligated or repaired. Remember that ligation of a jugular vein interrupts an important venous channel returning blood from the brain. Ligation of both jugular veins should be avoided at all costs, because this may result in cavernous sinus thrombosis.

If the jugular vein needs to be repaired, it should be accomplished with fine vascular monofilament sutures. The lumen may be narrowed, and the vein may thrombose. No evidence suggests that pulmonary embolism occurs with a greater frequency in primarily repaired jugular veins.

26. How are laryngotracheal injuries managed?

All injuries incurred by the laryngeal complex should be managed with close consultation with otorhinolaryngologists. Many injuries require opening the thyroid cartilage and repair of the vocal cords.

Laryngotracheal injuries are defined as simple or complex. *Simple tracheal injuries* in which there has been no tissue loss may be primarily repaired by approximating the mucosa and cartilage using fine absorbable sutures. An endotracheal tube passed distally to these injuries helps to protect the repair. In *complex tracheal injuries,* in which segments of the trachea need to be resected, a tension-free anastomosis that is well vascularized may be performed using fine nonabsorbable sutures. The blood supply of the trachea enters laterally and must be meticulously preserved. Tracheostomies are usually needed to protect these repairs.

27. How are thyroid gland injuries managed?

Thyroid gland injuries are uncommon and are usually the result of gunshots wounds. Control of hemostasis is important because the thyroid gland is quite vascular. The damaged gland must be débrided with meticulous attention toward preservation of glandular tissue. If a lobe is severely injured, a lobectomy is performed in the usual fashion after identification and preservation of the ipsilateral recurrent laryngeal nerve.

28. How are parathyroid injuries managed?

Parathyroid injuries are less common than thyroid gland injuries. Because the glands are quite delicate, they are generally severely damaged and require extirpation.

29. Is there such a thing as thoracic duct injury?

Thoracic duct injuries are rare and are usually associated with injuries to the jugular or subclavian veins. In general, they occur from penetrating injuries to the left side of the neck. If detected intraoperatively, the thoracic duct should be identified and doubly ligated using fine nonabsorbable sutures.

A milky, white fluid drains from the incision if injuries are missed at the initial procedure. The fluid should be sent to the laboratory for cell count and pH determinations and for protein, fat, and triglyceride levels. These patients can be managed nonoperatively with hyperalimentation or low-fat diets. If the fistula does not heal in 2 weeks, repeat operative intervention is usually necessary for ligation of the transected duct.

30. What are complex and combined injuries, and how are they managed?

Complex and combined injuries have an extensive transcervical trajectory and harbor combined tracheoesophageal injuries, tracheal plus vascular injuries, esophageal plus vascular injuries, or injuries to all three systems. They sometimes require bilateral neck explorations and extensive débridement.

These injuries carry extremely high morbidity and mortality rates because of complications, chiefly failure of vascular repairs, abscesses, and tracheoesophageal fistulas. Management includes primary repair of all injuries if feasible, débridement as necessary, interposition of muscle flaps between all suture lines, and avoiding tracheostomies whenever possible. All of these injuries should be drained using closed systems.

BIBLIOGRAPHY

1. Asensio JA, Berne J, Demetriades D, et al: Penetrating esophageal injuries. Time interval of safety for preoperative evaluation—How long is safe? J Trauma 43:319–324, 1997.
2. Asensio JA, Chahwan S, Forno W, et al: Penetrating esophageal injuries: Multicenter study of the American Association for the Surgery of Trauma. J Trauma 50:289–296, 2001.
3. Asensio JA, Valenziano CP, Falcone RE, Grosh JD: Management of penetrating neck injuries: The controversy surrounding zone II injuries. Surg Clin North Am 71:267–296, 1991.
4. Demetriades D, Asensio JA, Velmahos G, Thal E: Complex problems in penetrating neck trauma. Surg Clin North Am 76:661–683, 1996.

13. SPINAL INJURIES

Duncan Q. McBride, M.D.

1. What is a Jefferson's fracture?

Jefferson's fracture is a blow-out fracture of C1. Due to an axial blow to the head that applies direct downward force on the skull, the lateral masses of the C1 ring are driven away from the spinal cord. This type of injury may occur if a heavy object falls onto the patient's head or if a person falls and lands on the top of his or her head. Typically, patients are neurologically intact.

2. What is a hangman's fracture?

A hangman's fracture is fracture of the posterior elements of C2. This is usually caused by extreme extension of the head and neck but is typically a stable injury.

3. Describe the three types of odontoid fracture.

A **type I odontoid fracture** is a fracture involving the tip of the dens. It is an avulsion of the tip with the ligamentous structures attached there. This is a stable injury, treatable with a cervical collar.

A **type II odontoid fracture** is a fracture across the base of the dens where it attaches to the body of C2. This fracture will heal with immobilization alone if the dens is displaced less than 5 or 6 mm. Otherwise, C1–2 fusion or an odontoid screw fixation is required to stabilize this injury.

A **type III odontoid fracture** is a fracture that includes the body of the C2 vertebra. This fracture will heal with immobilization alone.

4. In spinal cord injury, what is the nomenclature for the level of the injury?

Standard nomenclature identifies the injury by the lowest functional spinal cord level. For example, the cervical spine injury of a patient with biceps muscle (C6 innervated) that can contract, a triceps muscle (C7) that cannot contract, and a C6 dermatome that has some sensation is identified as a C6 spinal cord injury.

5. Describe the functions present for the different mid and lower complete cervical spinal cord injuries.

C1–C4: These injuries result in ventilator dependent quadriplegia. There is no motor sensory function of the upper extremities.

C5: Deltoid function permits abduction of the shoulder, and sensation is present in the lateral upper arm.

C6: Biceps and brachioradialis have contraction ability, wrist extension functions, and there is sensation to the thumb and index finger.

C7: Triceps and wrist flexion and sensation to the middle finger are present.

C8: Hand intrinsic function is present with sensation to the entire hand.

T1: There is lumbrical function and sensation in the entire arm.

6. Describe the difference between a complete and an incomplete spinal cord injury.

In a complete spinal cord injury, the cord is irreparably damaged, and there is no discernible motor, sensory, or electrical function (somatosensory evoked potentials) below the level of injury. In incomplete injury, some function is preserved, a twitch of movement, an anal wink, or some other reliable reproducible sensory finding.

7. What is the difference between plegia and paresis?

Plegia describes complete motor loss. Paresis describes weakness with some preservation of motor function.

8. How is paresis classified?

Paresis, or motor weakness, is classified on a scale of 0–5.

0: No contraction (plegic).

1: Contraction noted in the muscle by seeing or feeling but no motion of the joint in question.

2: Able to move the joint when gravity is eliminated.

3: Able to move the joint against gravity but not against resistance.

4: Able to move against resistance but not at full power.

5: Normal strength. Able to overcome resistance normally.

Because the scale is heavily weighted toward the weak end, many examiners scale power using 4+ and 5− categories. A designation of 4+ is where the joint can contract against moderate resistance but can be overcome by the examiner. The scale of weakness is typically given as a ratio with the amount of power that the muscle has over 5.

9. What is a Brown-Séquard injury?

A Brown-Séquard injury is an incomplete spinal cord injury that involves one side of the spinal cord and often results from a stab in the back or neck. The typical findings in this hemicord injury are *ipsilateral* motor loss and diminution of light touch sensation combined with *contralateral* loss of pain and temperature sensation starting two or three levels below the injury. This is due to the decussation of the pain and temperature fibers one or two levels above their root entry. Ipsilateral vibration and position sense may be lost if the posterior columns are involved. The prognosis for a Brown-Séquard injury patient to recover distal motor function is good owing to an uncrossed anterior corticospinal tract.

10. What is an anterior spinal cord injury?

This injury is an incomplete spinal cord injury that typically occurs with a flexion type of injury causing damage to the anterior spinal cord or the anterior spinal artery. In this circumstance, motor function and pain and temperature sensation are lost, but light touch and vibration and position senses are preserved. The prognosis for motor recovery is poor.

11. What is a central spinal cord injury?

In this incomplete cervical spinal cord injury, the motor dysfunction of the hands and arms is disproportionately worse than that of the lower extremities. This is probably due to injury to the central portion of the spinal cord, damaging the gray matter and synapses with relative preservation of the myelinated long tracts that go distally. These patients will usually recover most of their function, but fine hand movements may remain poor.

12. Besides motor and sensory loss, what systemic findings are typically present when a patient with spinal cord injury presents to the emergency room?

Hypotension is present due to distal vasodilatation. Bradycardia occurs due to unchecked vagal stimulation. Hypothermia can be present due to distal vascular dilatation. Urinary retention is present due to damaged bladder innervation. Priapism may be present in severe cord injuries.

13. What is the current medical management for spinal cord injury?

It is currently recommended to infuse 30 mg/kg of methylprednisolone over 1 hour followed by 5.4 mg/kg/h for the following 23 hours. Systemic hypotension and bradycardia can be treated with fluid infusion initially, plus dopamine or dobutamine. Atropine is given for symptomatic bradycardia.

14. What are some long-term consequences of spinal cord injury?

Respiratory depression occurs when the unassisted diaphragm fatigues in patients with cervical injuries below C4. Due to the lack of sensation, the patient's skin is highly susceptible to breakdown and pressure sores (decubitus ulcers). Intestinal ileus occurs. Commonly, patients also develop pancreatitis due to spasm of the sphincter of Oddi. Urinary tract infections and pneumonia are extremely common after these injuries, as well. Deep vein thrombosis occurs in immobile extremities.

15. How does one differentiate between an injury of the cauda equina and the conus medularis?

Cauda equina injury involves the lumbar and sacral nerve roots. This can have a highly variable presentation and may show patchy lower extremity dermatomal sensory losses and motor weaknesses. Pain in the legs is a common feature.

A conus medularis injury involves the gray matter supplying innervation to the sacral region. This injury typically includes sensory loss in the sacral dermatomes (saddle anesthesia) with loss of anal and bladder sphincter control, erectile function, and other sacrally innervated functions. Pain and weakness in the legs may not be present.

16. How does one define stability of the spine?

In general, spinal instability is defined as the inability of the spine to bear weight without anatomic deformation or pain.

17. Are there specific definitions of spinal bony stability?

Yes. The stability of the bony spine is defined in two different ways, both involving a three-column concept. The presence of injury to two of the three columns establishes instability.

The spinal structure can be thought of as having three columns, from anterior to posterior. The anterior column is the front half of the vertebral body and the anterior longitudinal ligament, the middle column is the posterior vertebral body and posterior longitudinal ligament, and the third column is the posterior elements including the pedicles and facets.

The other way to think of the three columns are the vertebral body and disc being one column and each of two facets posterolaterally being a separate column.

18. Does any vertebral body fracture constitute instability?

No. If a vertebral body is less than 50% compressed, instability is not present.

19. Can you list some stable spinal vertebral injuries?

- Teardrop avulsion fractures of the cervical vertebral bodies
- Clay-shoveler's (C6) or other spinous process fractures
- Compression fractures of less than 50% of the vertebral height
- Unilateral laminar, facet, or pedicle fractures
- Bilateral cervical locked facets where the inferior facets have jumped over the superior facets of the body below is also considered stable, if unreduced.

20. What is the typical mechanism of an L1 compression fracture?

When a person falls from a height and lands on his or her feet, legs, or coccyx, the axial compression load is centered over the upper lumbar spine owing to the double S curvature of the spinal column. The compressive forces typically are translated to the L1 body, which fractures.

21. What is a Chance fracture?

A Chance fracture is another type of L1 compression fracture. This is typically seen following a motor vehicle accident in which a passenger was restrained only at the waist and not at the shoulder. The resultant extreme anterior flexion causes an unstable compression fracture of the L1 vertebral body and disruption of the posterior ligaments and facets.

22. What neurologic injury is typical for L1 fractures?

Because of the anatomy in the spinal canal, a wide variety of injuries might result from an L1 fracture. A patient could be completely intact or have a complete injury of all lumbar and sacral functions. There is also a spectrum in between including partial or complete conus medularis injuries and partial or complete nerve root avulsions or transections.

23. What is appropriate emergency room management of a patient with suspected unstable spine injury?

The patient should be immobilized and stabilized as much as possible to prevent secondary injury to nervous structures. This would include cervical immobilization with a collar or sand bags and spinal support using a backboard. As soon as possible, appropriate radiographic studies need to be taken. Initially, these include a cervical spine x-ray series including open mouth view and, in a patient with a known spinal column or spinal cord injury, a whole x-ray series of the spine. In patients with known cervical spine injuries, the cervical spine needs to be immobilized; this is best performed with cervical traction. Approximately 5 lbs per level of cervical injury should be used. Computed tomography (CT) scan is the next diagnostic test of choice to assess bony injuries at all levels.

To prevent skin breakdown, a patient should be removed from the backboard as soon as it is deemed safe. Medical management should be initiated as described in question 13.

24. What is spinal shock?

Spinal shock is a condition found in patients who have significant spinal cord injuries. Within the first 24 hours, a patient with a spinal cord injury can manifest a complete lack of deep tendon reflexes and anal reflexes. This condition usually begins to reverse itself within one day. The first reflexes that typically return are the bulbocavernosus, or anal wink, reflexes.

25. What is neurogenic shock?

Neurogenic shock is a name for the profound hypotension that results from significant cervical or high thoracic spinal cord injury and resulting loss of sympathetic function.

26. Do children manifest differences in spinal injury as compared with adults?

Yes. Due to differences in developmental anatomy, children show a disproportionate amount of spinal cord injuries at the C1–2 levels or at the water shed zones (approximately upper thoracic). Because the child's spinal column is more flexible than the spinal cord and neurologic elements, children tend to manifest spinal cord injury without radiographic abnormalities (SCIWORA) on x-ray and CT scan. This condition occurs because the soft tissues are damaged, and the more flexible bones and ligaments do not suffer fractures or tears.

27. What are the general guidelines for spinal surgery after trauma?

Patients with incomplete spinal cord injury with evidence of foreign material (bone, disc, foreign body) in the spinal canal should be decompressed immediately and stabilized. Any patient with evidence of a nerve root injury due to disc herniation or other compressive force should be decompressed. All patients with unstable spinal injuries require either surgical stabilization or immobilization in a rigid orthosis such as a halo vest.

CONTROVERSIES

28. Should patients with complete spinal cord injuries undergo surgery acutely to decompress or stabilize the spine?

Historical evidence would argue that early surgery in a patient with complete spinal cord injury has no beneficial effect on spinal cord recovery. This is due to the irreversible nature of the complete spinal cord injury. However, a patient with a severe incomplete injury might present with spinal shock and have no discernible function initially, but may begin to recover some function within 24 hours. Therefore, if there is a compressive mass in the spinal canal, removal of this compressive force might benefit the patient's recovery. Currently, a prospective national study is being conducted to try to answer this question scientifically.

29. What is the best way to stabilize L1 compression fractures?

Many different regimens have been instituted to treat this instability successfully. These include long-term immobilization in a brace with the patient in the recumbent position and internal fixation with hardware, with short posterior fusion of one or two levels versus longer fusions. Anterior fusion has also been performed successfully. This may include partial or complete vertebrectomy with strut graft fusion and fixation with a plate. Finally, some clinicians recommend both anterior and posterior fixation and fusion.

BIBLIOGRAPHY

1. Greenberg J (ed): Handbook of Head and Spine Trauma. New York, Marcel Dekker, 1994.

III. Thoracic Trauma

14. PENETRATING CHEST TRAUMA

Demetrios Demetriades, M.D., Ph.D., and Javier Romero, M.D.

1. How is the diagnosis of tension pneumothorax made?
- Severe respiratory distress, panicky patient
- Tachycardia, hypotension, distended neck veins
- Absent breath sounds, hyperresonance or percussion, trachea shifted to opposite side
- Diagnosis is clinical, and no radiologic confirmation should be attempted.

2. What is the treatment of a tension pneumothorax?
A needle thoracostomy is both diagnostic and therapeutic. Placement of a thoracostomy tube should follow.

3. What is the anatomic site of insertion of thoracostomy tube?
In the midaxillary line, above the level of the nipple (to avoid accidental injury to the diaphragm), insert the tube aiming toward the apex and posteriorly. A subcutaneous tunnel is unnecessary, painful, and does not reduce the incidence of intrathoracic infections.

4. Should the thoracostomy tube be removed during deep inspiration or deep expiration?
It does not matter.

5. What is the role of prophylactic antibiotics with thoracostomy tubes?
Review of all prospective, randomized studies showed that prophylactic antibiotics used in cases of penetrating trauma reduce intrathoracic infections. The role of prophylactic antibiotics in blunt trauma is not clear. Anecdotally, most surgeons give antibiotics.

6. What is the duration of prophylactic antibiotics for chest trauma treated with a thoracostomy tube?
The only available prospective, randomized study concluded that a single dose was as good as prolonged prophylaxis.

7. What are the risk factors for development of empyema after thoracostomy tube insertion?
- Poor technique
- Residual hemothorax
- Duration of thoracostomy tube
- Violation of the diaphragm and gross peritoneal contamination
- Lack of antibiotic prophylaxis

8. Do all small pneumothoraces require a thoracostomy tube?
Many small pneumothoraces (<20%) do not need drainage. However, if the patient requires mechanical ventilation, the presence of any pneumothorax is a strong indication for thoracostomy tube insertion. Failure to insert a tube may result in tension pneumothorax.

9. How should retained hemothorax be managed?

If there is a persistent hemothorax after thoracostomy tube insertion, a computed tomography (CT) scan should be obtained on days 2 to 4; it is essential to differentiate between hemothorax and atelectasis or parenchyma hematoma. If there is significant clot, an early operative evacuation (within 4 to 5 days of admission) is recommended. Thoracoscopic evacuation is very effective. If this technique is not available, a limited thoracotomy may be necessary.

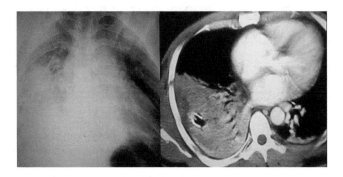

Chest x-ray is suspicious for residual hemothorax. However, the CT scan shows a large atelectasis and intrapulmonary hematoma.

10. What factors determine prognosis in penetrating cardiac injuries?

- Time from injury to operation. Every minute counts! Scoop and run to the nearest trauma center by any means—cab, ambulance, helicopter—whatever is available.
- Mechanism of injury. Gunshot injuries are about three times more lethal than stab wounds.
- Site of cardiac injury. Intrapericardial aortic injuries have the worst prognosis. Left ventricular injuries have a worse outcome than right ventricular injuries. The relatively thick wall with relatively low pressures in the right ventricle make a favorable combination.
- Size of cardiac injury.
- Cardiac tamponade. The presence of tamponade improves prognosis by preventing exsanguination.
- Associated injuries. The presence of associated injuries, especially to vascular structures, makes the prognosis worse.
- Experience of the trauma center and trauma team.

11. What are the clinical signs and symptoms of cardiac tamponade?

- Restless, confused patient (often mistakenly attributed to alcohol or illicit drug use).
- Shock, tachycardia, weak peripheral pulses.
- Beck's triad (i.e., shock, distended neck veins, and distant cardiac sounds) is found in about 90% of patients with tamponade.
- Pulsus paradoxus is present in only about 10% of patients with cardiac tamponade.
- Every penetrating injury to the chest associated with shock is a cardiac injury until proved otherwise.

12. Which investigations are useful for the diagnosis of cardiac injury?

No investigation. Do not waste valuable time if the diagnosis is obvious!

Cardiac ultrasound (FAST), which can be performed by emergency medicine physicians or surgeons, is the investigation of choice in modern trauma centers.

Chest x-ray film is helpful in about 50% of patients. Suspicious findings include an enlarged cardiac shadow, pneumopericardium, and widened upper mediastinum.

Electrocardiogram (ECG) is helpful in about 30% of patients. Usual findings include low QRS, elevated ST, and inverted T waves.

Central venous pressure (CVP) measurements. Suspect tamponade if the CVP is less than 12 cm H_2O. Remember that other conditions, such as restlessness, tension pneumothorax, fluid overload, mechanical ventilation, or a misplaced catheter, can produce an elevated CVP. However, cardiac tamponade associated with significant blood loss may not give a high CVP.

Pericardiocentesis is of limited value and has been abandoned by most trauma centers.

Subxiphoid window is used by some trauma centers but not used at all by others. It has a limited role in modern trauma centers.

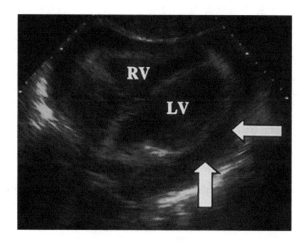

Trauma ultrasound shows a large cardiac tamponade (*arrows*).

13. What is the incision of choice for repair of cardiac injury?

It is a matter of personal preference and experience. Many trauma surgeons prefer a median sternotomy for most cardiac injuries, reserving a left thoracotomy for posterior injuries or emergency room thoracotomies. Other surgeons prefer a left thoracotomy for all cases.

14. Is it essential to close the pericardium after repair of a cardiac injury?

The pericardium should be closed if it can be done without tension. An opening should be left at the upper part (i.e., base of the heart) to avoid retamponade. Pericardium closure is not always possible because of cardiac enlargement due to fluid overloading or failure. In these cases, the pericardium should be left open.

15. What postoperative test should be performed after successful repair of a cardiac injury?

Routinely, an ECG and echocardiogram are obtained. The patient should be reevaluated a few weeks later because of the high incidence of late cardiac sequelae. Reported late complications include septal defects, valvular lesions, dyskinesias, hypokinesias, and pericardial effusions.

16. What are the indications for emergency room thoracotomy in cases of penetrating chest trauma?

Liberal indications are applied because there are sometimes unexpected survivors, the patient sometimes becomes an organ donor, and the procedure has excellent educational value for the trauma team. Every patient with loss of vital signs before or after arrival at the hospital and those with imminent cardiac arrest should undergo emergency room thoracotomy.

17. What options are available to control cardiac wounds in the emergency room after a thoracotomy?
- Your finger
- Sutures
- Staples
- Foley balloon catheter

18. What are the indications for emergency thoracotomy?
- Severe shock due to blood loss or cardiac tamponade. A trauma ultrasound scan and chest radiograph are extremely helpful.
- Initial blood loss in the thoracostomy tube exceeding 1000 to 1500 mL.
- The rate of blood loss in the thoracostomy tube is not always a reliable indication of the severity of cardiovascular injuries. Cardiac tamponade, a clotted hemothorax, or an improperly placed tube may not be associated with significant blood loss through the tube. On the other hand, fairly benign injuries such as a peripheral lung laceration or an intercostal venous injury may be associated with significant bleeding during the first hours, but it usually stops on its own. The decision to operate or observe should be based on the hemodynamic condition of the patient and the trend of bleeding in the thoracostomy tube.
- Endoscopic or contrast swallow evidence of tracheal or esophageal injuries.
- Air leak in the presence of a normal endoscopy is rarely an indication for surgery.

19. How often do patients with penetrating chest trauma require emergency thoracotomy?
Only about 15% of those with stab wounds and 15% to 20% of those with gunshot wounds to the chest reaching the hospital require an emergency thoracotomy.

20. Do all transmediastinal gunshot wounds require surgery?
More than 70% of patients who are hemodynamically stable do not require an operation.

21. What is required for evaluation of patients with transmediastinal gunshots wounds who are hemodynamically stable?
- Trauma ultrasound to rule out pericardial effusion.
- Chest x-ray film.
- Spinal CT scan to evaluate the direction of the bullet tract. If the tract is away from the major vessels and the aerodigestive tract, no further investigations are needed. For suspicious bullet tracts, an aortogram or esophagram or endoscopy may be performed. Spiral CT can eliminate the need of angiography or esophageal studies in two thirds of hemodynamically stable patients.

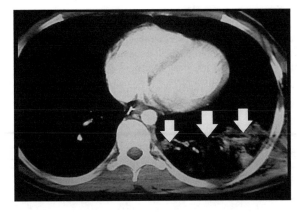

Spinal CT scan for transmediastinal gunshot wound: The bullet tract (*arrows*) is away from the aorta and the esophagus. No further investigations are required.

22. **Which injuries tend to bleed less: lung injuries or liver injuries?**

Lung injuries bleed less than liver injuries for two reasons. The lung vessels are low-pressure systems, and the lung tissues are rich in thromboplastin.

23. **What is the operative management of continuous bleeding from a bullet tract in the lung parenchyma and away from the hilum?**

Bleeding is managed by tractotomy with gastrointestinal anastomosis (GIA) stapler and direct control with sutures.

24. **What is the best technique for emergent pneumonectomy or lobectomy?**

En masse stapled resection, which includes vessels and bronchi, is safe and fast. No need for isolation and division of individual hilar structures.

25. **What is the mortality rate and the most common cause of death after pneumonectomy for trauma?**

The mortality rate is usually higher than 50%, and the most common cause of death is acute right cardiac failure. It is essential to avoid fluid overloading.

26. **Which trauma conditions predispose to air embolism?**

Injuries to low-pressure cardiac chambers, lung, and major veins.

27. **What is the diagnosis and treatment of air embolism?**

The diagnosis is based on a high index of suspicion for patients with high-risk injuries. Sometimes, air bubbles can be seen in the coronary veins. Management should include isolation of the source of air (i.e., venous or lung hilum cross-clamping) and aspiration of the heart. Postoperatively, a hyperbaric chamber may be beneficial.

28. **What is the diagnosis of thoracic esophageal perforation based on?**

- Perforation may be suspected because of the direction of bullet or knife tract.
- Mediastinal emphysema is a suspicious radiologic finding.
- The diagnosis is confirmed by contrast swallow studies or esophagoscopy.

29. **How important is early diagnosis of perforation of the thoracic esophagus?**

Extremely important! If the diagnosis is delayed for more than 12 to 16 hours, severe mediastinitis occurs, making the repair difficult, and it carries a very high mortality rate because of uncontrollable sepsis.

30. **What is the diagnosis of traumatic chylothorax after a penetrating injury to the chest?**

Chylothorax usually follows injury to the left supraclavicular region (i.e., junction of thoracic duct and left subclavian vein) or a mediastinal injury. It may manifest as milky fluid in the pleural cavity. The fluid may not have the characteristic milky appearance, especially if the patient is not fed enterally. The diagnosis is confirmed by the high protein content (>3g/dL), a total fat content (>0.4 g/dL), alkaline pH, triglyceride level of more than 200 mg/dL, and a marked lymphocytic predominance, although these findings are not always present. Lymphangiography may confirm the site of thoracic duct injury.

31. **How do you manage traumatic chylothorax?**

Nonoperative management with thoracostomy tube drainage and a low-fat diet or total parenteral nutrition is almost always successful. Somatostatin accelerates the resolution of a chyle leak.

32. **What are the indications for surgical intervention in traumatic chylothorax?**

Surgical intervention is indicated if a major chyle leak persists without signs of improvement after 10 to 14 days of conservative treatment.

33. What are the operative procedures for persistent chylothorax?
1. Right posterolateral thoracotomy and mass ligation of the tissues between the aorta and the esophagus above the diaphragm
2. Thoracoscopic ligation of the thoracic duct

34. What investigation should be performed in asymptomatic patients with penetrating injuries to the left thoracoabdominal area?
- Chest radiograph (look for hemothorax, pneumothorax, or an elevated diaphragm).
- CT scan in selected cases of gunshot wounds to evaluate the bullet tract direction and assess possible solid organ injuries in the abdomen.
- On the basis of the bullet tract direction, further studies such as angiography or esophagography may be required.
- Routine laparoscopy to evaluate for left diaphragmatic injuries. About 28% of asymptomatic stab wounds and 14% of asymptomatic gunshot wounds to the left thoracoabdominal area have diaphragmatic injuries.

BIBLIOGRAPHY

1. Asensio JA, Steward MB, Murray J, et al: Penetrating cardiac injuries. Surg Clin North Am 76:685–724, 1996.
2. Demetriades D, Breckon V, Breckon C, et al: Antibiotic prophylaxis in penetrating injuries of the chest. Ann Royal Coll Surg Engl 73:348–351, 1991.
3. Demetriades D, Rubinowitz B: Indications for thoracotomy in stab injuries of the chest: A prospective study of 543 patients. Br J Surg 73:888–890, 1986.
4. Demetriades D: Cardiac wounds: Experience with 70 cases. Ann Surg 203:315–318, 1986.
5. Hanpeter DE, Demetriades D, Asencio JA, et al: Helical computed tomographic scan in the evaluation of mediastinal gunshot wounds. J Trauma 49:689–694, 2000.
6. Richardson DJ, Miller FB, Carrillo EH, Spain DA: Complex thoracic injuries. Surg Clin North Am 76: 725–748, 1996.

15. BLUNT CHEST TRAUMA

George C. Velmahos, M.D., and Areti Tillou, M.D.

1. Which are the most common injuries after blunt chest injuries?
- Thoracic cage fractures
- Lung contusion and tears
- Myocardial contusion
- Aortic rupture

2. How useful is the initial plain chest radiograph?
The initial plain chest radiograph is usually performed with the patient in the supine position and with poor technique under emergency conditions. Exclusive reliance on it may be misleading. However, it is routinely obtained in most trauma patients as a screening rather than a definitive diagnostic test. Fractures, hemopneumothorax, and mediastinal abnormalities may be missed at the initial radiograph. For suspicious symptoms, repeat radiographs or a chest computed tomography (CT) scan should be ordered.

3. What is the *widened mediastinum*?
A mediastinal width of more than 8 cm seen on the supine chest radiograph is considered abnormal and should be investigated further. It occurs in 85% of cases with aortic injury.

4. What are the causes of mediastinal widening?
- Aortic rupture in 10% to 15% of cases
- Thoracic spinal fractures in 5% to 10% of cases
- Sternal fractures, soft tissue injuries, or cardiac tamponade in 5% of cases
- No abnormalities in the remaining 65% to 70% of cases

5. Are there other radiographic signs suggestive of a ruptured aorta?
- Indistinct aortic knob (25% of cases)
- Apical cap (20%)
- First and second rib fractures (15%)
- Tracheal deviation (10%)
- Nasogastric deviation (10%)
- Depressed left mainstem bronchus (5%)
- Widened mediastinum
- Loss of aortopulmonary window

Other nonsensitive signs such as rib, sternal, scapular, and clavicular fractures or pleural effusion may exist. The most specific finding is nasogastric tube deviation. In 7% of cases, the plain radiograph may be completely normal.

6. How do you evaluate a widened mediastinum?
- Repeat plain chest radiograph in the upright position. Although approximately 50% of suspected cases can be ruled out by this simple method, elevation of the blunt trauma patient may be contraindicated because of shock or concerns about the spine.
- Aortic angiogram. This is the gold standard for the diagnosis of aortic rupture, with a sensitivity and specificity of 97%. However, it is invasive, expensive, time and labor consuming, and associated with complications in up to 5% of cases.
- Chest CT scan. It is rapid, noninvasive, and may provide additional information for associated injuries. Especially in cases that require CT scanning of other body regions, as is often the case with blunt trauma victims, it is the test of choice to confirm or exclude the ex-

istence of mediastinal hematoma. Helical CT has in many centers replaced conventional aortography. The role of aortography tends to be limited to cases in which the helical CT findings are equivocal (see Figures).

- Transesophageal echocardiography. The test has varying degrees of accuracy (60% to 98%) because of operator dependency. It may be an excellent alternative for the unstable patient who should not be transported out of the intensive care unit. Its use should be individualized according to the existing experience in each institution.

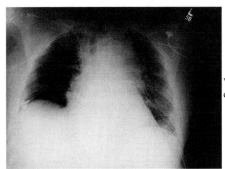

Widened mediastinum with loss of the aortic knob and deviation of the trachea to the right.

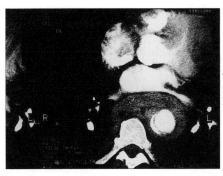

The helical CT scan shows an aortic injury with contrast filling outside the proper lumen. Notice the periaortic hematoma.

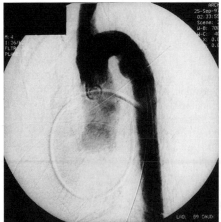

Aortography shows an aortic pseudoaneurysm at the classic site distal to the left subclavian artery.

7. Where is the typical site of aortic injury?

Aortic injury occurs distal to the left subclavian take-off in 93% of cases. The transition of the fixed ascending to the more mobile descending aorta creates significant shearing forces around the ductus arteriosum. Ascending aorta and arch injuries occur in the remaining 7% of the cases.

8. What is the mortality rate of thoracic aortic injury?

About 85% of patients die at the accident scene. The mortality rate for patients reaching the hospital alive is 30%. Most of these patients arrive in extremis or rupture before operation. For stable patients undergoing planned aortic repair, the mortality rate is 15%.

9. What operative techniques are used for aortic repair?
- Clamp and sew
- Bypass (e.g., Gott shunt, full bypass, partial bypass, centrifugal pump)

10. What are the major complications after aortic surgery?
- Respiratory complications (e.g., pneumonia, empyema)
- Renal failure
- Suture line failure (dehiscence, aneurysm)
- Paraplegia (10% of cases)

11. What are risk factors for development of paraplegia?

Intraoperative hypotension, duration of aortic cross clamping and technique. It seems that if the aorta is clamped for less than 30 minutes, both techniques (clamp and sew or bypass) are equally safe. However, for repairs lasting longer than 30 minutes, bypass techniques offer better spinal protection. Hypotension resulting in hypoperfusion of the spinal cord should be avoided at all times before and during repair.

12. What is the spectrum of blunt cardiac trauma?
1. Asymptomatic myocardial contusion (electrocardiogram [ECG] abnormalities only)
2. Symptomatic myocardial contusion (cardiogenic shock or arrhythmias)
3. Free wall or septal wall rupture
4. Valvular tears
5. Coronary artery thrombosis

13. What are the symptoms of blunt cardiac trauma?

Most myocardial contusions are asymptomatic, but most patients with cardiac rupture do not reach the hospital alive. Hemodynamic instability or cardiac arrhythmias are common manifestations of clinically significant blunt myocardial injury.

14. What are possible mechanisms of cardiac rupture?
- Acute deceleration (e.g., falls from a height, motor vehicle accidents)
- Forceful anteroposterior compression
- Lacerations from ribs or sternal fractures
- Sudden massive return of venous blood to the heart after blunt abdominal trauma (rare)

15. How is the diagnosis of myocardial contusion established?

There is no highly sensitive or specific diagnostic test, but the following points should be considered:

1. Suspicious mechanism of injury (e.g., significant steering wheel damage, anterior chest blows) with associated sternal fractures, multiple rib fractures, or precordial bruises. However, some believe that these injuries are not significant risk factors for blunt cardiac trauma.

2. Clinical signs and symptoms such as cardiogenic shock or arrhythmias.

3. Cardiac enzymes such as creatine phosphokinase (CPK), lactate dehydrogenase (LDH),

and CPK-MB have been used but are not predictive of myocardial contusion because the dam-aged skeletal muscle, which contains all of these enzymes, may obscure the small amounts re-leased by injured myocardial cells. Troponin levels, which have a high sensitivity and specificity for myocardial infarcts, are increasingly used for blunt cardiac injury and have replaced CPK-MB in most centers.

   4. ECG. Although the initial ECG may not be conclusive, it is rare to have blunt heart trauma without ECG changes within 12 hours of admission. Unfortunately, these changes are nonspecific and consist of rhythm disturbances (predominantly sinus tachycardia) or conduction abnormali-ties (predominantly right bundle branch block).

   5. The combination of a normal admission ECG, a repeat ECG at 8 hours after admission, and three normal troponin levels (2 hours apart) has a negative predictive value of 100% for clin-ically significant blunt myocardial injury. If results of these two tests are normal, the patient will not manifest any cardiac abnormalities and, in the absence of other injuries, can be discharged.

   6. Echocardiogram. It is sensitive in diagnosing wall motion abnormalities or anatomic de-fects, and it is the recommended investigation in patients with ECG abnormalities or unexplained hemodynamic instability.

   7. Radionuclide scan (MUGA). It is specific in detecting serious abnormalities but cannot be used as a screening test.

16. What is the proper way of evaluating a patient with suspected blunt myocardial trauma?

   1. Obtain an admission ECG and troponin levels in patients with suspicious symptoms or mechanism of injury.

   2. Repeat the ECG 8 to 12 hours after admission.

   3. Repeat troponin levels every 2 hours for a total of three levels.

   4. Observe the patient during this period in a monitored bed (not necessarily in intensive care unit).

   5. Perform echocardiogram in case of unexplained hemodynamic instability or cardiac ar-rhythmias.

   6. Discharge after 12 hours in the absence of suggestive symptoms, abnormal test findings, or associated injuries.

17. What is the treatment of blunt cardiac trauma?

   Most patients with blunt cardiac trauma do not require any treatment other than observation. ECG waves and enzyme levels almost always return to normal within a week. Between 2% and 5%) of patients may develop significant arrhythmias with hemodynamic compromise, requiring antiarrhythmics (usually intravenous lidocaine). Patients with echocardiographically or MUGA-confirmed myocardial contusion should be kept in the hospital until a repeat test shows no ab-normal findings.

   The survival of patients with cardiac rupture depends on prompt recognition and surgical repair.

   Although delayed complications after untreated blunt cardiac trauma have been reported in the literature, they are rare.

18. What types of tracheobronchial and lung injuries occur after blunt chest trauma?

   Pneumothorax or hemothorax after blunt trauma is usually a result of direct injury from frac-tured ribs. Persistent high-volume air leaks should raise the possibility of tracheobronchial injury, requiring bronchoscopic evaluation.

   Lung contusion may be a result of direct blunt trauma with or without a component of acute deceleration (see Figure). It may not be apparent radiographically at the initial stage, which may allow a false sense of security. Deterioration of the respiratory status over the ensuing hours is not uncommon in such cases and may catch the unprepared physician by surprise. A high index of suspicion supported by appropriate tests (e.g., sequential chest radiographs, blood gases), ad-equate monitoring (e.g., oxygen saturation), and close clinical surveillance is the only way to avoid significant problems.

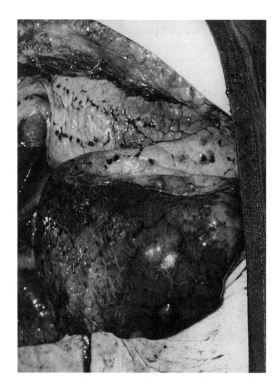

Notice the difference in appearance of the contused lower lobe of the left lung compared with the normal upper lobe.

19. What is the significance of rib fractures?

Upper rib fractures (i.e., first and second ribs) may be associated with aortic rupture. Lower rib fractures are associated with injuries to the spleen and liver. Multiple rib fractures may result in significant pain, muscle splinting, inadequate lung expansion, and development of respiratory failure. Adequate analgesia and physiotherapy are essential to avoid such complications.

20. What are methods of pain control for patients with multiple rib fractures?

- Epidural analgesia (i.e., catheter placed in epidural space).
- Intercostal analgesia (i.e., frequent injections in corresponding intercostal spaces close to intercostal nerves).
- Patient-controlled analgesia (PCA).
- Conventional analgesia (IM, IV, or PO analgesics).
- Epidurally placed catheters provide the most effective pain control with few adverse effects. This method is the treatment of choice for patients with significant pain and risk of respiratory complications.

21. What is flail chest?

Flail chest is defined as three or more consecutive ribs that are each fractured in at least two sites. A flail chest is associated with mechanical malfunction of the corresponding hemithorax, which becomes evident by paradoxical respiration. In this condition, the affected hemithorax moves inward as the opposite hemithorax expands during inspiration. Approximately 40% to 80% of patients with flail chest require mechanical ventilatory support. The underlying lung contusion contributes to the development of respiratory failure more than the lack of coordinated chest movement. Voluntary "splinting" of the chest because of pain is also a major factor of respiratory failure.

22. How do you treat patients with flail chest?

1. Monitor closely the respiratory rate and oxygen saturation.

2. Supply additional oxygen by mask or nasal cannula.

3. Maintain a low threshold for mechanical ventilatory support before the patient decompensates.

4. Provide adequate pain control, ideally by means of epidural analgesia.

Internal stabilization by operative rib fixation has been used in some centers, claiming good results. There is not extensive experience with this method.

23. What is traumatic asphyxia?

Traumatic asphyxia is caused by an acute increase in the intravascular pressure of the upper torso, head, and neck due to sudden compression of the chest. Diffuse reddening above the site of compression is characteristic of this entity and attributed to rupture of small vessels and blood extravasation. Subconjunctival hemorrhage is also typical. Increased intracranial pressure may occur because of microhemorrhages.

24. What are the most common pitfalls in the diagnosis and treatment of patients with blunt chest trauma?

- Failure to include causes other than aortic injuries in the differential diagnosis of widened mediastinum (especially thoracic spinal fracture)
- Underestimation of a significant lung contusion because the initial radiographic appearance is misleadingly unimpressive
- Failure to maintain a reasonably high index of suspicion for aortic trauma in patients with high-energy mechanisms of injury even when plain chest radiographs are normal
- Failure to recognize myocardial contusion as the reason of hemodynamic instability in the absence of bleeding
- Failure to provide adequate analgesia and early ventilatory support to patients with flail chest or multiple rib fractures

BIBLIOGRAPHY

1. Cachecho R, Grindlinger G, Lee VW: The clinical significance of myocardial contusion. J Trauma 33: 68–73, 1992.
2. Durham RM, Zuckerman D, Wolverson M, et al: Computed tomography as a screening exam in patients with suspected blunt aortic injury. Ann Surg 220:699–704, 1994.
3. Fabian TC, Richardson JD, Croce MA, et al: Prospective study of blunt aortic injury: Multicenter trial of the American Association for the Surgery of Trauma. J Trauma 42:374–383, 1997.
4. Harman PK, Trinkle JK: Injury to the heart. In Moore EE, Mattox KL, Feliciano DV (eds): Trauma, 2nd ed. Norwalk, CT, Appleton & Lange, 1991, pp 373–391.
5. Salim A, Velmahos GC, Jindal A, et al: Clinically significant blunt cardiac trauma: Role of serum troponin levels combined with electrocardiographic findings. J. Trauma 50:237–43, 2001.
6. Smith MD, Cassidy JM, Souther S, et al: Transesophageal echocardiography in the diagnosis of traumatic rupture of the aorta. N Engl J Med 332:356–362, 1995.

IV. Diaphragm and Abdominal Trauma

16. DIAPHRAGM INJURIES

James A. Murray, M.D., and Demetrios Demetriades, M.D., Ph.D.

1. What are the external landmarks that correspond to the diaphragm during full expiration?

The position of the hemidiaphragms in the thorax is dynamic. During unlabored exhalation, the right leaflet rises to the fourth intercostal space, and the left leaflet rises to the level of the fifth intercostal space. Both diaphragms ascend to the level of the eighth intercostal space posteriorly. Roughly, this correlates to the level of the nipple line anteriorly and the tip of the scapulae posteriorly.

2. What are the three major openings (apertures) in the diaphragm and which structures pass through each of these?

1. The aortic hiatus is at the level of T12 and allows the passage of the aorta, thoracic duct, and azygous vein.

2. The esophageal hiatus is located at the level of T10 and contains the esophagus and the vagus nerves.

3. The caval hiatus is at the level of T8 and contains only the inferior vena cava.

3. What is the pressure gradient across the diaphragm between the abdominal cavity and thoracic cavity?

The pressure in the abdominal cavity varies during normal respiration from 2 to 10 cm H_2O. The intrapleural pressure may vary from -5 to -10 cm H_2O. In the supine position, the pleuroperitoneal gradient fluctuates from 7 to 20 cm H_2O. With maximal inspiration, this gradient can exceed 100 cm H_2O. A corresponding increase in intra-abdominal pressure can obtain a pressure gradient of 150 to 200 cm H_2O.

4. What is the innervation of the diaphragm?

The diaphragm is innervated by the phrenic nerves. These arise from the third, fourth, and fifth cervical nerve roots. They course along the anterior scalene in the neck and along the posterolateral mediastinum on the pericardium. The phrenic nerve inserts on the diaphragm at the junction of the pericardium and the central tendon. It then splays out laterally and divides into anterior and posterior branches that pass circumferentially through the peripheral ring of muscle.

5. How do blunt and penetrating injuries of the diaphragm differ?

Penetrating injuries of the diaphragm usually produce 1- to 2-cm perforations in the diaphragm. Penetrating injuries can cause larger lacerations because of the curved nature of the diaphragm. If the penetrating object takes a more tangential course, the perforation can be longer.

Blunt injuries usually result in a larger laceration (7 to 10 cm), tearing in a radial fashion involving the posterolateral diaphragm. However, all areas of the diaphragm can be involved in blunt injuries. Seventy-five percent of blunt diaphragm injuries involve the left hemidiaphragm. In penetrating trauma, gunshot wounds involve both hemidiaphragms equally, but stab wounds involve the left hemidiaphragm more commonly, presumably because of the right-handedness of the assailant.

Overall, the incidence of diaphragm injuries from blunt trauma is 5%. For blunt abdominal trauma, the incidence ranges from 2.5% to 5%. For blunt thoracic trauma, incidence is about 1.5%. From autopsy studies, an incidence of 7.5% has been reported.

6. What are the physical findings associated with diaphragmatic injuries?

The diagnosis of diaphragmatic injuries can be difficult. Penetrating injuries may not produce any symptoms in the absence of herniation. The physical findings or hemodynamic alterations are usually caused by associated injuries. In the absence of these associated injuries, the diagnosis of diaphragmatic injury may not be considered. If herniated viscera are present, there may be prominence and immobility of the chest, absence of breath sounds, auscultation of bowel sounds in the chest, or tympanic percussions over the thorax.

7. What are the radiographic features associated with diaphragmatic injuries in blunt and penetrating injuries?

The radiographic findings associated with diaphragmatic injuries can vary from normal to obvious herniation of intestinal viscera. The chest radiograph may be normal in up to 50% of patients. Others may demonstrate nonspecific changes such as an elevation, an irregular contour, or haziness to lack of visualization of the hemidiaphragm. It is not uncommon to see small pleural effusions or associated hemothoraces or pneumothoraces. None of these findings is diagnostic of diaphragmatic injuries but must heighten the examiner's concern. Obvious diaphragmatic herniation in the acute setting is more common in blunt trauma because of the larger size of the defect. A radiolucency near the base of the lung probably represents a viscus, which may or may not be associated with an air-fluid level, in the hemithorax. If a nasogastric tube is inserted and does not pass below the diaphragm, gastric herniation has occurred through the defect. A pneumothorax associated with free air in the abdomen could result from a ruptured viscus in association with a diaphragm perforation.

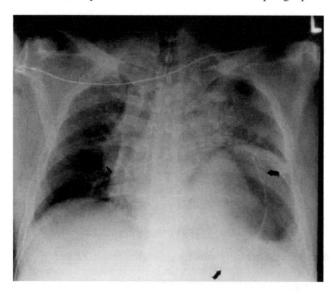

Colonic and gastric herniation can be diagnosed with contrast studies. Computed tomography (CT) is helpful if herniation is present. Bowel or omentum within the thoracic cavity can be well visualized with this modality. CT scans are not be able to identify the small perforations associated with penetrating injuries in the absence of herniation. Magnetic resonance imaging (MRI) and spiral CT scans with thin sections through the diaphragm and with the use of reformatted images have been used to help visualize the defect and determine the anatomic location and extent of the injury. Remember that adjuvant studies should not be performed in the hemodynamically unstable patient.

8. What other conditions in trauma may be associated with an elevation of the diaphragm?

Other traumatic conditions that are often associated with an elevated hemidiaphragm include a diaphragm injury, a subpulmonic hemothorax, splinting due to pleuritic chest pain from associated rib fractures, a subphrenic hematoma, or paralysis of the phrenic nerve.

9. What other conditions may appear radiographically similar to a diaphragm injury?

Other conditions that appear radiographically similar to a diaphragm injury and must be included in the differential diagnosis include atelectasis, pleural effusions, pulmonary contusion, loculated pneumothoraces, eventration, and phrenic nerve paralysis.

10. Which diaphragm is more likely to perforate from blunt trauma?

The left hemidiaphragm is the most commonly involved diaphragm in blunt trauma. Approximately two thirds of the injuries are isolated to the left hemidiaphragm. In the remaining one third, the right hemidiaphragm is involved alone or in bilateral ruptures. It is postulated that the liver provides protection to the right hemidiaphragm. Experimental studies have suggested that the left diaphragm may have some intrinsic weakness compared with the right.

11. What is the incidence of diaphragmatic injuries in penetrating injuries to the left lower chest?

Penetrating injuries to the left lower chest have an over all incidence of injury to the diaphragm of 42%. The incidence was 59% for gunshot wounds and 32% for stab wounds. For patients who were hemodynamically unstable or had peritonitis, the incidence of diaphragmatic injury was 60%. Asymptomatic patients had an incidence of 24% to 26%.

12. What other injuries are associated with diaphragmatic injuries?

In penetrating injuries, the thoracic and abdominal cavities may contain injured organs. The hemodynamic or respiratory compromise usually results from the associated injuries. Most penetrating thoracic injuries can be managed without an operation. If the patient has abdominal tenderness or hemodynamic instability, the abdomen must be explored.

The incidence of associated intra-abdominal injuries in penetrating trauma to the diaphragm is 75%, whereas 25% of diaphragm injuries are isolated. Most of the injured organs are the upper abdominal viscera (i.e., spleen, liver, stomach, esophagus, and small bowel). A thorough examination of the entire abdominal cavity is required.

In blunt trauma patients, extensive injuries are likely to exist within and outside the abdomen and chest. In patients with blunt diaphragmatic rupture, associated intra-abdominal injuries occur in 100% of cases if the right hemidiaphragm is involved. Rupture of the left hemidiaphragm is associated with intra-abdominal injuries in 77% of cases. Other associated injuries include head injuries and fractures of the pelvis and long bones. There is also an increased risk for thoracic aortic injuries in blunt diaphragmatic injuries.

13. What other modalities are available for evaluating patients for diaphragmatic injuries?

Diagnostic peritoneal lavage (DPL) has been used extensively for the evaluation of patients with blunt abdominal trauma. It is a very good diagnostic tool in the evaluation of potential intra-abdominal injuries. However, it is not a reliable method for the diagnosis of isolated diaphragmatic injuries. Isolated injuries to the diaphragm, especially from penetrating trauma, may not be associated with significant intraperitoneal bleeding. DPL may be falsely negative in these cases. Organs that herniate into the chest may be bleeding into the thoracic cavity, and DPL results may be falsely negative. In penetrating injuries, DPL is again, unreliable. The red blood cell count has been lowered in some studies to improve the sensitivity of the study. This may lead to a higher incidence of negative laparotomies from a falsely positive lavage.

Pneumoperitoneum, contrast studies of the peritoneal or pleural cavities, nuclear scanning, ultrasonography, and many other modalities have been explored to assist with diagnosing diaphragmatic injuries, but none has proved to be reliable.

Some physicians suggested mandatory laparotomy for patients suspected of having diaphragmatic injuries. However, this could lead to a significant number of negative celiotomies, which can be associated with significant complications.

The only method available to ensure adequate evaluation of the diaphragm is by direct visualization. Current minimally invasive surgical techniques provide reliable methods to examine the diaphragm. Laparoscopy and thoracoscopy are being used for the evaluation of stable patients suspected of having diaphragmatic injuries. Each has advantages and disadvantages, but each provides a thorough examination of the diaphragm without the need for a formal open operation.

14. What is the best diagnostic modality for diagnosing an occult injury to the diaphragm?

Diagnostic laparoscopy allows for direct visualization of the left hemidiaphragm. This minimally invasive technique allows early diagnosis of occult diaphragmatic injuries before development of lethal complications. It should be performed in all patients with penetrating injuries to the left thoracoabdominal region, regardless of clinical signs or radiographic findings. The chest radiograph often is normal or demonstrates nonspecific findings.

15. What complications are associated with diaphragmatic hernias?

Patients with diaphragmatic hernias may be asymptomatic, with the diagnosis made during a routine examination if hernias are not identified in the acute setting. Gastrointestinal complaints associated with obstructive symptoms are common and may be caused by incarceration of stomach, colon, or small bowel. Intestinal strangulation, bowel necrosis, and perforation can occur. These patients may have cardiac and respiratory embarrassment. Cardiac function can be compromised because compression of the ventricles can prevent adequate filling. A mass effect may cause a shift of the mediastinum, impairing venous return to the heart. The respiratory status of the patient may be affected by compression of the ipsilateral parenchyma. In chronic cases, the patients may have aspiration due to a gastric hernia resulting in chronic pneumonia. Other complications commonly associated with diaphragmatic hernias include sepsis, respiratory failure, pneumonia, empyema, and wound infections. The overall rate of complications can be as high as 60% in blunt injuries, compared with 40% in penetrating trauma.

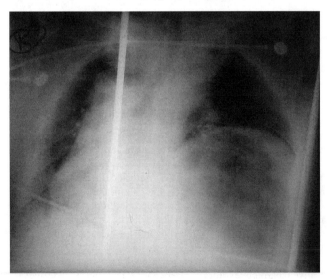

16. When do delayed diaphragmatic hernias present?

A diaphragmatic injury, if not repaired in the acute setting, may develop complications and herniation hours to years after the initial injury. In cases of delayed hernias, the diagnosis of a di-

aphragmatic hernia is often not suspected because the history of trauma is not elicited or so remote that the patient does not think it to be significant enough to volunteer the information.

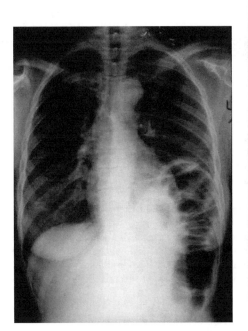

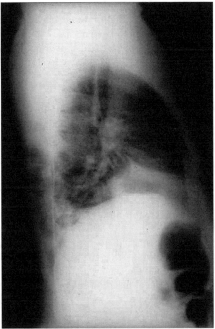

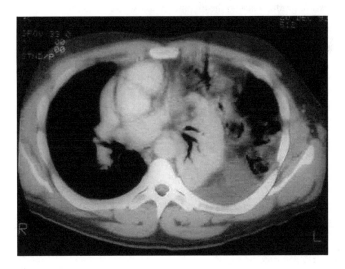

17. What operative approach should be used in the repair of diaphragmatic injuries?

In the acute setting, diaphragm injuries should be repaired through the abdomen to assess for
associated intra-abdominal injuries. This is true for penetrating and blunt ruptures of the diaphragm.
Evacuation of the thoracic cavity can be performed through the diaphragmatic perforation or a separate thoracotomy if necessary. The thoracic cavity must be evaluated for ongoing bleeding at the

time of operation. In the case of chronic, delayed herniation, a debate remains over which incision should be performed: celiotomy or thoracotomy. Many surgeons prefer an abdominal approach. A celiotomy allows adequate evaluation of the bowel for viability after reduction. If resection is required, this is best done with the intestines in the abdomen rather than in the chest. A thoracotomy allows lysis of adhesions, which may have formed on the thoracic wall, to be performed safely for chronic hernias. This prevents inadvertent injuries to the bowel and contamination of the thorax that may occur when manual reduction from the abdomen is attempted. Thoracoscopic and laparoscopic techniques have been used to reduce acute and chronic diaphragmatic hernias.

18. What is the best method for surgical repair of penetrating diaphragmatic injuries acutely?

The traditional open approach has been accepted as the gold standard for repair of diaphragmatic injuries. Two animal studies compared the open technique of suturing with laparoscopic stapling and suturing techniques. Both studies looked at the histology and strength of the repairs after a 6-week healing period. Laparoscopic techniques (i.e., suturing or stapling) resulted in equivalent healing of the diaphragm compared with the open technique. Equivalent studies in humans with long-term follow-up of patients with laparoscopic repairs are not yet available.

19. What techniques are available if primary closure of a diaphragmatic injury is not be possible?

Most diaphragmatic injuries can be repaired primarily. Occasionally, large defects require prosthetic material to assist with closure of the diaphragm. When the diaphragm is avulsed from its insertion to the chest wall, no tissue is left for anatomic reconstruction. In these cases, the rib above the site of insertion can be used. A stitch is placed around the rib and then through the diaphragm to secure it to the chest wall.

20. What factors prevent diaphragm injuries from healing?

- Healing may be impaired by the constant motion of the diaphragm.
- The pressure gradient across the diaphragm allows a constant flux of peritoneal fluid from the abdomen to the chest, preventing healing of an injury.
- Aportion of omentum or viscus may occlude to perforation and prevent healing, "putting a foot in the door."

21. Which organs are most likely to herniate through a perforation of the diaphragm?

The stomach is the most common organ involved in diaphragmatic hernias, followed in decreasing order of frequency by the colon, spleen, small intestine, liver, and kidney. The omentum is often involved in these defects.

BIBLIOGRAPHY

1. Asensio JA, Demetriades D, Rodriguez A: Injuries to the diaphragm. In Feliciano DV, Moore EE, Mattox KL (eds): Trauma, 3rd ed. Norwalk, CT, Appleton & Lange, 1996, pp 461–486.
2. Degiannis E, Levy RD, Sofianos C, et al: Diaphragmatic herniation after penetrating trauma. Br J Surg 83:88–91, 1996.
3. Demetriades D, Kakoyiannis S, Parehk D, et al: Penetrating injuries to the diaphragm. Br J Surg 72: 824–826, 1988.
4. Fabian TC, Croce MA, Stewart RM, et al: A prospective analysis of diagnostic laparoscopy in trauma. Ann Surg 217:557–565, 1993.
5. Feliciano DV, Cruse PA, Mattox KL, et al: Delayed diagnosis of injuries to the diaphragm after penetrating wounds. J Trauma 28:1135–1144, 1988.
6. Ivatury RR, Simon RJ, Stahl WM: A critical evaluation of laparoscopy in penetrating abdominal trauma. J Trauma 34:822–828, 1993.
7. Ivatury RR, Simon RJ, Weksler B, et al: Laparoscopy in the evaluation of the intrathoracic abdomen after penetrating injury. J Trauma 33:101–108, 1992.

8. Jackson AM, Ferreira AA: Thoracoscopy as an aid to the diagnosis of diaphragmatic injury in penetrating wounds of the lower chest: A preliminary report. Injury 7:213–217, 1976.
9. Kozar RA, et al: Laparoscopic repair of traumatic diaphragmatic injuries. J Surg Res 97:164–171, 2001.
10. Murray JA, Cornwell EE, Velmahos GV, et al: Healing of traumatic diaphragmatic injuries: Comparison of laparoscopic versus open techniques in an animal model. J Surg Res 100:189–191, 2001.
11. Murray JA, Demetriades D, Asensio JA, et al: Occult injuries to the diaphragm: Prospective evaluation of laparoscopy in penetrating injuries to the left lower chest. J Am Coll Surg 187:626–630, 1998.
12. Murray JA, Demetriades D, Cornwell EE, et al: Penetrating left thoracoabdominal trauma: The incidence and clinical presentation of diaphragmatic injuries. J Trauma 43:624–626, 1997.
13. Oschner MG, Rozycki GS, Lucente F, et al: Prospective evaluation of thoracoscopy for diagnosing diaphragmatic injury in thoracoabdominal trauma: A preliminary report. J Trauma 34:704–710, 1993.
14. Spann JC, Nwariaku FE, Wait M: Evaluation of video-assisted thoracoscopic surgery in the diagnosis of diaphragmatic injuries. Am J Surg 170:628–631, 1995.
15. Uribe RA, Pachon CE, Frame SB, et al: A prospective evaluation of thoracoscopy for the diagnosis of penetrating thoracoabdominal trauma. J Trauma 37:650–654, 1994.

17. PRINCIPLES OF ABDOMINAL TRAUMA

Frederic S. Bongard, M.D.

1. What are the three regions of the abdomen?
The three distinct regions of the abdomen are the peritoneal cavity, the retroperitoneal space, and the pelvis.

2. What constitutes the upper abdomen?
The upper abdomen is the portion of the peritoneal space covered by the bony thorax. It includes the diaphragm, liver, spleen, stomach, and transverse colon.

3. What constitutes the lower abdomen?
The lower abdomen contains the small bowel and the remainder of the intra-abdominal large bowel.

4. What is contained in the retroperitoneum?
The retroperitoneum contains the aorta, vena cava, pancreas, kidneys, adrenal glands, ureters, and parts of the duodenum and colon.

5. What is contained in the pelvis?
The pelvis contains the rectum, bladder, iliac vessels, and, in females, genitalia.

6. What is the most commonly injured abdominal solid organ?
In blunt trauma, the spleen. The liver is the most commonly injured in penetrating trauma.

7. What is the most commonly injured abdominal hollow viscus?
The small bowel.

8. Hemoperitoneum causes "peritoneal" findings in what percentage of patients?
About 80% of patients with acute hemoperitoneum have acute abdominal findings on examination. About 20% of patients with acute hemoperitoneum have a benign physical examination on initial presentation.

9. On inspiration, the diaphragm ascends to what intercostal space?
With deep breathing, the diaphragm may reach upward to the fourth intercostal space. This is of particular concern because patients with penetrating injuries below the level of the nipple may harbor intra-abdominal injuries.

10. What is the most common cause of abdominal distention after surgery?
Aerophagia and unintentional insufflation of the stomach with a bag-mask breathing device are the most common causes of posttraumatic abdominal distention.

11. When should a nasogastric tube be inserted?
A nasogastric (NG) tube is useful both for diagnosis and treatment and should be inserted as quickly as possible after the patient's neck and airway are secured and intravenous access is obtained. Decompressing the stomach of ingested air will make the patient more comfortable. Blood obtained from the tube should alert the clinician to the possibility of gastrointestinal injury. When facial trauma is present, blood obtained from the NG tube may have been swallowed. If severe facial fractures are present, the NG tube should be placed through the mouth (orogastric) to prevent the possibility of placing the tube into the brain through a fracture in the cribriform plate.

12. Lower rib fractures are typically associated with what intra-abdominal injuries?
Liver and spleen.

13. Lower thoracic spine injuries are typically associated with what abdominal injuries?
Pancreas and small bowel.

14. Lumbar vertebral transverse process fractures are typically associated with what abdominal injuries?
Abdominal viscera and kidneys.

15. Pelvic fractures are typically associated with what injuries?
Pelvic organ or vessels and retroperitoneal structures, particularly genitourinary.

16. Which abdominal or pelvic organs are most commonly injured following blunt trauma?
The liver, spleen, and kidneys are most commonly injured after blunt abdominal trauma. However, the incidence of bowel injury and lumbar spinal fractures increases with incorrect seat belt usage.

17. Following blunt trauma, which part of the diaphragm is most commonly injured?
Although injuries to the diaphragm may be located anywhere in its substance (and may be associated with cardiac or pericardial trauma), the most common location is in the left postero-lateral portion.

18. What are the characteristic findings of diaphragmatic rupture on chest radiograph?
Elevation of the left hemidiaphragm and a bubble of air in the left chest are common findings. A hemothorax or blunting of the left costophrenic angle may also be present. Placement of an NG tube may be helpful because the chest x-ray may show it "curled" in the left hemithorax.

19. Does a normal serum amylase exclude pancreatic injury?
Serum amylase levels may be normal in the face of pancreatic injury and do not necessarily exclude trauma of the pancreas.

20. Is elevation of the serum amylase concentration indicative of pancreatic injury following blunt trauma?
No. It is not unusual for blunt trauma victims to sustain multiorgan trauma, including injuries of the head and neck that may cause elevation of the serum amylase from a salivary gland source.

21. Following a motor vehicle accident, a patient presents with a linear ecchymosis across the abdominal wall. What is the most likely cause?
Incorrectly worn seat belts that lie high across the abdomen usually cause this finding. Of concern is the potential for underlying intra-abdominal hollow viscus injuries.

22. What is a Chance fracture?
A Chance fracture is a transverse fracture of a low thoracic or lumbar vertebral body usually produced by a distracting flexion-extension mechanism. Chance fractures are common with seat belt use and are associated strongly with intestinal injury. Some authors even state that unless an alert patient has a completely benign abdomen on physical examination, the presence of a Chance fracture mandates abdominal exploration or diagnostic peritoneal lavage.

23. Which abdominal organs are most commonly injured by penetrating trauma?
The liver, small bowel, colon, and stomach are the abdominal viscera most commonly injured by penetrating trauma.

24. Should knife and gunshot wounds be managed differently?
Because of the effects of cavitation, energy dissipation, and change in trajectory, the damage caused by a gunshot wound cannot be predicted reliably. For this reason, many experts will explore all patients with all but the most superficial gunshot wounds. When doubt exists regarding whether the bullet entered the abdominal cavity, laparoscopy can be used. Although laparoscopy is becoming a common *diagnostic* modality, at this time, few would rely solely on laparoscopy to exclude a visceral injury following penetrating (especially gunshot wound) trauma.

25. Why are penetrating injuries of the flank and back of particular concern?
Injuries in these areas may cause perforation of retroperitoneal viscera such as the kidneys, duodenum, pancreas, or portions of the colon. While bleeding from a renal injury may be apparent on a computed tomography (CT) scan, violation of the hollow viscera in this location is difficult to detect and may lead to significant morbidity if not diagnosed and treated in a timely fashion.

26. What is the mortality rate of open pelvic fractures?
Very high, near 50%.

27. Pelvic fractures most commonly are associated with what other injuries?
Genitourinary (especially in men) and vascular injuries, although gastrointestinal injuries occur occasionally. Bleeding from the fractured pelvic bones or disruption of associated vessels can cause extensive blood loss and hypotension.

28. What is the preferred method of management of bleeding from pelvic fractures?
The key to management is reduction of the pelvic volume, which decreases the space into which the injured vessels can bleed. This is best accomplished with fixation of the pelvis, usually requiring the placement of an external fixator. Embolization via angiography is a useful adjunct when bleeding continues. Surgery for bleeding from a pelvic fracture is a last resort.

29. Major bleeding occurs from which type of pelvic fractures?
Those lying posteriorly, typically involving the sacroiliac joint.

30. If an external fixator cannot be placed rapidly in a patient with bleeding from a pelvic fracture, what alternative therapy exists?
A M.A.S.T. suit (military antishock trousers), or pneumatic antishock garment (PASG), may be placed until definitive external fixation can be accomplished.

31. What are some general indications for celiotomy in a patient who is suspected of having an abdominal injury?
1. Hypotension with evidence of an abdominal injury
2. Peritonitis
3. Recurrent hypotension despite adequate resuscitation
4. Extraluminal air on abdominal or chest x-ray
5. Diaphragmatic injury
6. Intraperitoneal perforation of the urinary bladder on cystography
7. CT scan evidence of intra-abdominal or retroperitoneal injury
8. A contrast study of the upper or lower gastrointestinal tract indicating injury
9. Persistent hyperamylasemia in a patient with abdominal physical findings

32. How did Harry Houdini die?
Houdini was 52 years old when he was struck four times in the abdomen by a boxer attending one of his magic shows. He died from peritonitis on October 31, 1926, in Detroit, Michigan. He promised that his greatest illusion would be to return "from the other side." We're still waiting.

33. How do you assess the abdomen for suspected injury in an unconscious patient, a paraplegic, or a quadriplegic patient?
As they may not present with the usual acute abdomen, imaging studies such as ultrasound and computer tomography are used. Peritoneal lavage or even laparoscopy may be needed to exclude injury.

BIBLIOGRAPHY

1. American College of Surgeons: Advanced Trauma Life Support Course for Physicians, 5th ed. Chicago, American College of Surgeons, 1993.
2. Blaisdell FW, Trunkey DD: Trauma Management, Vol 1. Abdominal Trauma. New York, Thieme-Stratton, 1982.
3. Fabian TC, Croce MA: Abdominal trauma, including indications for celiotomy. In Feliciano DV, Moore EE, Mattox KL (eds): Trauma. Stamford, CT, Appleton & Lange, 1996.
4. Wilmore, Cheung, Harkin, et al: ACS Surgery: Principles and Practice. New York, 2002.

18. ABDOMINAL COMPARTMENT SYNDROME

Jonathan R. Hiatt, M.D.

1. What are the defining features of a compartment syndrome?

Compartment syndrome is the consequence of elevated pressure in a confined or limited space. Pressures are elevated because of an increase of interstitial fluid or of cell swelling. Space is limited because of a decrease in the size of the compartment or an increase in its contents. As a result, circulation and function and viability of the tissues or structures within the space are compromised.

2. List common sites where compartment syndromes occur.

Compartment syndromes occur most commonly in the extremities, usually in the legs. However, they may occur in any confined space, including the skull, orbit, kidney, or abdomen.

3. What are the common causes of compartment syndromes?

Most compartment syndromes are related to trauma. Traumatic causes include fractures, crush and blast injuries, and operative trauma. Compartment syndromes also may follow ischemia and subsequent reperfusion, such as may occur with an arterial injury to an extremity. For example, prolonged ischemia to the lower extremity from an injury to the femoral artery may produce a compartment syndrome in the compartments of the leg, distal to the femoral artery distribution.

4. List the five key features of the abdominal compartment syndrome (ACS).

1. Elevated ventilatory pressures
2. Elevated central venous pressure
3. Decreased urine output
4. Massive abdominal distention
5. Reversal of these derangements with abdominal decompression

5. What is the normal intraperitoneal pressure, and why is this important?

Intraperitoneal (abdominal) pressure, usually expressed in millimeters of mercury (mmHg), is approximately zero, although it may be slightly positive or negative. Surgeons create conditions of increased intraperitoneal pressure with insufflation of the abdomen for laparoscopic operations. When abdominal pressure becomes elevated to pathologic levels, described below, ACS may occur.

6. What are ways in which abdominal pressure may be measured, and which are most applicable in the clinical setting?

Intra-abdominal pressure (IAP) may be measured using direct and indirect techniques. With direct techniques, a measuring device, such as a needle connected to a manometer system, is placed directly into the peritoneal cavity. The most commonly used direct technique is the electronic insufflator system, used for measurement of the pressures produced with carbon dioxide pneumoperitoneum for laparoscopic operations. With indirect techniques, pressures are measured across the wall of an intra-abdominal structure via an indwelling device. While inferior vena cava (IVC) and transgastric pressures may be used, the bladder pressure is used most commonly today. The bladder serves as a passive diaphragm for volumes of 50–100 ml, and bladder pressures have been shown to correlate with IAP for pressures ranging from 5–70 mmHg. Operationally, the indwelling bladder catheter is connected to the manometer system, and IAP may be measured at the bedside in a rapid and simple system. Note that a pressure transducer will provide readings in mmHg, while a water manometer reads cm H_2O, which may be converted (1 mmHg = 1.36 cm H_2O).

7. Classify and list the causes of ACS.

Causes may be acute or chronic (see table). Acute causes are spontaneous, postoperative, traumatic, and iatrogenic. Mortality of ACS is as high as 40% in collected reports.

Causes of ACS

ACUTE	CHRONIC
Peritonitis	Ascites
Intra-abdominal abscess	Tumors
Ileus or intestinal obstruction	Pregnancy
Ruptured abdominal aortic aneurysm	Peritoneal dialysis
Intra-abdominal bleeding	
Tight abdominal closure	
Abdominal packing	
Mesenteric vascular occlusion	
Pneumoperitoneum	

8. Identify the major clinical setting in which ACS is most often encountered, and describe the major factors that contribute to development of ACS in this setting.

Most cases of ACS occur in association with major trauma; multifactorial mechanisms are responsible for posttraumatic ACS. These mechanisms include hypoperfusion of the viscera with hemorrhagic shock; large-volume fluid resuscitation; tight abdominal closures, sometimes with packing, in patients who have undergone exploratory laparotomy; and the use of positive pressure ventilation. The contents of the abdominal compartment may be increased markedly with swollen intestines, ongoing coagulopathic hemorrhage, and the use of packs for tamponade of bleeding surfaces.

9. Describe the major pathophysiologic effects of increased IAP on: (1) abdominal wall, (2) venous return, (3) mesenteric visceral perfusion, (4) renal function, (5) pulmonary function, and (6) hemodynamics.

All are markedly deranged with significant increases of IAP.

1. **Abdominal wall.** With increasing IAP, the abdominal wall becomes stiffer, and compliance falls in a linear fashion.

2. **Venous return.** Venous return is diminished. Causes of decreased venous return include decreased IVC flow and elevation of the diaphragm. IVC flow is decreased as a consequence of retroperitoneal pooling of blood, obstruction by diaphragmatic crura, and decreased venous outflow from the legs. Diaphragmatic elevation produces increased ventricular filling pressures and decreased cardiac compliance, hindering return of blood to the heart.

3. **Mesenteric visceral perfusion.** Visceral blood flow declines linearly with increasing IAP. Perfusion of mesenteric arteries, intestinal mucosa, and liver are diminished, with resultant visceral ischemia that may be quantified using gastric tonometry.

4. **Renal function.** Renal blood flow, glomerular filtration rate, and urine output are diminished. Oliguria is a hallmark of ACS and occurs as a consequence of decreased cardiac output and compression of the aorta, and renal arteries and veins, but not of the ureter. Classic experimental work has shown that the effect on urine output is graded: Oliguria is seen with IAP of 15–20 mmHg, while IAP greater than 20 mmHg will produce anuria. Effects of urine output are not reversed by correction of cardiac output deficits alone; IAP must be lowered by abdominal decompression.

5. **Pulmonary function.** The thoracic cavities are compressed by the abdominal distention, and lung compliance falls. Elevated ventilatory pressures, such as oliguria, are hallmarks of the syndrome. Pulmonary artery pressures and pulmonary vascular resistance are increased. Arterial blood gas derangements include hypoxemia, hypercarbia, and acidosis; this is a combined acidosis, with respiratory (hypercarbia) and metabolic (hypoperfusion) components. Note that these pulmonary derangements may be exacerbated by addition of positive end-expiratory pressure

(PEEP, used to treat hypoxemia by opening collapsed airway), because PEEP will further increase the intrathoracic pressure.

6. **Hemodynamics.** Cardiac output is depressed because of markedly diminished stroke volumes, despite compensatory tachycardia. Preload is decreased, because of decreased venous return and increased intrathoracic pressure, and afterload is increased, because of elevated systemic vascular resistance. The table below shows the usual effects of ACS that would be seen using modern monitoring tools (arterial and pulmonary artery catheters; ventilatory pressures).

Hemodynamic and Ventilatory Effects of ACS

↑	↓	↔
Heart rate	Cardiac output	Mean blood pressure
Systemic vascular resistance (SVR)		
Pulmonary artery (PA) pressure		
Pulmonary capillary wedge (PCW) pressure		
Central venous pressure (CVP)		
Peak airway pressure		

10. Provide a grading system for ACS according to the measured bladder pressure and describe the implications of such as a system for treatment.

Pressure elevations may be described as mild, moderate, and severe. In the most recent major review, Burch and coauthors propose a system shown in the table below.

Grading System for ACS

GRADE	BLADDER PRESSURE		MANAGEMENT
	cm H$_2$O	mmHg	
I	10–15	7–11	Normal postoperative pressures
II	15–25	11–18	Close monitoring indicated
III	25–35	18–26	Most require decompression
IV	> 35	> 26	All require decompression

Adapted from Burch JM, Moore EE, Moore FA, Franciose R: The abdominal compartment syndrome. Surg Clin North Am 76:833–842, 1996.

ACS is rare for grade II elevations and may develop insidiously with grade III. Grade IV is a surgical emergency, with progression to fatal organ dysfunction and cardiac arrest if the abdomen is not decompressed.

11. List compounding factors that may exacerbate the organ system effects of ACS.

Premorbid illnesses (cardiac, pulmonary, renal)

Massive fluid volumes, which increase the abdominal contents

Trendelenburg positioning, which increases diaphragmatic compression by the abdominal contents

PEEP, described above

Associated injuries, particularly those that produce bleeding and coagulopathy

12. State the two major surgical interventions that are required for treatment of ACS.

1. Abdominal decompression
2. Closure of the abdominal wall

13. What are the major physiologic consequences of abdominal decompression, and how do these relate to management of the patient before and during the actual operative decompression?

The effects of abdominal decompression in the patient with ACS are dramatic. Cardiac, respiratory, and renal function are improved markedly. Cardiac output increases, systemic vascular resistance declines, and urine output improves. The anesthesiologist often will report substantial improvements in ventilatory mechanics, as well as a brisk diuresis. It must be recognized that a transient fall in blood pressure secondary to peripheral vasodilatation may occur, and asystole secondary to reperfusion injury has been reported.

Prior to decompression, aggressive efforts are directed to restoration of intravascular volume with blood and blood products and maximization of oxygen delivery. Invasive hemodynamic monitoring and large-bore vascular access are essential. Coagulation defects and hypothermia should be corrected insofar as possible; however, ACS may develop during massive resuscitation after operation for major injury. When clinical deterioration is marked, with anuria, ventilatory dysfunction, and hemodynamic instability, abdominal decompression may be needed before the therapeutic goals have been reached.

14. What are the options for abdominal closure at the time of decompression?

These include open packing, skin closure, or prosthetic closure. Open packing has risks of fistulization, evisceration, and massive fluid loss. The skin may be closed over open fascia using sutures or towel clips, but the risk here is of recurrent compression. Prosthetic closures are used most frequently. Various types of prosthetic mesh are available, but because these are quite expensive, the use of a sterilized, open 3-liter irrigation bag, sutured to fascia or skin, is preferred by many surgeons.

15. Describe timing of and options for delayed abdominal closure.

Abdominal reclosure is performed 4–7 days following decompression. Hemodynamics should be stable at this point, and diuresis should have occurred, with body weight near the premorbid level. The patient is returned to the operating room, and the prosthesis is removed. The abdomen is explored, with gentle inspection of suture lines and a search for any purulent fluid collections. It may be appropriate to measure bladder pressure at this point, if there is any question that recurrent compression might be created with abdominal wall closure. Surgical options include definitive closure of the abdominal wall at this time. Alternatively, a staged closure may be chosen, with mesh or skin grafts used at the present operation. If the closure is staged, definitive closure is performed at a minimum of 3–6 months postoperatively. The patient should be essentially healthy, with good nutrition, and the abdominal wall should be soft and pliable; "woody" edema should have resolved, and the skin and stomas, if present, should be loose and protuberant. Because flaps and tissue expanders are sometimes needed, the assistance of a surgeon expert in major reconstruction may be of benefit.

16. Summarize the critical decisions in management of ACS.

1. Recognizing the clinical syndrome in a patient with risk factors
2. Measuring IAP when the diagnosis is in question
3. Identifying the patient for whom abdominal decompression will be a potentially life-saving intervention
4. Preparing the patient operative decompression
5. Selecting a method for temporary closure of the abdominal wall after decompression
6. Timing of reoperation for abdominal reclosure
7. Selecting a technique for secondary closure or later definitive reconstruction.

ACS is a challenging condition for which judicious critical care and operative management have the potential to salvage an otherwise often fatal condition.

BIBLIOGRAPHY

1. Barnes GE, Laine GA, Giam PY, et al: Cardiovascular responses to elevation of intra-abdominal pressure. Am J Physiol 248:R208–R213, 1985.
2. Burch JM, Moore EE, Moore FA, Franciose R: The abdominal compartment syndrome. Surg Clin North Am 76:833–842, 1996.

3. Cullen DJ, Coyle JP, Teplick R, Long MC: Cardiovascular, pulmonary, and renal effects of increased intra-abdominal pressure in critically ill patients. Crit Care Med 17:118–121, 1989.
4. Harmon PK, Kron IL, McLachlan HD, et al: Elevated intra-abdominal pressure and renal function. Ann Surg 196:594–597, 1982.
5. Kashtan J, Green JF, Parsons EQ, Holcroft JW: Hemodynamic effects of increased abdominal pressure. J Surg Res 30:249–255, 1981.
6. Perry MO: Compartment syndromes and reperfusion injury. Surg Clin North Am 68:853–864, 1988.
7. Richardson JD, Trinkle JK: Hemodynamic and respiratory alterations with increased intra-abdominal pressure. J Surg Res 20:401–404, 1976.
8. Richards WO, Scovill W, Shin B, Reed W: Acute renal failure associated with increased intra-abdominal pressure. Ann Surg 197:183–187, 1983.
9. Schein M, Wittmann DH, Aprahamian CC, Condon RE: The abdominal compartment syndrome: The physiological and clinical consequences of elevated intra-abdominal pressure. J Am Coll Surg 180:745–753, 1995.

V. Gastrointestinal Tract

19. LIVER AND BILIARY INJURIES

Hernan I. Vargas, M.D.

LIVER INJURIES

1. Are injuries to the liver common?

Yes. The liver is the most commonly injured solid organ.

2. What are the common mechanisms of liver trauma?

About 80% of liver injuries are the result of penetrating abdominal trauma, and about 20% are the result of blunt trauma. Solid organ injuries may be difficult to diagnose. Blunt injuries to the liver can occur by direct trauma or compression to the torso. Patients with right-sided rib fractures have a higher incidence of liver injuries. Rapid deceleration may be responsible for the avulsion of the hepatic veins or retro-hepatic inferior vena cava injuries.

3. Does the mechanism of injury influence the means of diagnosis of liver injuries?

Yes. Victims of penetrating abdominal injury generally require an exploratory laparotomy. This is how liver injuries are discovered in these patients.

Patients who suffer blunt trauma to the abdomen are only explored if they are hemodynamically unstable. The patients who are hemodynamically stable are subjected to less invasive means of diagnosis, such as diagnostic peritoneal lavage (DPL), computed tomography (CT), or ultrasound (US).

4. What is the preferred diagnostic modality in the hemodynamically stable patient with blunt abdominal trauma?

Tests are selected according to individual circumstances and availability at different centers. CT is the most commonly used test. It provides high sensitivity and specificity in the diagnosis of abdominal trauma, particularly for the management of solid organ injury. DPL has a sensitivity of 98% for intraperitoneal blood, but it is poorly specific. The rate of nontherapeutic laparotomy based on a positive DPL varies from 25 to 67%. US evaluation is becoming more popular because it is noninvasive, quick, inexpensive, and frequently available. It has a specificity of 80% and is highly sensitive (99%), but it requires an experienced operator and is thus operator-dependent.

5. Are liver injuries always life threatening?

No. The mortality from liver injuries is less than 10%. Liver injuries may be stratified according to their severity into six classes as outlined in the table below.

Liver Injury Scale

GRADE	INJURY DESCRIPTION	FREQUENCY
I	< 10% subcapsular. Laceration < 1 cm	15%
II	10–50% subcapsular. Laceration 1–3 cm	55%
III	> 50% subcapsular or ruptured or expanding. Large intraparenchymal hematoma	25%
IV	Parenchymal disruption (25–75% liver)	3%
V	> 75% parenchymal disruption. Major vascular injury	2%
VI	Hepatic avulsion	< 1%

6. Is it possible to manage a blunt liver injury nonoperatively?

Yes. Twenty percent to 50% of patients with blunt liver injury require operative intervention. Patients treated nonoperatively must be hemodynamically stable, and peritoneal signs should be absent. Liver injury–related transfusion requirement should be minimal. CT should delineate the liver injury, and there should not be any associated hollow visceral injuries. Patients with higher severity of injury on CT scan are more likely to fail nonoperative management and should be monitored very closely.

7. What are some of the perils of nonoperative management?

- Hemorrhage may occur as a consequence of a prolonged observation period. The surgeon must be very careful not to attribute the bleeding to a second source (bone fracture, external bleeding). If there is any evidence of bleeding, a repeat CT scan may show an enlarging liver hematoma.
- Occasionally embolization via angiography may provide vascular control and arrest bleeding in the stable patient.
- Infrequently ($<$ 5%), an enteric or other intra-abdominal injury may be missed.
- Commonly, biliary ductal disruption with formation bile collection may occur, but it is rarely clinically significant (1%).
- Intrahepatic abscess formation.

8. Are most patients with a penetrating liver injury candidates for nonoperative care?

No. Most patients with a penetrating abdominal injury require an exploratory laparotomy to evaluate the entire peritoneal cavity (examine the solid organs as well as viscera) and retroperitoneum. Exceptionally, a stable, asymptomatic patient with a right thoracoabdominal injury may be successfully managed with laparoscopy, thus avoiding open surgery.

9. What are the principles of operative management?

Adequate exposure and exploration of the abdomen; use of a midline incision with an appropriate subcostal retractor

Control of bleeding by packing of the abdomen and direct compression on the liver

Volume resuscitation

Assessment of the injury

10. What is the Pringle maneuver?

It consists of occlusion of the hepatic inflow, by cross clamping the portal triad. The safety of this maneuver over prolonged periods of time is uncertain. Occlusion times of 30–60 minutes are commonly seen. Experimentally, up to 90 minutes of normothermic ischemia have been well tolerated by the liver under controlled conditions. Some surgeons have empirically used local hypothermia and systemic steroids in an attempt to avoid further liver injury in cases when prolonged cross clamp (over 20 minutes) is required.

11. What are some of the conventional technical maneuvers used to control hepatic bleeding?

Use of electrocautery or argon beam laser to control superficial lacerations or raw surfaces

Use of liver sutures (mattress stitch with an absorbable suture)

Hepatorrhaphy with finger fracture and control of individual bleeding vessels and injured ducts

Debridement of devascularized and friable liver parenchyma

Patch with a pedicle omental flap

12. How often is bleeding from a hepatic injury not controlled with conventional techniques?

In approximately 5% of patients undergoing operative management of a liver injury, bleeding is not controlled with conventional techniques. In patients who develop a coagulopathy, or in those who are hemodynamically unstable, perihepatic packing is used to control bleeding. Other indications for perihepatic packing are massive subcapsular hematoma or severe bilobar injuries.

13. What is the diagnosis of a patient with dark venous bleeding in the back of the liver after Pringle maneuver and compression and packing the liver have been performed? How is the injury managed?

Retrohepatic vena cava or hepatic vein injury. Options for treatment include:

Complete mobilization of the liver and repair of the venous injury

Transparenchymal approach of the hepatic veins

Placement of an atrio-caval shunt. An atrio-caval shunt is an intraluminal shunt that temporarily procures caval return from the kidneys and lower half of the body to the right atrium. It is placed operatively through the right atrium into the IVC, generally through a median sternotomy. If considered, this is a maneuver to be performed early, before severe hemodynamic or metabolic complications start.

14. A patient developed jaundice, an upper gastrointestinal bleed and hematochezia, and colicky abdominal pain 2 weeks after a motor vehicle accident. What is the clinical diagnosis?

Hematobilia. It represents hemorrhage into the biliary tree. It is generally confirmed on upper endoscopy by seeing bleeding through the ampulla of Vater. These patients are further studied and treated during angiography by embolization of the bleeding vessel(s) or pseudoaneurysm. If embolization is not successful, hepatotomy with direct exposure of the bleeding vessel or hepatic resection may be necessary. However, there is significant blood loss and high operative morbidity and mortality associated with this procedure.

BILIARY INJURIES

15. What are the common mechanisms of biliary injuries?

Penetrating injury is the most common cause of biliary injuries. Stab wounds cause transection or laceration of the biliary tree and gallbladder. Gunshot wounds cause lacerations or crushing injuries and are commonly associated with vascular injuries.

The biliary tree may be injured by direct injury with compression over the spine or during rapid deceleration events at the points of fixation. The gallbladder may be contused, lacerated, or avulsed when a direct or shear force is applied to the peritoneal cavity or by sudden increase in pressure of the duct and "blowout."

16. What is the most significant predictor of outcome in patients who suffer gallbladder trauma?

The prognosis is predicated on their associated injuries. If a gallbladder injury is recognized early, the prognosis is excellent in the absence of other associated injuries.

17. How are biliary injuries found in patients with penetrating abdominal trauma?

These injuries will generally be identified at the time of exploratory laparotomy. Occasionally an injury may be missed on initial exploration. In such a case, patients may present with evidence of obstructive jaundice, biliary ascites, or sepsis. Varying with the clinical syndrome, a biliary injury may be documented by paracentesis, hepato-iminodiacetic acid (HIDA) scanning, or endoscopic retrograde cholangiopancreatography (ERCP). ERCP allows anatomic definition of the level of the injury and provides a road map for subsequent reconstruction.

18. True or false: Blunt biliary tree injuries have symptoms early in their course and are easy to recognize.

False. Patients present with a retroperitoneal or an intraperitoneal leak of bile. In either case, the lack of irritation caused by sterile bile may be responsible for the paucity of symptoms. An abdominal CT that shows a fluid collection in the retroperitoneum, around the duodenum or ascites, is often interpreted as blood.

19. What is the most common site of extrahepatic biliary duct injury in blunt trauma?

The injury occurs most often at the suprapancreatic area, at the junction of the pancreas and common bile duct.

20. What is the necessary preoperative work-up for intrahepatic biliary disruption?

CT of the abdomen is important to identify any possible hepatic parenchymal injury with intrahepatic biliary disruption. If no evidence of parenchymal injury is seen, other potential sources of biliary leakage are the gallbladder or the extrahepatic biliary tree. A preoperative ERCP is valuable to provide information useful in planning the operative approach.

21. What are the surgical principles in the management of the patient with a bile duct injury?

Stabilize the patient and treat immediately life-threatening vascular and solid and hollow viscus injuries first.

Carefully examine the biliary tract at surgery. Use cholangiography to assist with definition of the anatomy.

If safe and possible, perform the biliary repair or reconstruction immediately. In the unstable patient or in the patient with severe associated injuries, the safest approach is to mark the duct ends and to exteriorize the bile outflow by draining the area.

22. What is the preferred mode of reconstruction in a completely transected bile duct after a stab wound?

A primary end-to-end anastomosis is appropriate if there is no devascularization or damage to the edges of the transected duct. It is probably one of the few occasions when this mode of reconstruction is acceptable. If there is segmental loss of biliary duct, devascularization, or injury to the transected duct, the preferred approach is a Roux-en-Y choledoco- or hepaticojejunostomy.

BIBLIOGRAPHY

1. Feliciano DV: Biliary injuries as a result of blunt and penetrating trauma. Surg Clin North Am 74:897–908, 1994.
2. Patcher HL, Feliciano DV: Complex hepatic injuries. Surg Clin North Am 76:763–782, 1996.

20. SPLENIC INJURIES

Gideon P. Naudé, M.B.Ch.B.

1. Is the spleen commonly injured in trauma?

Splenic rupture is the most common cause of major abdominal injury. Motor vehicle accidents are the most common cause of blunt splenic injury.

2. Is splenic injury only associated with severe trauma?

No. The injury is occasionally so trivial that the patient presents without a history of trauma.

3. What clues are there to suspect splenic injury in blunt trauma?

- History of trauma involving the left upper abdomen or lower chest
- Abdominal pain and tenderness
- Rib fractures of the left lower chest
- Pain referred to the left shoulder tip
- Progressive anemia by serial hematocrit determinations
- Signs of shock such as tachycardia and hypotension

4. How is the diagnosis of ruptured spleen confirmed?

Seriously injured patients are taken to surgery promptly, and the exact cause of intraperitoneal bleeding (e.g., ruptured spleen) is made at surgery.

Less acute injuries are diagnosed clinically. Hematologically, declining hemoglobin and hematocrit values and a rising leukocyte count (e.g., above 15,000 u/L) can indicate a ruptured spleen. Intraperitoneal blood and injury to the spleen may be visualized sonographically. Plain abdominal radiographs often are noncontributory. Positive signs include enlargement of the spleen, fractured ribs in the left lower chest, and displacement of gas in the transverse colon inferiorly and the gastric air bubble medially. Rarely, serrations of the greater curvature of the stomach are seen because of dissection of blood into the gastrosplenic ligament. Arteriography is accurate and is used particularly in the evaluation of nonoperatively treated patients and in cases of delayed rupture. Computed tomography (CT) with contrast enhancement has become the most valuable tool in evaluating patients for nonoperative management of injured spleens. The diagnosis of patients requiring surgery can be made early before hemodynamic instability occurs. Paracentesis revealing intraperitoneal blood can point to the diagnosis.

5. How does the Organ Injury Scaling (OIS) Committee grade blunt splenic injuries?

The OIS system is based on hematoma and laceration size from grade 1 to grade 5, in escalating order of severity.

Grade	Hematoma	Laceration
1	Subcapsular: nonexpanding, <10% depth, nonbleeding	Capsular tear: <1 cm parenchymal surface area
2	Subcapsular: nonexpanding, 10–50% surface area. Intraparenchymal: nonexpanding, <2 cm in diameter	Capsular tear: active bleeding, 1–3 cm parenchymal depth, not involving a trabecular vessel
3	Subcapsular: >50% surface area or expanding; ruptured subcapsular hematoma with bleeding. Intraparenchymal: >2 cm or expanding	Tear: >3 cm parenchymal depth or involving trabecular vessels
4	Ruptured intraparenchymal hematoma with bleeding	Involving segmental or hilar vessels, producing major devascularization (>25% of the spleen)
5	Completely shattered spleen	Hilar vascular injury that devascularizes the spleen

6. What are the indications for splenectomy after trauma?

- Irreparable injury to the spleen, such as grade 4 and 5 injuries
- Severe blood loss leading to hemodynamic instability
- Multiple injuries obviating time-consuming repairs
- Coagulopathy, hypothermia, and associated medical or surgical conditions that preclude lengthy surgery

7. Is penetrating splenic injury managed in the same manner as blunt trauma?

No. Because of danger of injury to adjacent and nearby organs such as the stomach, colon, small bowel, pancreas, and chest cavity, exploration is carried out in almost all patients with penetrating injuries. Definitive treatment of the splenic injury depends on the operative findings, and splenectomy or repair of the spleen is then carried out.

8. Do surgeons ever harm the spleen?

Yes. About one fifth of all splenectomies are performed for iatrogenic injury to the spleen during surgery on neighboring organs such as the stomach, colon, pancreas, and hiatus or during vagotomy.

9. Is splenectomy the only management option for a splenic injury?

No. Nonoperative management is frequently employed (particularly in children) if life-threatening hemorrhage is not present. Among those requiring laparotomy, the less severely injured may receive spleen-preserving procedures.

10. Describe the alternatives to total splenectomy.

Minor lacerations and capsular tears can be managed by electrocautery, by argon beam coagulation, and by applying hemostatic gel (i.e., topical thrombin, oxidized cellulose, or microfibrillar collagen) or covering the injury with absorbable mesh.

Larger injuries are managed by debridement and suture repair with careful ligation of the vessels to the injured area to prevent further bleeding. Partial splenectomy is performed if severe injury has destroyed one part of the spleen with preservation of the remaining spleen. Absorbable mesh may be used to wrap the entire spleen and tamponade any further bleeding. To preserve full splenic function, 30% to 40% of the splenic mass must be retained as well as the hilar blood supply. Splenic fragments wrapped in omentum (and other forms of autotransplantation) have survived.

11. How common is delayed rupture of the spleen, and when does it occur?

Delayed rupture of the spleen occurs in approximately 5% of blunt trauma splenic injuries. Most cases (80%) occur within the first 2 to 3 weeks of injury, but some patients present months or even years later.

12. What is the mechanism of delayed splenic rupture?

Minor injury to the spleen results in intraparenchymal hemorrhage, or bleeding contained by peritoneal folds or omentum. With breakdown of the hematoma and liquefaction of the cells, the osmotic pressure leads to an increase in water in the hematoma, expanding its size and increasing the pressure, leading to rupture and hemorrhage.

13. How frequently is nonoperative management of a ruptured spleen performed and how frequently is it successful?

About 50% of ruptured spleens are treated nonoperatively in adults. The patients are observed for signs of hemorrhage and taken to surgery if they occur. Serial CT scans are performed to ensure that extracapsular bleeding is not excessive. Of the patients treated nonoperatively, about one fourth eventually require surgery. In children, 90% of splenic injuries are treated nonoperatively, with a success rate of more than 90%.

14. **Which patients are most suited to be treated nonoperatively for a ruptured spleen?**
   - Patients suffering blunt trauma with subcapsular bleeding or very small amounts of intraperitoneal bleeding.
   - Patients in whom the spleen is the only organ injured and there are no other injuries requiring laparotomy.
   - Children younger than 6 years of age and particularly those younger than 2 years of age should have every effort made to preserve the spleen. Immunodepressed adults should have their spleens preserved if possible.

15. **What is the blood picture after trauma splenectomy?**
   - *Red blood cell* numbers do not change significantly, but inclusion bodies such as Howell-Jolly bodies appear (a useful sign that splenectomy is complete and that no splenunculi are present).
   - *White blood cell* numbers increase immediately after splenectomy, with granulocytes being increased initially. After several weeks, the granulocytes normalize, and monocytes and lymphocytes increase.
   - *Platelets* usually increase modestly to about 500,000 for a prolonged period. If hypersplenism was present before injury and splenectomy, the count may go higher than 1 million, making the patient more susceptible to thrombosis.

16. **What are the complications of splenectomy?**
   - Postoperative bleeding
   - Atelectasis, pneumonia, and pleural effusion, because the operation is in the left upper quadrant, decreasing breathing and coughing effort
   - Pancreatitis and damage to the tail of the pancreas
   - Gastric injury or necrosis on the greater curvature, leading to peritonitis or a gastric fistula, which may be caused by direct injury or devitalization during ligation of the short gastric vessels
   - Increased platelet count, occasionally causing thrombosis
   - Fulminant postsplenectomy infection
   - Subphrenic abscess

17. **What is the mortality of splenectomy and splenorrhaphy?**
   Splenectomy has a mortality rate of 12% to 23%, and splenorrhaphy has a rate of 0% to 10%. Splenectomy patients have more severe associated injuries, including intracranial, chest, pelvic, and additional intra-abdominal injuries. Splenectomy alone is responsible for very few deaths.

18. **What factors in the splenectomized patients render them susceptible to postsplenectomy sepsis?**
   - Young children are most susceptible (80% of cases).
   - The incidence is increased if the patient had a hematologic condition.
   - Decreased removal of bacteria from the blood after splenectomy is a factor because the spleen is the site of the many fixed macrophages necessary to clear bacteria from the circulation.
   - The spleen is the site of maturation of natural killer cells, helper T cells, and cytotoxic or suppressor T cells.
   - Production of opsonins, properdin, and tuftsin is deficient, rendering certain bacteria more resistant to the body's defenses.
   - Patients have decreased levels of IgM and IgG.

19. **Which organisms are most frequently involved in postsplenectomy sepsis?**
   Sepsis after splenectomy is most often caused by *Streptococcus pneumoniae, Haemophilus influenzae,* and *Neisseria meningitides.*

20. How frequently and when does postsplenectomy sepsis most commonly occur?

Sepsis occurs in 1.5% of postsplenectomy patients. Among children, the greatest incidence is within the first 2 years after splenectomy. Among adults, most cases occur after 1 year, and more than one half of cases occur after 5 years.

21. How would you clinically describe overwhelming postsplenectomy sepsis?

The condition starts with mild, prodromal flulike symptoms and progresses to shock and high fever from unopposed sepsis, usually a septicemia, often leading to disseminated intravascular coagulation and death.

22. What is the mortality rate for postsplenectomy sepsis syndrome?

The mortality rate for overwhelming postsplenectomy infection varies between 25% and 50%, with children being at greatest risk.

23. How is postsplenectomy sepsis prevented?

- Every effort is made (especially in children) to preserve as much of the spleen as possible.
- Polyvalent pneumococcal vaccine (Pneumovax) is administered as soon as possible.
- Prophylactic antibiotics given over a prolonged period may be effective in preventing infection.
- Patients are cautioned to present for treatment very early in the course of suspected infection.

24. When is the ideal time to administer pneumococcal vaccine?

The vaccine should be administered as soon as possible after splenectomy and repeated every 4 to 5 years. In cases of elective splenectomy, the vaccine is given before surgery.

25. Does polyvalent pneumococcal vaccine (Pneumovax) give complete protection against postsplenectomy sepsis?

No. It is effective against 80% of the causative organisms, and prophylactic antibiotics are necessary for prolonged periods to prevent infection, particularly in young children.

26. In what circumstances would you perform a splenorrhaphy?

- The patient does not have an injury that has totally destroyed the spleen or completely disrupted the splenic blood supply.
- The patient is not in danger of dying from exsanguination.
- There are not multiple additional injuries, and time is available for this time-consuming procedure.
- The patient is in good general condition and does not have hypothermia or coagulopathy.

27. How would you describe the procedure of splenorrhaphy?

The splenic injury is debrided, the blood clot removed, the vessels to the injured area ligated, and the splenic capsule repaired. Complete hemostasis is essential, and electrocautery, argon beam coagulation, and fibrin glue application may be used to this end. The spleen is often wrapped in absorbable mesh to further ensure hemostasis. Drains should be avoided in cases of isolated splenic injuries because they correlate with a higher incidence of infection. If multiple additional injuries (e.g., gastric, pancreatic, colonic) are present, drains may be unavoidable.

BIBLIOGRAPHY

1. Bongard FS, Stamos MJ, Passaro E: Surgery: A Clinical Approach. New York, Churchill Livingstone, 1997.

2. Nyhus LM, Baker RJ: Mastery of Surgery, 2nd ed. Boston, Little, Brown, 1992.
3. Pickardt B, et al: Operative splenic salvage in adults. J Trauma 29:1386, 1989.
4. Pitcher ME, Cade RJ, Mackay JR: Splenectomy for trauma: Morbidity, mortality and associated abdominal injuries. Aust N Z J Surg 59:461, 1989.
5. Way LW: Current Surgical Diagnosis and Treatment, 10th ed. Norwalk, CT, Appleton & Lange, 1994.
6. Wilmore DW (ed): ACS Surgery: Principles and Practice. New York, WebMD Professional, 2002.

21. GASTRIC INJURIES

Gideon P. Naudé, M.B.Ch.B., and Francois H. Van Zyl, M.B.Ch.B.

1. Is blunt trauma to the stomach common?

No. Perforation of the stomach due to blunt trauma comprises only about 1% of intra-abdominal injuries. It usually only occurs when the stomach is full and direct force is applied to it, such as in a motor vehicle accident or a fall from a height.

2. Why is blunt trauma to the stomach uncommon?

The relatively protected position of the empty stomach and its pliability protect it from most blunt trauma. The force required to rupture an empty stomach is usually enough to cause fatal injuries in other organs, which is why we rarely see patients with ruptured stomachs due to blunt injury. A full stomach ruptures with less force applied to it.

3. How common is penetrating injury to the stomach?

Of all patients with penetrating intra-abdominal organ injury, the stomach is injured in 20%. Stab wounds and gunshot wounds usually involve several organs, such as the stomach, transverse colon, omentum, small bowel, spleen, and liver.

4. What are the causes of gastric necrosis?

- Ingested corrosives may cause gastric necrosis.
- Surgical trauma during a highly selective vagotomy, as well as antireflux fundoplications, can lead to lesser curve necrosis.
- Devascularization during trauma is a rare cause.

5. Are gastric perforations usually easy to diagnose?

Generally, gastric perforations are easy to diagnose. The mechanism of injury, whether stab wound, gunshot wound, or blunt trauma, suggests the diagnosis. An acute abdomen with tenderness, guarding, and rebound usually develops early because leaking gastric juice causes severe peritoneal irritation. The liver dullness may disappear as free gas overlies the liver. Imaging studies confirm the diagnosis. Peritoneal lavage may show blood or gastric contents. Perforation may be an incidental finding at laparotomy in patients with multiple abdominal injuries.

6. Under what circumstances is clinical examination unreliable?

For unconscious patients, patients with spinal injury, and patients intoxicated with alcohol or narcotic analgesics, other diagnostic modalities are required, such as computed tomography (CT), peritoneal lavage, and diagnostic laparotomy.

7. Which diagnostic modalities are commonly used to diagnose gastric perforation?

Chest (erect) and abdominal (lateral decubitus) radiographs often reveal free gas in the abdomen. Peritoneal lavage may reveal blood and gastric contents in the peritoneal cavity. CT with contrast accurately indicates gastric perforation and extraluminal air and fluid.

8. What would prompt surgery in a patient who ingested corrosives?

Generalized peritonitis, if gastric perforation has occurred, should prompt surgery. Surgery can prevent the caustic material from spreading all over the abdominal cavity and causing caustic injury to other intra-abdominal organs.

9. How would you manage a caustic perforation of the stomach?

Laparotomy should be performed, and peritoneal toilet with copious irrigation to remove all caustic material is essential. The perforation is then managed by excising various amounts of necrotic stomach, depending on the size of the injury.

10. What incision is used to explore the abdomen in cases of suspected gastric perforation?
A midline or left paramedian upper abdominal incision is used. This incision can be extended if other injuries are present that cannot be reached through a transverse or oblique incision.

11. When exploring the stomach, what maneuvers are performed?
The greater curvature is held firmly and pulled downward to visualize the entire anterior aspect of the stomach. The lesser sac is opened below the greater curvature of the stomach to inspect the posterior aspect of the stomach for signs of injury.

12. How is a blunt perforation of the stomach repaired?
Blunt injuries of the stomach are frequently crushing in nature, and care must be exercised to ensure that the wound edges are viable. This process entails excising the wound edges until healthy bleeding is encountered. The wound edges are then repaired in two layers with an absorbable suture. A nasogastric tube is left in the stomach to prevent postoperative gaseous distention and undue stress on the anastomosis. In very severe injury, a partial or even total gastrectomy may be necessary. Hematomas of the gastric wall are deroofed and drained.

13. How is a sharp perforation of the stomach managed?
At laparotomy, the stomach is inspected to identify entrance and exit wounds. Both wounds are repaired. Peritoneal toilet is carried out, and the abdomen is irrigated with copious amounts of saline until it is clean. A nasogastric tube is left in place to prevent postoperative distention with tension on the suture line. Broad-spectrum antibiotics are administered to prevent postoperative infection.

14. How does a patient who has a traumatic injury to the diaphragm with stomach and other abdominal viscera in the chest usually present?
The patient usually has a history of severe blunt trauma, often with a fractured pelvis (i.e., an indication of the severity of the injury), or a history of penetrating trauma to the chest with injury of the diaphragm. The trauma might have occurred months or even years before the patient presents. Presentation may be prompted by intestinal obstruction, which frequently causes pressure in the chest leading to respiratory insufficiency or to perforation of the stomach or bowel, causing an infected pleural effusion.

15. How is the diagnosis made of a traumatic injury of the diaphragm with stomach and other abdominal viscera in the chest?
Clinical examination may reveal dullness in the left chest with diminished breath sounds. Sometimes, bowel sounds are heard in the chest. The chest radiograph may reveal the stomach or bowel in the chest, particularly if a nasogastric tube has been passed, and it goes into the chest as well. Contrast-enhanced radiography or CT can confirm the diagnosis.

16. In esophageal injury, how can the stomach be used?
If a significant amount of esophagus is lost and a primary repair cannot be carried out, the stomach may be used to replace the lost esophagus, and an esophagus-to-stomach anastomosis may be carried out in the chest or even in the neck.

17. Are postoperative complications common after gastric injury and repair?
Postoperative complications are relatively uncommon after gastric injury and repair. The stomach has a very rich blood supply, and gastric anastomoses heal well and rarely break down and leak. The gastric contents have relatively few bacteria compared with the bowel, particularly

the distal colon. When laparotomy and repair, as well as peritoneal toilet, are carried out in a timely fashion, infection is uncommon.

18. What are the complications of gastric perforation?

Generalized peritonitis follows untreated gastric perforation. This may lead to septicemia and disseminated sepsis. Subphrenic abscesses occur after inadequate treatment and even occur in a small percentage of patients who have been adequately treated. Leaking gastric suture lines occur but are uncommon, as are gastric fistulas. Wound infection occurs with higher frequency in patients in whom gastric or intestinal contents contaminate the wound.

19. How are complications of gastric perforation diagnosed?

Clinically, the patient may have signs of peritonitis or ongoing infection with a raised temperature and a high white blood cell count. Subphrenic and other intra-abdominal fluid collections may be diagnosed with ultrasound or CT. Fluid leaking through the wound or drainage site should be tested for pH. An acid result indicates a gastric fistula. Contrast-enhanced radiography and CT may demonstrate a gastric fistula.

20. What is the approach to a subphrenic abscess?

Small, newly developing subphrenic collections have been treated successfully with antibiotics only. In general, however, subphrenic abscesses are drained by placing a needle or catheter in the abscess, which is guided by ultrasound or CT visualization. If this relatively noninvasive method is not successful, surgical drainage, usually through an extraperitoneal approach, is used.

21. What is the approach to an acute gastric fistula?

An acute gastric fistula may be treated successfully by keeping the stomach empty and decompressed with a nasogastric tube on suction while the patient is nourished with total parenteral nutrition through a central line. Most fistulas close with this method of treatment. Signs of peritonitis or failure of medical treatment should prompt surgical exploration with repair.

22. When is clinical examination of the abdomen with radiographs unreliable for diagnosing gastric injury?

Radiographs are unreliable for detecting penetrating wounds of the back where perforation of the posterior wall of the stomach has occurred without injury to the anterior wall or without spillage of gastric contents into the general peritoneal cavity. CT is valuable in this situation to indicate injury of the posterior abdominal wall and fluid in the lesser sac. Continued observation may also elicit signs that were originally absent.

23. What diagnostic test would best indicate the need for surgery in the case of a gunshot wound that penetrates the peritoneal cavity?

A gunshot wound that penetrates the abdominal cavity requires a laparotomy to evaluate and treat the damage.

24. How are tangential gunshot wounds treated?

If the patient has peritoneal signs, a laparotomy is performed. In the absence of peritoneal signs, peritoneal lavage, CT, or laparoscopy may be carried out to demonstrate intra-abdominal penetration and injury.

25. How would you grade gastric injuries?
1. Intramural hematoma less than 3 cm and a partial-thickness laceration
2. Intramural hematoma greater than 3 cm and a full-thickness laceration less than 3 cm
3. Laceration greater than 3 cm
4. Large laceration involving the vessels on the lesser or greater curvature
5. An extreme rupture of more than 50% of the stomach with a devascularized stomach

BIBLIOGRAPHY

1. Ivatury RR, Cayten CG (eds): The Textbook of Penetrating Trauma. Media, PA, Williams & Wilkins, 1996.
2. Moore EE, Mattox KL, Feliciano DV (eds): Trauma, 2nd ed. Norwalk, CT, Appleton & Lange, 1991.
3. Read RA, Moore EE, Moore FA, Burch JM: Blunt and penetrating abdominal trauma. In Zinner MJ, Schwartz SI, Ellis H (eds): Maingot's Abdominal Operations. Stamford, CT, Appleton & Lange, 1997.
4. Wilmore DW (ed): ACS Surgery: Principles and Practice. New York, WebMD Professional, 2002.
5. Wilson RF, Walt AJ: Management of Trauma: Pitfalls and Practices, 2nd ed. Baltimore, Williams & Wilkins, 1996.

22. DUODENAL AND PANCREATIC TRAUMA

Mary-Anne Purtill, M.D., and Bruce E. Stabile, M.D.

1. What is the frequency of injury to the duodenum? What mechanisms contribute to these injuries?

Although duodenal injuries are relatively uncommon, they do account for 3–5% of all abdominal injuries. Penetrating trauma accounts for approximately three fourths of these injuries. Blunt duodenal injury usually is caused by abrupt deceleration, crushing the retroperitoneal duodenum against the spine or by causing a blow-out of an air-filled, closed duodenal loop. Sharp blows to the epigastric region, such as a steering wheel injury in drivers or handlebars in children, are the most common cause of duodenal injury from blunt trauma. Combined duodenal-pancreatic injuries are usually secondary to penetrating trauma, and comprise one quarter of all duodenal injuries.

2. What is the mortality associated with duodenal injury?

Because duodenal injuries are relatively rare, few studies are available to elucidate their true incidence and mortality. However, historically, they have a very high mortality rate. Reported noncivilian mortality rates from duodenal injuries between the Civil War and the Korean War were 40–100%. Recent data from large urban trauma centers have shown a progressive decrease in mortality over the last 20 years, from 35% to 17%.

3. What are the anatomic landmarks of the duodenum? With what anatomic variations should the trauma surgeon be familiar?

The duodenum is the beginning of the small intestine and measures about 21 cm in length. It is located roughly between the first and third lumbar vertebrae. The duodenum consists of the superior, descending, transverse, and ascending portions; they are also known as the first, second, third, and fourth portions, respectively. The first portion of the duodenum is located intraperitoneally, while the other three are retroperitoneal. The duodenum is fixed where it enters and exits the retroperitoneum, just beyond the pyloric sphincter and at the ligament of Treitz, respectively. The duodenal bulb constitutes the first portion. The common bile duct enters the duodenum medially in the second portion via the ampulla of Vater and serves as the landmark that divides the second and third portions. The superior mesenteric artery and vein are the landmarks dividing the third and fourth portions, and the inferior mesenteric vein lies near the fourth portion at the duodenojejunal flexure. The duodenum shares its somewhat tenuous blood supply with the pancreas, with perforating vessels originating from the gastroduodenal artery and the arcades formed by the inferior and superior pancreaticoduodenal arteries. There are a number of anatomic variations in this area with which the trauma surgeon should be familiar. The gastroduodenal artery originates from the common hepatic artery in 82% of the population, from the left hepatic artery in 11% of the population, from the right hepatic artery in 7%, and rarely from the celiac or superior mesenteric arteries. An anomalous retroduodenal right hepatic artery originates from the superior mesenteric artery in 25% of the population.

4. How much fluid is processed or managed by the duodenum daily?

The volume of fluid traversing the duodenum ranges between 5 and 10 L per day. This large volume of fluid, with its activated digestive enzymes and bile, is responsible for the profound inflammatory response associated with duodenal injuries.

5. How are duodenal injuries diagnosed?

Duodenal injuries from penetrating trauma are most commonly diagnosed intraoperatively. The duodenum's retroperitoneal location deep within the abdomen makes it a relatively protected organ, and exploratory laparotomy is usually undertaken for other more apparent injuries. Blunt trauma to the duodenum is even more difficult to diagnose. A high index of suspicion based on mechanism of injury and physical exam findings may lead to further diagnostic studies. Complaints of severe epigastric pain out of proportion to the physical findings should raise the question of duodenal injury.

6. Is peritoneal lavage useful in diagnosing duodenal injuries?

Although diagnostic peritoneal lavage (DPL) is an invaluable tool for the early detection of intra-abdominal injury, it has a limited role in evaluating the retroperitoneal duodenum. Studies have shown a positive DPL in 50–70% of patients with duodenal injuries, although most of these were associated with other intra-abdominal injuries.

7. Should plain x-rays of the abdomen be obtained when duodenal injury is suspected?

Flat plate and cross-table lateral x-rays of the abdomen are useful in suggesting duodenal perforation when gas bubbles are present in the retroperitoneum adjacent to the right psoas muscle, around the right kidney, or anterior to the upper lumbar spine. Fractures of the transverse processes of the lumbar vertebrae are indicative of forceful retroperitoneal trauma and serve as a predictor of duodenal or pancreatic injury.

8. How accurate is computed tomography (CT) versus an upper gastrointestinal series for diagnosing duodenal injuries?

No randomized trials have assessed the two tests; however, both are reasonably accurate in diagnosing duodenal injury. Accuracy figures range from 57% to 88%. For either study to be adequate, contrast must be visualized at some point within all portions of the duodenum without extravasation. Retroperitoneal air or extravasated oral contrast medium constitute proof of injury.

9. Is ultrasound useful in diagnosing duodenal trauma?

There has been little experience with this modality for diagnosing duodenal trauma. The recent use of ultrasound by trauma surgeons in the emergency department should provide useful information in the near future.

10. What injury severity classification system is used for duodenal injuries?

The Organ Injury Scaling Committee of the American Association for the Surgery of Trauma has developed grading systems for specific organ injury to facilitate clinical research and continued quality improvement. Increasing number indicates increasing complexity of injuries.

Grade		*Injury Description*
I	Hematoma	Involving single portion of the duodenum
	Laceration	Partial thickness, no perforation
II	Hematoma	Involving more than one portion
	Laceration	Disruption < 50% of circumference
III	Laceration	Disruption 50–75% of circumference of D2
		Disruption 50–100% circumference of D1, D3, D4
IV	Laceration	Disruption > 75% of circumference of D2
		Involving ampulla or distal common bile duct
V	Laceration	Massive disruption of duodenopancreatic complex
	Vascular	Devascularization of duodenum

11. How is operative exposure of the duodenum best achieved?

All abdominal injuries should be explored through a midline incision extending from the xiphoid process to the symphysis pubis. Thorough exploration of the duodenum consists of visualization of all four portions of the organ. Intraoperative findings that suggest duodenal injury in-

clude bile staining or crepitance of the tissues around the duodenum and right-sided retroperitoneal hematoma. Complete mobilization of the duodenum should be performed using the Kocher
or Cattell maneuvers. These allow full visualization of the anterior and posterior portions of the
duodenum. Keep in mind that many important vascular structures are in the vicinity of the duodenum, including the inferior vena cava (IVC), aorta, hepatic artery, portal vein, and splenic and
mesenteric vessels. If bleeding is identified in the right retroperitoneum, it is prudent to ensure
that proximal and distal control of the aorta and distal control of the IVC are readily available before exploration of the region is undertaken.

12. How is the Kocher maneuver performed?
    A Kocher maneuver is performed by incising the lateral peritoneal attachments of the duo-
denum and mobilizing both the second and third portions of the duodenum medially with a combination of sharp and blunt dissection. The first assistant should provide gentle traction on the
duodenal C-loop while the surgeon performs the dissection. If a large hematoma is present in
the region, good visualization may be very difficult. Under these circumstances, it is useful to
advance the nasogastric tube (NGT) through the pylorus into the C-loop, so that palpation can be
used to assist in identifying the duodenal wall.

13. How is the Cattell maneuver accomplished?
    More appropriately referred to as the Cattell and Braasch maneuver, it is useful for thorough
inspection of the third portion of the duodenum. It requires mobilization of the hepatic flexure of
the colon and upward mobilization of the small bowel. The small bowel mobilization is undertaken by sharply incising its retroperitoneal attachments from the lower right quadrant to the ligament of Treitz, with cephalad reflection of the small bowel and right medial visceral rotation.
    Alternatively, the third and fourth portions of the duodenum can be well visualized and pal-
pated by performing an extended Kocher maneuver and incising the ligament of Treitz.

14. Do all duodenal hematomas require surgical intervention?
    Duodenal hematomas are typically injuries of childhood play or child abuse but can also oc-
cur in adults. Approximately 50% of all duodenal hematomas in children are attributable to child
abuse. The symptoms of gastric outlet obstruction that occur can take up to 48 hours to present;
this is the result of fluid shifts into the hyperosmotic duodenal hematoma. The diagnosis can be
made by double contrast CT or upper gastrointestinal contrast x-rays that show the "coiled spring"
or "stacked coin" sign. The injury usually is considered a nonsurgical problem, and best results
are obtained with conservative management. However, in 20% of cases, there are associated injuries, and these must be ruled out before committing to a nonoperative approach. Conservative
treatment consists of nasogastric decompression and parenteral nutrition. The average time for
hematoma resolution is 10–14 days. After 2 weeks of conservative therapy, reevaluation and exploratory laparotomy for evacuation of the hematoma should be considered.

15. When should primary repair of duodenal lacerations be undertaken?
    Approximately 80% of all duodenal injuries can be repaired safely using simple surgical prin-
ciples and techniques. Debridement of injuries back to viable tissue and secure double-layered
closure should provide satisfactory results for most grade I, II, and III lacerations.
    For extensive grade III and all grade IV and V injuries, more complex surgery is required.
Judgment regarding the type of operation needed is based on the patient's presentation, mechanism of injury (blunt vs. penetrating), time elapsed from injury to repair, associated injuries, blood
loss, hemodynamic stability, and the surgeon's familiarity with the available procedures. The more
commonly used procedures include duodenorrhaphy with external drainage; duodenorrhaphy
with either transduodenal or antegrade tube duodenostomy; triple ostomy technique with gastrostomy and antegrade and retrograde jejunostomies; and duodenal resection with duodenoduo-
denostomy or duodenojejunostomy. Less commonly used procedures include jejunal serosal
patches and omental pedicle grafts.

16. Should all duodenal injuries be drained?

Most experienced surgeons agree that in the face of traumatic duodenal injury, at a minimum, external drainage should be provided, because this affords early detection and control of duodenal fistulas. The drain is preferably a simple, soft silicone rubber, closed system placed adjacent to the repair. The drain should not be placed in contact with the suture line because this can facilitate fistula formation.

17. What does "diverticulization" of the duodenum mean?

Duodenal diverticulization involves primary closure of the duodenal wound, lateral tube duodenostomy, vagotomy, antrectomy and end-to-side gastrojejunostomy (Billroth II), and T-tube drainage of the common bile duct. The goal is to completely divert the gastric and biliary contents away from the repaired duodenum. Also, a potentially uncontrolled lateral duodenal fistula would be converted to a controlled end duodenal fistula.

18. What is "pyloric exclusion"?

Currently, this conservative approach is the favored procedure for diverting gastric secretions away from an area of severe duodenal or combined duodenal and pancreatic injury. First suggested by Vaughn in 1977, it consists of internal suture closure of the pylorus (via gastrotomy), followed by gastrojejunostomy. A vagotomy usually is not performed. The closure of the pylorus reopens within 2 weeks to 2 months, allowing the duodenal injury time to heal. Functionally, the gastrojejunostomy closes in time. This procedure is a less technically involved, quicker operation than diverticulization of the duodenum and appears to be equally effective as long as the ampulla of Vater is intact.

19. What is the incidence of pancreatic injury from trauma?

As with duodenal injuries, pancreatic trauma is uncommon, with a recently reported incidence of 7% from large trauma centers. The majority of injuries to the pancreas are from penetrating trauma (75%), with the remainder from sharp blows to the epigastrium in blunt trauma.

20. What is the mortality associated with pancreatic injuries?

The reported mortality from pancreatic injuries during the Korean War was 22%. More recent studies have shown an approximate 18% overall mortality, although the rate drops to 3% when injury is limited exclusively to the pancreas.

21. What is the average number of additional abdominal organs injured when pancreatic trauma is identified? What additional organs are usually injured?

The three most commonly injured organs associated with pancreatic trauma are the liver (50%), the stomach (48%), and major vascular structures (43%). Other frequently injured organs include the small bowel and colon (39%), spleen (21%), kidney (20%), duodenum (20%), and the biliary tract (5%). Over 90% of patients with pancreatic injuries have at least one other intra-abdominal injury, with the mean number being 3.4.

22. Is serum amylase level a good indicator of pancreatic injury?

Although the highest concentration of amylase in the body is in the pancreas, serum amylase or isoamylase levels have not been found to be reliable indicators of pancreatic injury. The positive predictive value of an elevated amylase for pancreatic injury in blunt trauma is only 10%. However, with a normal amylase after blunt trauma there is a 95% likelihood that there is no injury to the gland. The value of serial amylase determinations is that a rising level signals a need for further studies.

23. What are some important anatomic considerations for managing pancreatic injuries?

While the pancreas has a relatively protected position deep within the retroperitoneal abdomen, it is intimately associated with a number of major structures. Behind the pancreas are the inferior vena cava, aorta, left kidney, both renal veins, and the right renal artery. The head of the pancreas lies within the sweep of the duodenum, the body overlies the spine, and the tail is in the hilum of the spleen. The splenic artery has a serpiginous route across the upper border of the pancreas, and the splenic vein lies behind the gland, just above its lower edge.

The main pancreatic duct of Wirsung usually traverses the entire length of the gland just above its center. The duct of Wirsung usually ends by joining the common bile duct and emptying into the duodenum through the ampulla of Vater. The minor duct of Santorini usually branches from the main pancreatic duct in the neck of the pancreas and empties into the duodenum through a minor papilla located about 2.5 cm above the major papilla. There are many variations on the anatomy of the pancreatic ductal system, and familiarity with the common variations is advisable.

The arterial supply and venous drainage of the pancreas are fairly constant. However, anomalous origins off the superior mesenteric artery and of the common hepatic and the right hepatic arteries make them prone to injury during pancreatic manipulation. Importantly, much of the blood supply to the duodenum is dependent on a pancreatic vascular source. It is important to note that exocrine and endocrine functions of the pancreas are reasonably well maintained after resection of up to 80% of the gland.

24. What is the anatomic landmark dividing the head from the body and tail of the pancreas?

The anatomic landmark used to divide the proximal from the distal pancreas is the superior mesenteric vessels passing behind the neck of the pancreas. There are no actual anatomic distinctions within the gland itself.

25. How are the pancreatic injuries classified?

According to the Organ Injury Scaling Committee of the American Association for the Surgery of Trauma, pancreatic injuries are classified according to severity.

Grade		Injury Description
I	Hematoma	Minor contusion without duct injury
	Laceration	Superficial laceration without duct injury
II	Hematoma	Major contusion without duct injury or tissue loss
	Laceration	Major laceration without duct injury or tissue loss
III	Laceration	Distal transection or parenchymal injury with duct injury
IV	Laceration	Proximal transection or parenchymal injury involving ampulla of Vater
V	Laceration	Massive disruption of the pancreatic head

26. What diagnostic studies are used to evaluate pancreatic injuries?

As with duodenal injuries, most penetrating injuries to the pancreas are discovered intraoperatively when the patient undergoes emergent exploratory laparotomy for penetrating abdominal trauma. Blunt trauma to the pancreas is unreliably diagnosed by plain abdominal x-rays or DPL. CT scanning of the abdomen may reveal an abnormality of the pancreas or adjacent to the pancreas, although the injury of the gland may take days to appear on CT scan.

27. Does endoscopic retrograde cholangiopancreatography (ERCP) have a role in the diagnosis of pancreatic duct injuries?

ERCP has no role in the evaluation of a hemodynamically unstable patient. However, it can be very useful in determining the etiology of persistent hyperamylasemia or unexplained abdominal symptoms related to trauma of the pancreas.

28. How is the pancreas exposed intraoperatively?

In a thin patient, the body of the pancreas usually can be adequately visualized and palpated by retracting the stomach downward; this exposes the pancreas through the somewhat transparent gastrohepatic ligament. To completely assess the pancreas, the lesser sac must be entered by incising the gastrocolic ligament. For visualization of the posterior aspect of the pancreas, the following maneuvers should be undertaken: mobilization of the hepatic flexure of the colon, wide Kocherization, incision of the inferior retroperitoneal attachments of the pancreas, and mobilization and medial rotation of the spleen. Incision of the ligament of Treitz may also be useful.

29. What operative techniques are used to repair or treat pancreatic injuries?

If after careful and delicate exploration the major ductal system of the pancreas is found to be intact, the pancreatic injury can be managed with simple external closed drainage. Leakage from minor ducts in grade I and II injuries will cease within a few days or weeks if drainage is adequate. Grade III injuries are distal to the superior mesenteric vein and are managed by distal pancreatectomy. Injuries of grade IV and V require alternative, more complex procedures to ensure good outcomes.

30. What are some of the options available intraoperatively to assess the integrity of the pancreatic duct?

Major ductal injuries occur in about 15% of pancreatic trauma injuries and are usually readily apparent by visual inspection. Ductal injuries may not be apparent with penetrating injuries to the head, neck, or central portion of the pancreas. After complete mobilization and inspection of the pancreas, pancreatography can be performed if a major ductal injury is suspected.

Because most patients with severe pancreatic trauma have other injuries and are frequently hemodynamically unstable, it is inappropriate to perform time-consuming intraoperative studies that can be done later. Frequently, wide drainage of the pancreatic injury is best for the patient.

When the need to assess the pancreatic duct is present, it is prudent to obtain a cholangiogram of the common bile duct to ensure its integrity. This can be performed with a needle cholangiogram through the gallbladder. The puncture hole can be closed by oversewing with an absorbable suture. In cases of abnormal pancreatic ductal anatomy (i.e., the pancreatic duct drains directly into the duodenum), the cholangiogram will not be useful for assessing the pancreatic duct. If there is an associated open duodenal injury, the ampulla can be cannulated directly and a retrograde cholangiopancreatogram performed. A transection of the tail can also be performed for direct cannulation of the ductal system. However, the duct may be very small and difficult to identify, incurring the risk of fistula formation. Intraoperative ERCP has been reported but is rarely done.

31. What are the management options if a distal pancreatic duct injury is identified?

If a distal ductal injury is identified, the safest option is a distal pancreatectomy. After the devitalized distal pancreas has been removed, the main duct should be identified and closed with a U-stitch. Drains should be placed in the region to control any fistula that may form at the surgical site.

Procedures for salvage of the distal pancreas, such as a pancreaticojejunostomy, have had unacceptably high rates of fistula formation. Because exocrine and endocrine function are well preserved with up to 80% resection of the gland, these procedures are no longer recommended.

32. When a distal pancreatectomy is performed, is it advisable to attempt splenic preservation?

Although concern over postsplenectomy sepsis may make splenic preservation appealing, the additional operative time (about 1 hour), potentially greater blood loss, and need for transfusion usually outweigh the benefits. In the setting of pancreatic trauma, it can be technically challenging to isolate the splenic artery and vein from the gland. It is, therefore, not generally recommended to attempt splenic preservation in complicated pancreatic trauma.

33. When is a Whipple procedure indicated?

Pancreatoduodenectomy as an emergency operation carries a very high mortality rate. In general, the only indication for a Whipple procedure for trauma is when the traumatic injury has already nearly performed the operation (i.e., the pancreatic head is transected or destroyed).

34. What are some of the principles and procedures used to treat combined pancreatico-duodenal injuries?

Combined pancreatic and duodenal injuries are uncommon. They are usually secondary to penetrating trauma and are associated with other intra-abdominal injuries. Review of a large series of combined pancreatic and duodenal injuries determined that 24% of patients underwent simple repair and drainage, 50% underwent repair and pyloric exclusion, and 10% required pancreatoduodenectomy. Surgical management of these injuries is dictated by the status of the distal common bile duct and ampulla of Vater, as well as the grade of the duodenal trauma. Thus, a cholangiogram should be performed in all patients with combined duodenal-pancreatic injuries. If the common bile duct and the ampulla of Vater are both intact, primary repair of the duodenum can be performed and appropriate treatment of the pancreas undertaken. This will suffice in most patients. However, when disruption of the pancreatic duct cannot be assessed (hemodynamic instability on the operating table), wide drainage of the pancreas should be performed rather than pancreatic resection. If such a patient develops a postoperative enterocutaneous fistula, pancreatic fistula, or intra-abdominal abscess, further studies, such as an hepato-iminodiacetic acid (HIDA) scan, ERCP, transhepatic or magnetic resonance cholangiogram can be performed to rule out major duct injury. Based on this assessment, further nonoperative or appropriate operative management can be instituted.

With severe duodenal injury in conjunction with a pancreatic injury, it is prudent to protect the duodenal repair by either pyloric exclusion or diverticulization of the duodenum.

35. When is the best time to remove drains placed for a pancreatic injury?

Different durations of pancreatic drainage are used depending on the mechanism and degree of injury. In general, the drainage fluid should be tested for amylase level. If the level is higher than the serum level, the drain should be left in place until the patient is eating, drainage is minimal, and the amylase content is no greater than that of the serum.

36. What is the role of somatostatin analogues in pancreatic trauma?

Somatostatin and its analogues have an inhibitory effect on both basal and stimulated pancreatic exocrine secretion. Although the use of somatostatin analogue has not been proven to change the closure rate or the time to closure of pancreatic fistulas, it may be helpful in the overall management of patients with pancreatic trauma. In pancreatic injuries of a magnitude that have a high potential for pancreatic fistualization (grades III–V), use of somatostatin prophylaxis should be considered. In lower grade injuries where postoperative drainage output is high in amylase, somatostatin therapy should be started.

37. What are some of the common complications associated with pancreatic trauma?

Between 20% and 40% of patients sustaining pancreatic trauma suffer associated complications. Pancreatic and duodenal fistulas are the most common problems and occur in up to 20% of patients with duodenal and 35% of those with combined pancreaticoduodenal injuries. An intra-abdominal abscess develops in up to 25% of such patients. Pancreatitis complicates the injury in 18% of patients. Postoperative hemorrhage generally requires reoperation, although it sometimes can be managed by arteriographic transcatheter embolization. Pseudocyst formation is generally associated with blunt pancreatic injury that is managed nonoperatively. Assuming the gland was normal before injury, pseudocyts often can be managed by simple percutaneous drainage. However, it first should be established by ERCP that no major ductal injury has been overlooked. A major ductal injury requires either operative intervention or endoscopic ductal stenting.

38. When is it okay to feed someone who has a pancreatic injury?

The postoperative course of the patient with pancreatic trauma can be unpredictable. For this reason, recommendations regarding when to begin postoperative feeding must be individualized. Because of the frequency of associated injuries and prolonged paralytic ileus, many patients require parenteral nutritional support, at least initially. Occasionally, a patient with severe pancreatic injury will benefit from placement of a jejunostomy tube during the initial procedure to expedite postoperative enteral feeding.

BIBLIOGRAPHY

1. Asensio JA: Duodenum. In Ivatury RR, Cayten CG (eds): The Textbook of Penetrating Trauma. Media, PA, Williams & Wilkins, 1996.
2. Feliciano D, Martin T, Cruse P, et al: Management of combined pancreaticoduodenal injuries. Ann Surg 205:673, 1987.
3. Jones RC: Pancreas. In Ivatury RR, Cayten CG (eds): The Textbook of Penetrating Trauma. Media, PA, Williams & Wilkins, 1996, pp 631–642.
4. Jurkovich GJ: Injury to the duodenum and pancreas. In Feliciano DV, Moore EE, Mattox KL (eds): Trauma. Stamford, CT, Appleton & Lange, 1996, pp 573–594.
5. Kadell BM, Zimmerman PT, Lu DSK: Radiology of the abdomen. In Zinner MJ, Schwartz SI, Ellis H (eds): Maingot's Abdominal Operations. Stamford, CT, Appleton & Lange, 1997, pp 3–116.
6. Krige J, Beningfield SJ, Funnell IC: Pancreatic trauma. In Pitt HA, Carr-Locke DL, Ferrucci JT (eds): Hepatobiliary and Pancreatic Disease: The Team Approach to Management. Boston, Little, Brown, 1995, pp 421–435.
7. Moore EE, Cogbill TH, Malangoni MA, et al: Organ injury scaling. Horiz Trauma Surg 75:2, 1995.
8. Read RA, Moore EE, Moore FA, Burch JM: Blunt and penetrating abdominal trauma. In Zinner MJ, Schwartz SI, Ellis H (eds): Maingot's Abdominal Operations. Stamford, CT, Appleton & Lange, 1997, pp 763–786.
9. Ridgeway MG, Stabile BE: Surgical management and treatment of pancreatic fistulas. Surg Clin North Am 76:1159–1173, 1996.

23. TRAUMATIC INJURIES TO THE SMALL BOWEL, COLON, RECTUM, AND ANUS

Dat T. Nguyen, M.D., and Michael J. Stamos, M.D.

1. Name the three most commonly injured abdominal organs in penetrating trauma (stab and gunshot wounds) in decreasing order of frequency.

Small bowel, liver, and colon. The incidence of small bowel injury in penetrating trauma is highest (> 80%) in gunshot wound patients. For patients with abdominal stab wounds, the incidence is lower and is between 30% and 50%. The fact that the small bowel occupies most of the abdominal cavity explains its high incidence of injury.

2. Is small bowel injury common in blunt abdominal trauma?

The small bowel is not commonly injured in blunt abdominal trauma. Its incidence of injury ranges from 5–15%. The three most commonly injured organs in blunt abdominal trauma in decreasing order of frequency are the liver, spleen, and kidney.

3. Which segments of small bowel are usually injured in blunt trauma?

In motor vehicle accidents (MVA), the mechanism of injury is from shearing, crushing, or bursting. Proximal jejunum and terminal ileum are the most commonly injured areas because the small bowel is sheared away from its "anchoring points" (ligament of Treitz and cecum). Infrequently, the small bowel, especially the duodenum, is injured by being crushed against the spine or the pelvis. A compressed loop of small bowel may also be ruptured due to high intraluminal pressure.

4. Which type of abdominal trauma has the highest incidence of colon injury: stabbing, gunshot, or blunt?

Like the small bowel, the highest incidence of colon injury occurs in gunshot wounds (25–30%). For abdominal stab wounds, the incidence is approximately 5–10%. The lowest incidence of colon injury is associated with blunt trauma (3–10%).

5. How does blunt trauma produce colon injury?

The same mechanisms described for blunt small bowel injury also apply to blunt colon injury. Cecum (by bursting force), midtransverse (by crushing force), hepatic and splenic flexures, and sigmoid colon (by shearing force) are typical locations for these colon injuries.

6. What is the most common location of injured organs in patients with stab wounds?

Left-sided abdominal organs are more commonly injured than those on the right side because most assailants are right handed.

7. What is the best diagnostic test to rule out the possibility of intra-abdominal organ injury in a patient with a gunshot wound to the abdomen?

Regardless of the patient's hemodynamic status, a patient with a nontangential abdominal gunshot wound needs an exploratory laparotomy. For stable patients with tangential gunshot wounds to the abdomen, if there is a low suspicion of peritoneal violation and perhaps intra-abdominal organ injuries, laparoscopy or triple-contrast abdominal computed tomography (CT) may help to determine if a laparotomy is needed.

8. Is an exploratory laparotomy necessary for all patients with abdominal stab wounds?

If local exploration of the stab wound or laparoscopy shows no evidence of fascial or peritoneal violation, exploratory laparotomy is not necessary.

9. Should an exploratory laparotomy be performed in all stab wound patients with peritoneal penetration?

If intestinal or omental evisceration is found or if there is evidence of peritonitis or hemodynamic compromise, an exploratory laparotomy should be performed immediately. However, if the initial examination is deemed unreliable or showed no such findings, a diagnostic peritoneal lavage (DPL) may help determine if surgical intervention is needed.

10. Which DPL findings suggest an intestinal injury has occurred?

A white blood cell count > 500/cc or finding of fecal materials suggests an intestinal injury. Likewise, a large number of bacteria on Gram's stain also suggests a similar injury. Gross blood aspirate from a DPL catheter indicates intra-abdominal bleeding. Otherwise, a wide range of red blood cell thresholds—from > 10,000 to > 100,000/cc—have been used to determine the presence of intra-abdominal bleeding. An exploratory laparotomy should be performed if there is evidence of an intestinal injury or significant intra-abdominal bleeding on DPL.

11. Is there any special circumstance in blunt trauma where risk of hollow viscus injury should be highly suspected?

Although the incidence of small and large bowel injury is relatively small in blunt trauma, patients who are wearing only a lap belt at the time of a motor vehicle accident are at increased risk for a bowel perforation. Therefore, a high index of suspicion of bowel injury is needed when evaluating an MVA patient with a seat belt mark across his or her abdomen.

12. How should one evaluate the abdomen of a patient with a flank or back stab wound?

Retroperitoneal injury (duodenum, right and left colon) is often difficult to assess because the intact peritoneum may prevent blood and intestinal content spillage into the abdominal cavity. CT scan with triple contrasts (IV, oral, and enema) may help in this evaluation. In addition, a period of close observation with frequent vital sign and serial physical examination, amylase, and white blood cell count will allow early detection of these retroperitoneal intestinal injuries.

13. What physical examination or laboratory findings suggest possible bowel injuries?

If abdominal pain, tenderness, guarding, rebound tenderness, absence of bowel sound, increasing leukocytosis, elevated amylase, and fever are found on examination, especially during close observation of a patient with abdominal trauma, a strong possibility of a bowel injury exists.

14. In which situations may abdominal examination not be reliable for detection of intra-abdominal organs injuries?

If a patient has a head injury, spinal cord injury, severe distracting injury, or alcohol intoxication, abdominal examination may be unreliable. Therefore, additional diagnostic tests or procedures such as DPL, laparoscopy, or CT scan may be used to evaluate for intra-abdominal organ injuries.

15. Are plain abdominal radiographs helpful in evaluation of penetrating or blunt abdominal trauma?

Plain x-rays of the abdomen are usually not helpful in evaluating abdominal trauma. Free air usually is not seen on plain films in patients with a hollow viscus injury produced by stabbing or blunt trauma. Plain film is most often obtained to document the path of bullet wounds or the presence of intra-abdominal bullets or other foreign bodies.

16. If there is a high index of suspicion for hollow viscus injuries, what test should be performed to completely rule out such possibilities?

DPL is the best diagnostic test to evaluate for intestinal injuries, However, if DPL is negative and there is still a strong suspicion of a bowel injury, an exploratory laparotomy should be performed.

17. How are most colonic injuries detected?
Most colonic injuries are found at exploratory laparotomy. Therefore, the safe course is an abdominal exploration when there is a strong suspicion for hollow viscus injuries.

18. Name the indications for exploratory laparotomy in trauma patients.
Hemodynamic instability
Peritoneal signs or symptoms
Penetrating torso wounds below the nipple
Intraperitoneal free air
Bullet or pellet
Positive DPL
High index of suspicion of bowel injury

19. When should antibiotics be given to a patient with possible intra-abdominal organ injuries?
When a decision is made that a patient needs an exploratory laparotomy, antibiotics should be given intravenously. A broad-spectrum antibiotic with coverage of anaerobes and gram-negative aerobes should be chosen. A second generation cephalosporin such as cefoxitin or cefotetan is appropriate.

20. What are the goals or priorities of an exploratory laparotomy?
There is no point to repair intestinal injuries when the patient is exsanguinating and is on the brink of death. Therefore, hemostasis (control of exsanguination) should be the first priority. Temporary measures to control intestinal content spillage should be the next priority. Exploration for associated injuries should then be performed. Finally, the intestinal injuries are addressed.

21. Which of the following anastomotic techniques is best for repairing a small bowel injury: single-layer handsewn, double-layer handsewn, or closure with stapler?
All techniques are appropriate for repair of a single small bowel injury. The stapling technique is less time consuming and thus is best for a patient with multiple injuries. The single-layer technique has no inner hemostatic layer of suture; thus submucosal bleeding must be under control before closure.

22. How should multiple adjacent small bowel injuries be managed?
Resection of the entire short segment containing the injured areas with an anastomosis would be the most appropriate management. This approach would result in only one anastomotic line. In contrast, primary repair of multiple adjacent injuries would leave two or more anastomotic lines. The anastomosis can be performed with a single- or double-layer handsewn technique or with a stapling technique.

23. What is the risk with resection of a long segment of small bowel?
If too much small bowel is resected, the patient is at risk to develop short bowel syndrome. As a general rule, in an adult, at least 60 cm of small bowel and an intact ileocecal valve are needed to avoid short bowel syndrome.

24. Should a small bowel mesenteric hematoma be explored?
Not all mesenteric hematomas need to be explored. An expanding hematoma should be explored, and bleeding should be controlled. A large hematoma adjacent or abutting the wall of the small bowel should be explored to rule out bowel perforation.

25. What is the best management for most penetrating colonic injuries?
Most colonic injuries are best managed with primary repair. Primary repair has been shown to be associated with lower incidences of intra-abdominal abscess and wound infection than exteriorizing the injured colon as a colostomy.

26. Are there any contraindications for primary closure of penetrating colonic injuries?

There is no universally accepted absolute contraindication to primary closure of colonic injuries. In fact, studies have not consistently shown any correlation among the outcomes of colonic injuries and shock, number of blood transfusions, extent of stool contamination, extent and location of colon injuries, or mechanism of injury. Non–colon-related mortality of the patient, however, is related to severity of shock and number and extent of associated organ injuries.

27. Is there any situation when one should perform colon resection?

A large destructive injury to the colon or a devascularized colon secondary to mesenteric injury is best managed with a resection.

28. When should creation of a colostomy be considered?

In a patient with persistent intraoperative hemodynamic instability and major comorbidities (medical illnesses), a colocolostomy (a colon-to-colon anastomosis) after a colon resection may be at risk for anastomotic leak. Creation of a colostomy in this situation may be appropriate.

29. Is there another option beside primary repair, resection with anastomosis, and colostomy?

No. Reportedly, a primary repair can be exteriorized in the same manner as a colostomy and then returned to the abdominal cavity in 7–10 days if the repair is healed. However, this exteriorization is unnecessary and is associated with a high frequency of anastomotic breakdown. In addition, there is still a risk of anastomotic leak after the healed colon repair is returned to the abdomen.

30. How long should one wait before performing colostomy closure?

Colostomy can be taken down during the same hospitalization—within 1–2 weeks from the first operation if all colon injuries are proven to be healed and the patient has no complications. Reportedly, early colostomy closure is easier and quicker and sustains lower blood loss. However, most colostomies are closed after at least 6 weeks of recovery.

31. Is there any difference in the management of blunt versus penetrating colonic injuries?

In general, blunt colon injuries are managed as described previously for penetrating colon injuries. However, blunt colonic injuries usually require resection owing to the larger colon destruction produced by blunt mechanism. Again, the comorbidities and intraoperative hemodynamic of the patients are the most important factors in deciding whether colostomy should be created.

32. True or false: The mortality rate of patients with colon injury is mostly colon-related.

False. The mortality rate in these patients is usually related to the severity of associated injuries. Associated major abdominal vessel injuries result in the highest mortality.

33. Should the abdominal incision be closed if intestinal injuries are found and managed during exploratory laparotomy?

Although the abdominal fascia can be closed, the skin and subcutaneous tissue are usually left open. If very minimal soilage is found, the skin may be reapproximated with close postoperative observation of the incision. If any signs of infection appear, the skin should be re-opened promptly and packed with moist dressings.

34. How long should antibiotics be continued postoperatively?

Depending on the severity of contamination or soilage, intravenous antibiotics are usually continued for 2–5 days.

35. Are rectal injuries common in trauma?

Rectal injuries are rare and represent 3–5% of all colon injuries. They often occur as a result of a gunshot injury or a penetrating foreign object inserted into the rectum. However, rectal injuries also can occur as a result of blunt trauma. Pelvic fractures can lacerate the rectum. In addition, the high pressure produced by an MVA may blow out the pelvic floor and cause rectal and anal injuries.

36. Is a rectal examination necessary in trauma patients?

In addition to evaluation for spinal cord injury and genitourinary injury, a rectal examination is essential to rule out rectal and anal injuries. A perianal laceration in association with weak anal sphincter tone suggests an anal or sacral injury. Rectal blood suggests a rectal injury and needs further evaluation.

37. How should one further evaluate for rectal injury?

A rigid sigmoidoscopy should determine any rectal injury. However, the rectum usually is not prepared for this examination. A Gastrografin enema may be used to determine the presence of a rectal injury.

38. Should the rectum be mobilized intraoperatively for injury assessment during an exploratory laparotomy?

The rectal injury should be evaluated preoperatively if the patient is stable with proctoscopy or Gastrografin enema. Intraoperatively, these same diagnostic procedures may also be performed. The rectum usually should not be mobilized during a laparotomy for this evaluation because of the potential contamination of the peritoneal cavity with rectal spillage and because a potential devascularization of the rectum will impair its healing.

39. Should a rectal injury be repaired primarily?

In contrast to small bowel and colon injuries, primary repair of extraperitoneal rectal injuries usually is not recommended. The reasons include: The severity of rectal injuries may be difficult to adequately assess; the presence of other major pelvic injuries may complicate primary rectal repairs (such as major pelvic fractures and/or large pelvic hematoma); and adequate repair is difficult because of the anatomic constraints of the bony pelvis. Intraperitoneal proximal rectal injuries should be treated in a similar manner as colon injuries are.

40. How is an extraperitoneal rectal injury managed?

Due to the above reasons, an extraperitoneal rectal injury usually is managed by fecal diversion with proximal colostomy and distal rectal washout, with or without presacral drainage. The rectal injury is evaluated subsequently on an elective basis for healing with proctoscopy and/or barium enema. Once the injury is completely healed, the colostomy is taken down.

41. Is there any situation in which primary repair of rectal injury is feasible?

If a patient is stable and has minimal contamination and no other associated injuries, an accessible simple rectal injury may be repaired transanally. Presacral drainage may be placed if the repair is suboptimal. No difference in morbidity between patients with primary rectal repair and patients with proximal fecal diversion has been reported. In addition, the morbidity in patients with primary repair is usually not directly related to the repair.

42. What is the most common cause of anal injury?

The most common cause of anal injury is iatrogenic obstetric trauma (large episiotomies or puerperal anal injuries from large tears). Gunshot wounds and lacerations produced by a penetrating foreign body are other, much less common, causes of anal injury.

43. Should an anal injury be repaired primarily?

Obstetric anal injuries are often identified and repaired immediately. For anal injuries produced by gunshot trauma or associated with other pelvic injuries or with a large perineal wound, the primary goal of treatment is usually debridement of necrotic tissue and proximal fecal diversion. The anal injuries are repaired subsequently on an elective basis.

44. Name the postoperative complications in patients with small bowel, colon, rectal, and anal injuries.

The most common complication is wound infection, which occurs in approximately 15–20% of patients. Intra-abdominal abscesses also occur at a significant frequency (5–15%). Anastomotic leak, rupture, and fistula are infrequent. Of note, intra-abdominal abscess occurs at a higher incidence in patients treated with a colostomy than for patients with primary repair of the colon.

45. How is wound infection managed?

Re-opening the incision and frequent moist dressing changes are usually adequate. Intravenous antibiotics may be needed if systemic signs of infection or surrounding skin erythema (cellulitis) is found.

46. How should one treat an intra-abdominal abscess?

With the CT scan, many abscesses can be safely drained percutaneously. However, if the patient continues to have signs and symptoms of sepsis despite percutaneous drainage and IV antibiotics, an exploratory laparotomy should be performed.

47. What is the mortality associated with colon and rectal injuries?

Mortality rates for patients with colon and rectal injuries generally range from 2–12%. The mortality rate is expected to be higher in the presence of associated organ injuries, but most are the result of non–colon-related complications.

BIBLIOGRAPHY

 1. Beck DE, Opelka FG: Pelvic and perineal trauma. Persp Colon Rect Surg 6:134–155, 1993.
 2. Carrillo EH, Somberg LB, Ceballos CE, et al: Blunt traumatic injuries to the colon and rectum. J Am Coll Surg 183:548–552, 1996.
 3. Ivatury RR, Cayten CG: The Textbook of Penetrating Trauma. Baltimore, Williams & Wilkins, 1996.
 4. Jacobson LE, Gomez GA, Broadie TA: Primary repair of 58 consecutive penetrating injuries of the colon: Should colostomy be abandoned? Am Surg 63:170–177, 1997.
 5. Levine JH, Longo WE, Pruit C, et al: Management of selected rectal injuries by primary repair. Am J Surg 172:575–580, 1996.
 6. Levy RD, Strauss P, Aladgem D, et al: Extraperitoneal rectal gunshot injuries. J Trauma 38:273–277, 1995.
 7. Moore EE, Mattox KL, Feliciano DV: Trauma, 2nd ed. Norwalk, CT, Appleton & Lange, 1991.
 8. Sasaki LS, Allaben RD, Golwala R, Mittal VK: Primary repair of colon injuries: A prospective randomized study. J Trauma 39:895–901, 1995.
 9. Sasaki LS, Mittal V, Alladen RD: Primary repair of colon injuries: A retrospective analysis. Am Surgeon 60:522–527, 1994.
10. Schultz SC, Magnants CM, Richman MF, et al: Identifying the low-risk patient with penetrating colonic injury for selective use of primary repair. Surg Gynecol Obstet 177:237–242, 1993.
11. Steward RM, Fabian TC, Croce MA, et al: Is resection with primary anastomosis following destructive colon wounds always safe? Am J Surg 168:316–319, 1994.
12. Ulualp KM, Sirin F, Eyuboglu E, et al: Management of rectal trauma. Contemp Surg 44:37–41, 1994.
13. Velmahos GC, Degiannis E, Wells M, et al: Early closure of colostomies in trauma patients—A prospective randomized trial. Surgery 118:815–820, 1995.
14. Wilson RF, Walt AJ: Management of Trauma: Pitfalls and Practices, 2nd ed. Baltimore, Williams & Wilkins, 1996.

VI. Genitourinary Trauma

24. GENITOURINARY TRAUMA

Johannes H. Naudé, M.B.Ch.B.

PENILE INJURIES

1. How would you handle a zipper firmly attached to the foreskin of a young boy?
Cut the zipper free from the garment. Do a ring block of the penis, and sedate the child. If your best attempt fails to free the zipper, perform a circumcision, but always obtain parental consent.

2. How do you treat a dog bite of the penis?
Ensure that there is no possibility of rabies. Provide broad-spectrum antibiotic coverage, and do not suture the wound primarily. Secondary suturing can be performed 1 or 2 weeks later, if necessary.

3. What is a "fracture" of the penis, and how would you treat it?
Unlike the walrus, humans do not have a bone in the penis, and fracture of the penis is not an orthopaedic injury. The term refers to a tear of the fibrous wall of the corpus cavernosum (i.e., tunica albuginea). It is caused by forceful bending of the erect penis and usually results from a thrust executed with more enthusiasm than accuracy. A sudden pain is felt in the penis, which rapidly becomes swollen and deviates away from the side of the injury. The tear can extend into the urethra, in which case blood comes from the external meatus. Treatment is surgical repair of the laceration and, in the case of urethral involvement, suprapubic cystostomy.

4. How does a degloving injury of the penis occur, and how should it be treated?
This is usually an industrial or agricultural injury in which the patient's trousers and penile skin get caught in a moving belt or chain. The penile skin is often devitalized; skin, the cut edge of which does not bleed freely, should be excised and replaced by a split-skin graft.

TESTICULAR INJURIES

5. How do you manage a bullet wound of the testis?
The testis is explored and tested for vitality (i.e., color and free bleeding on incision). If viable, it is sutured; otherwise, it is removed. If the injury is bilateral, a conservative approach is advocated in case there be any doubt about who caused the castration: the assailant or the surgeon.

6. What is the management of traumatic hematocele?
A large hematocele (i.e., blood within the tunica vaginalis after trauma) may indicate rupture of the tunica albuginea of the testis. Ultrasound can confirm this condition, and the testis should be explored, hemostasis effected, and the tunica albuginea repaired. If in doubt, exploration is the safer option because testicular atrophy can follow conservative treatment.

144

URETHRAL INJURIES

7. After falling astride scaffolding, a man has a tender swelling of the perineum and is unable to pass urine. How would you manage the case?

An ascending urethrogram can be used to diagnose rupture of the bulbar urethra, which is best treated by suprapubic cystostomy and delayed repair.

8. What is the best approach to low-velocity (handgun) bullet wounds of the male distal urethra?

Immediate repair and suprapubic cystostomy have yielded the lowest incidence of stricture formation.

9. Is further imaging necessary to establish the diagnosis of posterior urethral rupture in a man with a fractured pelvis and blood at the external meatus?

No. These features are diagnostic of rupture of the urethra. Additional studies may yield information on the extent of the injury.

10. What is the minimal, essential, initial treatment of a patient with a fracture of the pelvis and rupture of the urethra?

Suprapubic cystostomy is the minimal treatment. The urologist can decide later about further management.

11. Why is fracture of the pelvis and rupture of the urethra associated with a significant mortality rate?

It takes great force to fracture the pelvis, and these patients often have associated abdominal, chest, and head injuries.

12. What makes rectal examination imperative in patients with fracture of the pelvis and ruptured urethra?

Unrecognized rectal injury can have disastrous consequences, such as gross pelvic sepsis, septicemia, and death.

13. How is rupture of the membranous urethra managed?

Rupture is managed in one of two ways: immediate realignment over a catheter or initial suprapubic cystostomy only, followed 3 to 6 months later by anastomotic repair.

Procedure	*Advantages*	*Disadvantages*
Realignment	Technically easy; micturition established early; early return to work	Very high stricture rate; repeated urethral instrumentation to maintain patency
Suprapubic cystostomy	Permanent cure rate of 90%	Needs a high degree of skill; catheter-bound patient for 4–6 months

BLADDER INJURIES

14. Which investigation is diagnostic of bladder rupture?

Cystography is used to diagnose bladder rupture. Full bladder and drainage films can demonstrate extraperitoneal and intraperitoneal bladder rupture.

15. How can routine serum chemistry alert the physician to a diagnosis of intraperitoneal bladder rupture?

A disproportionate increase occurs in the level of blood urea nitrogen compared with serum creatinine. Because urea is a smaller molecule, it is much more readily absorbed by the peritoneum than creatinine.

16. How is extraperitoneal bladder rupture treated in the absence of other abdominal injury?

Extraperitoneal bladder rupture is treated by simple urethral catheterization.

17. Can a patient sustain a traumatic intraperitoneal bladder rupture without a history of trauma?

Yes. An inebriated patient may sustain a blow to the bladder but have no recollection of the event the next day.

18. Can a cystogram yield a false-negative result in cases of intraperitoneal bladder rupture?

Yes. A plug of omentum or a knuckle of bowel can temporarily seal the bladder rupture if insufficient contrast is instilled. Persist with the instillation until the patient finds it intolerable or until leakage is seen. Remember the drainage film! A full bladder can obscure contrast in the pouch of Douglas.

19. How should a rectovesical bullet wound be treated?

Repair the bladder and catheterize. Repair the rectum, interpose omentum between bladder and rectum, do an end colostomy, and clear the distal colonic segment by irrigation. Full antibiotic coverage is given.

20. In the case of accidental bladder injury during hysterectomy, the formation of a vesicovaginal fistula should be prevented. How is this best done?

Prevent fistulas by careful bladder repair and the interposition of omentum between bladder and vagina.

URETERAL INJURIES

21. Most ureteral injuries are iatrogenic. Name the situations in which this can happen.
- Hysterectomy
- Removal of an ovarian mass
- Colectomy
- Aortic aneurysm surgery
- Extraction of a calculus from the ureter
- Ureteroscopic procedures

22. What is the most likely diagnosis in a post-hysterectomy patient who is pyrexic and drains a large amount of pus followed by watery fluid from the vagina 1 week after surgery?

The diagnosis is a urinary fistula to the vagina. It may be a ureterovaginal or vesicovaginal fistula.

23. Does ureteral ligation invariably lead to severe loin pain?

No. Most patients are asymptomatic.

24. Can fluid drainage from a wound readily be identified as urine?

Yes. If it is urine, its creatinine concentration is many times that of the serum. However, a large degree of equilibration can occur in the tissue or peritoneal cavity.

25. What is the procedure of choice in a patient with a bullet wound involving the lower third of the ureter?

The patient is treated by reimplantation of the ureter into the bladder (i.e., ureteroneocystostomy).

RENAL INJURIES

26. Which is the imaging modality of choice for a patient suspected of having suffered blunt injury to the kidney?

Contrast-enhanced spiral computed tomography accurately defines the extent of the injury and can differentiate viable from devascularized renal tissue.

27. An injured patient is not and has not been in a state of shock, and he has no rib fractures, loin contusions, or abrasions, but he has microscopic hematuria. Should this be investigated?

The yield of significant positive findings in this situation is so low that it is not cost effective.

28. What is indicated by minimal trauma that results in frank hematuria?

This condition indicates an abnormal kidney. The patient may have hydronephrosis or a renal tumor.

29. What are the indications for surgery in cases of blunt renal trauma?

- Persistent hemorrhage—you cannot allow the patient to bleed to death!
- A shattered kidney or one with multiple major lacerations
- Vascular injury

30. What follow-up studies should a renally injured patient have a few months later?

The patient should have renal ultrasound or excretory urography and a blood pressure check.

31. The American Association for the Surgery of Trauma grading system for blunt renal trauma is widely used. How would you grade a small cortical laceration with a perirenal hematoma?

Grade 2.

32. How would you grade a single renal parenchymal laceration with extravasation of contrast?

Grade 4.

33. Does a patient with a posterior renal stab wound (i.e., stabbed in the back) not actively bleeding, hemodynamically stable, and with a normal abdominal examination need surgical exploration?

No, but the patient must be carefully monitored. Any signs of peritoneal irritation demand urgent exploration, because there may be bowel injury.

BIBLIOGRAPHY

1. Cass AS (ed): Genitourinary Trauma. Cambridge, MA, Blackwell Scientific Publications, 1988.
2. Guerriero WG, Devine CJ (eds): Urologic Injuries. Norwalk, CT, Appleton-Century-Crofts, 1984.
3. Hinman F: Atlas of Urologic Surgery. Philadelphia, WB Saunders, 1989.
4. Mitchell JP: Urinary Tract Trauma. Bristol, Wright, 1984.
5. Smith RB, Ehrlich RM (eds): Complications of Urologic Surgery, 2nd ed. Philadelphia, WB Saunders, 1990.
6. Tanagho EA, McAninch JW (eds): Smith's General Urology, 4th ed. Norwalk, CT, Appleton & Lange, 1995.
7. Turner-Warwick RT: Prevention of complications resulting from pelvic fracture, urethral injuries and from their surgical management. Urol Clin North Am 16:335, 1989.
8. Walsh PC, Retik AB, Stamey TA, Vaughan ED (eds): Campbell's Urology, 6th ed. Philadelphia, WB Saunders, 1992.
9. Webster GD, Kirby RS, King LR, Goldwasser B (eds): Reconstructive Urology. Cambridge, MA, Blackwell Scientific Publications, 1993.

VII. Orthopaedic Trauma

25. SOFT TISSUE INJURIES IN PELVIC FRACTURES

Gideon P. Naudé, M.B.Ch.B.

1. What causes pelvic fractures?

Blunt trauma, especially in motor vehicle injuries, cause pelvic fractures. Falls, crushing injuries, and explosions are additional causes. Elderly, osteoporotic patients can sustain a fracture after a minor fall.

2. Are pelvic injuries serious?

Major pelvic fractures carry a very high mortality rate, because of the fracture, bleeding, and associated injuries.

3. What would lead you to suspect a pelvic fracture?

The patient may be unable to bear weight without pain, even with a less severe fracture. Severe deformity in extreme cases with bruising and hematoma formation also points to this diagnosis.

4. How would you test for stability of the pelvis?

Anteriorly, pressure should be placed over the symphysis pubis. Laterally, pressure should be placed over the iliac wings, and the hip joint should go through a full range of movement. If pain is felt or if difficulty is experienced with the movements, radiographs must be taken in three planes: anteroposterior, lateral, and oblique.

5. How is an uncomplicated, nondisplaced, closed fracture of the pelvis managed?

The anterior portion of the pelvis does not contribute to weight bearing. Uncomplicated fractures in this region are treated symptomatically, and the patients are kept on bed rest until the pain subsides. Patients are then mobilized as tolerated. In posterior fractures, injury to the lumbosacral plexus should be ruled out. Mobilization is more gradual because this is a weight-bearing area.

6. Are diaphragmatic ruptures associated with pelvic fractures?

Yes. If a crushing injury is severe enough to cause a pelvic fracture, it can also cause a diaphragmatic rupture, which should be ruled out with imaging studies.

7. What are the main causes of mortality in pelvic injuries?

Hemorrhage and shock due to the pelvic fracture or adjacent injuries are the main causes of mortality.

8. Where does the bleeding in a pelvic fracture come from?

Bleeding occurs from the fractured bones. Bleeding also occurs from torn and lacerated pelvic arteries and veins.

148

9. How much blood can be lost in a closed pelvic fracture?

In a closed, nondisplaced fracture, pelvic and retroperitoneal bleeding may amount to as much as 4 liters. This is a fatal bleed if fluid replacement does not take place. Displaced fractures may bleed much more, sometimes several blood volumes of transfused blood. Open fractures have no limit on the amount they can bleed and can continue bleeding until surgical hemostasis has been obtained.

10. What are the most common soft tissue injuries associated with pelvic fractures?

1. *Muscle.* This is the most common soft tissue injury and can lead to hematomas, pain, and an inability to ambulate.

2. *Urinary system.* The urethra and bladder can be ruptured, particularly with displaced pubic fractures.

3. *Genitals.* Male and female genital injuries sometimes occur with pelvic fractures.

4. *Intestinal tract.* Rectal injuries, as well as large and small bowel perforations, may occur.

11. What are the priorities in the treatment of a pelvic fracture?

Treat life-threatening associated respiratory and circulatory injuries first. Abdominal sources of bleeding, such as a ruptured spleen or liver, are managed next. Pelvic bleeding can be controlled by external fixators, angiography with embolization, or surgical packing at laparotomy. Definitive fixation of the fracture is not urgent and can wait until the patient has been stabilized.

12. Are MAST suits useful in the management of shock in pelvic fractures?

There is no absolute proof that military antishock trousers (MAST suits) have a place in the management of any lower body injuries. The suits are useful in the treatment of severe pelvic fractures with bleeding by allowing more time to perform arteriography and embolization. Disadvantages of MAST suits include respiration compromise due to the pressure on the abdomen leading to an elevated diaphragm and possible increase in blood pressure causing increased bleeding above the level of the MAST suit.

13. How would shock be managed in a patient with a pelvic fracture?

Initially, the patient is treated with crystalloid infusion. Blood may be given if the bleeding is fast or if the hematocrit becomes very low. In the absence of injuries requiring exploration of the abdomen or chest, an external fixator is applied. It reduces fractures and lessens the bleeding by increased pressure between the fractured ends of the bones. This action stops bleeding from the bone fragments and venous bleeding.

14. How is ongoing arterial bleeding managed?

If bleeding persists after an external fixator has been applied and there is no abnormality of the blood clotting mechanism, angiography with embolization of the bleeding arteries is performed. If bleeding persists, surgical control is carried out by operation and ligation or repair of the bleeding vessels.

15. What would lead you to suspect a urinary injury?

In any case of major blunt trauma, urinary injury must be ruled out. In patients with pelvic fractures, pubic fractures and diastasis of the symphysis pubis should alert the examiner to the likelihood of urethral or bladder injuries. Blood at the meatus strongly suggests a ruptured urethra. A high-riding prostate identified on rectal examination suggests a complete rupture of the urethra. Hematuria indicates urinary injury and should be investigated. Anuria may result from a ruptured bladder with extravasation of urine into the abdomen. Penile and scrotal edema may also be a sign of extravasation of urine.

16. How would a urinary injury associated with a pelvic injury be managed?

A suprapubic cystostomy is performed as an emergency procedure in the case of a urethral injury. The urethra is repaired at a later time. A ruptured bladder is repaired primarily if there is an intraperitoneal leak. For some extraperitoneal leaks of the bladder, catheter drainage is performed until the injury has healed.

17. What would lead you to suspect a bowel injury associated with a pelvic fracture?

Clinically, an acute abdomen after a pelvic fracture should alert the physician to the possibility of bowel injury. Blood in the rectum also indicates rectal or bowel injury. Free gas in the abdomen seen on an abdominal radiograph is virtually diagnostic of intestinal injury. Imaging studies with contrast can demonstrate intestinal injury. Diagnostic laparoscopy or laparotomy may be carried out if the suspicion is high.

18. What is the abdominal compartment syndrome?

Abdominal compartment syndrome is abnormally elevated pressure in the abdomen that may follow trauma to the abdomen and pelvis. Infection, tumors, pneumoperitoneum, ischemia, bleeding, and several other causes have been identified. The intra-abdominal pressure is usually measured through an indwelling bladder catheter (indirect method) or by an intravenous (IVC) or intraperitoneal measuring device, and elevated pressure may cause the following:

- Compromised respiration due to diaphragmatic elevation
- Decreased venous return and a consequent drop in cardiac output
- Decreased visceral perfusion (kidneys and bowel) with oliguria, anuria, and bowel ischemia

19. How is the abdominal compartment syndrome managed?

The management strategy is based on the severity of increased pressure:

- *Mild.* With minimal or no symptoms and a pressure below 25 cm H_2O, the patient is closely observed and the pressure monitored.
- *Moderate.* If symptomatic with borderline ventilation, blood pressure, renal and mesenteric flow, and a pressure between 25 and 35 cm H_2O, most patients require decompression.
- *Severe.* If intra-abdominal pressure is above 35 cm H_2O, this is a life-threatening condition, and all patients require decompression. In patients requiring decompression, the abdomen is decompressed and the causative condition managed. The abdomen is then packed (using prosthetic material) and left open or closed without increased pressure. Formal closing is performed later when the condition has stabilized.

20. What is the mortality rate for pelvic fractures?

The mortality rate is between 12% and 50% in most series. The mortality rate depends on whether the fracture is open or closed and on the presence and severity of associated injuries.

BIBLIOGRAPHY

1. Bongard FS, Stamos MJ, Pessaro E (eds): Surgery: A Clinical Approach. New York, Churchill Livingstone, 1997.
2. Jerrard DA: Pelvic fractures. Emerg Med Clin North Am 11:147, 1993.
3. Mitchell JP: Urinary Tract Trauma. Bristol, Wright, 1984.
4. Perry MO: Compartment syndromes and reperfusion injury. Surg Clin North Am 68:853–864, 1988.
5. Way LW (ed): Current Surgical Diagnosis and Treatment, 10th ed. Norwalk, CT, Appleton & Lange, 1994.

26. ORTHOPAEDIC TRAUMA

Charles Moon, M.D., and Jackson Lee, M.D.

LOWER EXTREMITY

1. What is the role of Gustilo-Anderson grading of open fractures?

Gustilo-Anderson grading is primarily an attempt to correlate prognosis based on initial wound size. It has recently been used to guide treatment, but it is still important to perform intraoperative grading after the entire zone of injury is visualized. Although reliability of the grading system has been called into question because of poor interobserver agreement, it remains useful:

Type I wounds usually are less than 1 cm long and associated with injury to the soft tissues from an inside-out mechanism. There is minimal soft tissue injury and minimal contamination.

Type II wounds are longer than 1 cm but usually less than 10 cm and have moderate contamination and soft tissue injury.

Type III wounds are longer than 10 cm and are further subdivided into A, B, and C categories according to the degree of soft tissue loss.

Type IIIA injuries do no need flap procedures for soft tissue coverage of the bone, but there is extensive periosteal stripping and considerable damage to the soft tissues.

Type IIIB injuries have soft tissue loss to the extent that soft tissue reconstruction or a flap procedure is necessary for bone coverage.

Type IIIC injuries have a vascular injury requiring repair for limb viability. All farmyard contamination is type III, regardless of wound size.

2. Describe the role of antibiotics in the management of open fractures.

Antibiotics play a crucial role in decreasing the infection rates in open fractures. Generally, a first-generation cephalosporin is indicated in a type I open fracture, with the addition of an aminoglycoside for types II and III. If there is farm contamination, penicillin is added to protect against *Clostridia*. No studies show an increased benefit for the use of antibiotics for longer than 48 hours. Although the literature is subject to interpretation, many physicians recommend this regimen for 48 hours and restarting the regimen before each débridement until wound closure is achieved.

3. What are the options for achieving soft tissue coverage for open tibia fractures?

The tibia is unique in that it is a long bone with a large subcutaneous border. When injured, this subcutaneous border presents problems with wound closure. If the defect caused by the injury is small, delayed primary closure is frequently possible as long as little tension is placed on the wound edges. If there is sufficient muscle overlying the defect, split-thickness skin grafting may be performed. In the proximal two thirds of most tibias, local rotational flaps such as a gastrocnemius or soleus flaps may be used as long as the muscle groups were not traumatized by the injury. In severe injuries or on the distal one third, free tissue transfer is necessary to achieve coverage.

4. Why is it important to perform scheduled, deliberate, serial débridements of high-grade open fractures?

During the initial débridement, the goal is to fully visualize the entire zone of injury. However, on achieving this visualization, it is often difficult to determine what tissue is viable, particularly at the margins. It is important to leave questionable tissue to allow it a chance to "declare" itself and to minimize excessive débridement of healthy tissues.

5. When should an open fracture wound be closed primarily?

An open fracture wound should never be closed primarily. In low-grade open fractures (type I), the small wound should be allowed to heal by secondary intention. In higher-grade injuries, primary wound closure at the time of initial débridement should *not* be performed for the following reasons:

- Closure can create an anaerobic environment that may lead to clostridia sepsis.
- Because of the large amount of injured surface area, these wounds tend to ooze a fair amount. Closure allows formation of a hematoma, which can subsequently become infected.
- Primary wound closure is not conducive to a mandatory second-look débridement.

6. What is the timing of wound closure in open fracture management?

Open fracture wounds should be closed when the wound is clean and free of necrotic tissue, which usually occurs after the second débridement. Achieving coverage of open fracture wounds by postinjury day 5 or 6 is important. Delaying this closure has been correlated with a higher infection rate.

7. What are the absolute indications for primary amputation of an open tibia?

- Anatomic transection of the posterior tibial nerve in an open tibia fracture with an arterial injury
- Severe crush injury with a warm ischemia time of more than 6 hours

8. What are the relative indications for primary amputation of an open tibia?

- Serious associated polytrauma
- Severe ipsilateral foot injuries
- An anticipated protracted course for salvage, advanced age, or physiologic condition
- Massive wound contamination
- Necrosis of a substantial intercalary segment of calf musculature

9. What is a floating knee, and what complications are often associated with this injury?

Fracture of the femur associated with an ipsilateral tibia fracture is known as a *floating knee*. This injury most commonly occurs in cases of multiple trauma. This combination is extremely difficult to manage in traction and requires immediate stabilization. There is a high risk of vascular injury and pulmonary decompensation (e.g., fat emboli). The most common postinjury complication is loss of range of motion of the knee, which leads to a poor functional outcome.

10. In a patient with a femur fracture caused by blunt trauma, why is it essential to have a good anteroposterior (AP) pelvis radiograph and a good AP radiograph of the ipsilateral hip?

In a patient with a femoral shaft fracture caused by blunt trauma, it is essential to have these AP views to rule out a concomitant ipsilateral femoral neck fracture. This rare injury, if missed, has devastating consequences for the patient. In published series, even with a high degree of vigilance, this injury continues to be missed in 30% of patients.

11. What controversies are associated with the management of an ipsilateral femoral neck–femoral shaft fracture?

The controversy involves the method of stabilization of this combination of injury. The femoral neck fracture is the injury with poor reconstruction options if healing or avascular necrosis occurs because of suboptimal stabilization or reduction. However, performing optimal reduction and stabilization of the femoral neck fracture first would compromise options for the stabilization of the femoral shaft fracture.

Stabilization of the femoral neck usually involves the use of lag screws or pins, making standard anterograde femoral nailing impossible. Traditionally, the femoral shaft then is managed with plate fixation, but more recently, retrograde femoral nailing has become an option. Reconstructive or cephalomedullary nailing is another option for fixing both fractures with one implant, but it is technically difficult to perform and may compromise the reduction of the femoral neck fracture.

12. What are the advantages of early stabilization of long-bone fractures in the patient with multiple injuries?

Long-bone fractures can be stabilized any time during the peri-injury period without significant compromise of function. However, early stabilization (within 24 hours after injury) contributes to decreased pulmonary complications, including pulmonary shunting caused by the forced supine position; better pulmonary toilet; decreased dependence on narcotic analgesia; and decreased incidence of adult respiratory distress syndrome (ARDS) and fat emboli syndrome. Johnson et al. showed retrospectively that the incidence of ARDS in patients with an Injury Severity Score (ISS) greater than 40 is five times greater in those whose femur fracture stabilization was delayed than in patients who underwent immediate stabilization. Bone et al. conclusively showed in a prospective, randomized study that patients whose femur fractures were stabilized immediately had statistically significant improvement in pulmonary function compared with the group that had delayed stabilization.

13. What controversies are involved in the management of a multiply injured patient with a pulmonary injury and a femur fracture?

Reports indicate an increased incidence of ARDS and mortality in patients with an associated severe pulmonary injury who underwent early (<24 vs. >24 hours after injury) reamed intramedullary nailing of femoral shaft fractures. Products released into the systemic circulation during the process of reaming may have deleterious effects on injured pulmonary tissues. The data do not suggest that early fracture stabilization should be avoided in this group of patients but that alternative fixation methods that do not require reaming of the intramedullary canal should be used. Such alternative fixation methods include unreamed intramedullary nailing and plate fixation. Adding fuel to this controversy are several studies that fail to substantiate the original observation. A multicenter study compared multiply injured patients (ISS >17) with femur fractures treated with plate fixation or reamed intramedullary nailing; no difference in ARDS, pneumonia, and mortality rate was found. No difference was found in patients with or without pulmonary injury or in those without a femur fracture and a pulmonary injury.

14. What controversies are involved with the use of reamed versus unreamed intramedullary nails in the treatment of a femur fracture?

Intramedullary nailing of a femur fracture can be performed with and without reaming. The process of reaming of the intramedullary canal allows the inner diameter of the femoral canal to be defined. This has several advantages, including allowing placement of a larger-diameter implant. This is important because the strength of the implant is proportional to the fourth power of its radius. Another advantage is that by reaming the normally conical intramedullary canal to a known diameter, the contact area between the implant and bone is increased, providing better fixation.

The safety of reaming has been questioned. The embolization of marrow contents into the venous circulation may have deleterious effects on injured lung parenchyma. This concern leads to the use of intramedullary nailing without reaming, necessitating the use of smaller-diameter implants with poorer implant-bone contact. In several comparative studies, a tendency to higher nonunion rate and implant failure was noted in certain groups of fractures, such as those affecting the distal one third of the femoral shaft. Some advantages of nailing without reaming are a shorter operative time and less blood loss, but these advantages appear to be marginal and may not outweigh the disadvantages.

15. What is a subtrochanteric femur fracture?

A subtrochanteric femur fracture is a fracture of the femoral diaphysis that occurs below the intertrochanteric line, and the term incorporates fractures that occur in the proximal one third of the femur. Their presence, especially in the young patient, implies a high-energy injury. Implant failure occurs more often than usual because of the higher physiologic forces present in this area combined with the slower healing of cortical bone.

16. What causes orthopaedic implants to break?

All orthopaedic implants that are cycled or repeatedly stressed will break. This is referred to as *fatigue failure*. When orthopaedic implants are used to fix fractures, a race occurs between fracture healing and implant failure. For most successful fracture fixations, when fracture healing is complete, the implant is protected from further cycling. If fracture healing fails, such as in a nonunion, the implant is continuously cycled until fatigue failure occurs.

17. What is the significance of a femoral neck fracture in a young patient?

The presence of a femoral neck fracture in a young adult implies high-energy trauma. Unlike the femoral neck fractures that typically occur in the elderly, resulting from trivial trauma and reflecting an osteopenic state, such a fracture in a young patient can only occur from high-energy transfer. These fractures are considered surgical emergencies because of the increased risk of avascular necrosis. The risk of avascular necrosis is correlated with the degree of displacement, energy of the injury, and time to reduction and fixation. In an elderly patient, prosthetic replacement is a common treatment option, but this is a poor choice in the young patient. With the higher energy transfer, there is a higher risk of injuring the tenuous blood supply to the femoral head.

18. Are gunshot wound fractures considered open?

Low-energy (<1000 ft/sec most handguns) gunshot wounds are not *per se* considered to be open fractures (i.e., in need of emergent débridement). It is recommended that they be treated with a prophylactic course of antibiotics and local débridement of skin wounds. Generally, a 3-day course of a fluoroquinolone or a cephalosporin and an aminoglycoside is recommended. Indications for operative fixation are similar to those for closed fractures. Special circumstances include bullets that transverse the large bowel and high-energy wounds (>2000 ft/sec, high-powered rifles and military weapons). These wounds should be aggressively débrided and treated like grossly contaminated fractures.

19. In pediatric trauma patients, what factors can lead to immobilization-associated complications such as pneumonia, pulmonary abscesses, sepsis, decubiti, or fever and hypertension of unknown origin?

Age older than 7 years and a modified abbreviated injury severity scale (MISS) score of greater than 40 have been found to be associated with the complications listed. Earlier fracture fixation to allow mobilization has shown a trend toward decreasing these complications, but a study with statistical significance is lacking in the literature. The MISS is calculated by scoring (0 to 5) musculoskeletal injury, neural injury, abdominal injury, chest injury, and head and neck injury and using the Glasgow Coma Scale. The square of the three highest scores are taken to give the MISS score.

20. How does pediatric femoral shaft fracture treatment vary with age?

In children with closed growth centers, standard antegrade femoral nailing is recommended. Because of reports of avascular necrosis, it is not recommended in children with open epiphyses. Depending on physician preference, children 6 to 11 years old are generally treated with classic open reduction and internal fixation (ORIF) with plates and screws; flexible nails (avoiding the physes); or external fixation. For children younger than 6 years of age, spica casting with or without a period of skeletal traction is generally recommended.

21. What are the drawbacks of the various treatments for femur fractures in children 6 to 11 years old?

Classic ORIF involves placement of plates and screws. This requires a large incision and more blood loss than other methods. A second surgery is generally recommended to remove the plate and screws in children. External fixation of pediatric femur fractures has been plagued by pin site problems (i.e., infections), bulkiness of the frame itself, and refracture. Flexible nails are somewhat unfamiliar to many physicians. They may not adequately control length and rotation of the femur fracture. They also may necessitate a return to the operating room for removal after fracture maturation.

COMPARTMENT SYNDROME

22. What is compartment syndrome?
When the pressure in a facial compartment rises to a level at which the function of the muscles, nerves, or blood vessels traversing that compartment are jeopardized, a compartment syndrome results.

23. What are some common causes of compartment syndrome?
Compartment syndrome may be caused by hemorrhage resulting from injury; exertional, prolonged external compression; and prolonged ischemia.

24. What is the most reliable sign of compartment syndrome in an awake patient?
Pain out of proportion is the most reliable sign. Placing the muscles of the suspected compartment on gentle passive stretch produces pain that is extremely severe and out of proportion to the injury.

25. How is compartment syndrome monitored in a comatose patient?
The accepted method is to use continuous wick catheter measurements of the compartments in question.

26. What is the delta P?
The delta P (ΔP) is the difference between the mean arterial blood pressure and the compartment pressure. If the pressure difference is less than 40, a fasciotomy is indicated.

27. What are some sequelae of missed compartment syndrome?
In the early stages, the patient may develop myoglobinuria, which can lead to renal failure. The extremity can become infected, leading to systemic sepsis. Both of these complications can lead to multisystem organ failure and death. Late sequelae can run the gamut from something as mild as a footdrop from peroneal nerve injury to something as severe as a completely insensate, nonfunctional extremity with muscle fibrosis and joint contractures.

UPPER EXTREMITY

28. What sensory deficit occurs with an anterior interosseous nerve palsy?
The anterior interosseous nerve is, for the most part, a pure motor nerve and has no sensory component that can be detected on routine physical examination.

29. Differentiate between a radial nerve palsy and a posterior interosseous nerve palsy.
In a radial nerve palsy, function of all of the radial innervated muscles is lost, including the wrist extensors and the sensory branch, which provides sensation to the first dorsal web space of the hand. The posterior interosseous nerve is the motor branch that exits after the supinator of the forearm, and wrist extensors therefore are functional, as is the sensation to the first web space. In a posterior interosseous nerve palsy, only the extensors of the metacarpophalangeal joints are affected.

30. Does the presence of polytrauma affect the treatment for a humerus fracture?
Humerus fractures that are treated nonoperatively in a functional brace or splint do very well, with a high rate of union and low complication rates; as such, this is the treatment of choice when

a humerus fracture occurs as an isolated injury. This treatment modality, however, depends in part on the ability of the patient to be upright and allow gravity to aid the reduction. In cases of polytrauma, ORIF or intramedullary nailing of these fractures may be advantageous. Lower extremity injury and bilateral humeral fractures are good indications. Stabilization of this fracture can help with earlier patient mobilization and facilitate nursing care.

31. What is a floating shoulder, and how is it treated?

A floating shoulder represents a separation of the glenohumeral joint from the trunk. Two fractures usually are needed for this to occur. Most commonly, there is a clavicle fracture and a scapular neck fracture. The traditional treatment has been to operatively fix the clavicle fracture, restoring a connection of the glenohumeral joint to the trunk. There is now evidence that nonoperative treatment is effective in patients who do not have a significant caudal dislocation of the glenoid.

32. What is scapulothoracic dissociation?

Scapulothoracic dissociation represents a "closed" forequarter amputation. The upper extremity is disconnected from the thorax beneath a closed skin envelope. Typically, there is a massive muscular, neurologic, and vascular injury to the extremity. This is a surgical emergency, and the patient is at high risk for a dysfunctional rather than amputated extremity. The diagnosis is made for a dysvascular upper extremity in a patient with abnormal neurologic examination results (generally) and an abnormal chest radiograph. On a nonrotated chest x-ray film, the involved side has a scapula that is displaced considerably more laterally than on the normal side.

PELVIC FRACTURES

33. What are the sources of bleeding in a patient with a pelvic fracture?

A patient who sustains a major pelvic disruption has been subjected to high-energy trauma, and associated injuries are common. It is not unusual for the patient to have intrathoracic and intraperitoneal sources of bleeding. Bleeding from the pelvic fracture itself can come from three major sources: exposed bone fracture surfaces, venous plexus disruptions, and arterial bleeding.

34. Describe the role of the retroperitoneal space in pelvic bleeding.

The retroperitoneal space is a potential space. In the event of pelvic bleeding, this space can accommodate up to 4 L of blood before tamponade can occur. Because of the spherical nature of the pelvis, if bony instability results from a fracture, the volume can increase. The amount of increase in this volume is proportional to the fourth power of the radius, showing how a small change can affect the potential blood loss.

35. What is the role of external fixation in a patient with a pelvic fracture?

External fixation is used for immediate, temporary stabilization in a patient who is hemodynamically unstable. The external fixator stabilizes the pelvic fracture to prevent further displacement, controlling retroperitoneal volume and allowing tamponade of the hematoma. By limiting fracture site motion, external fixation minimizes further bleeding from fracture sites and venous plexus. Unfortunately, it plays little role in controlling arterial bleeding. By providing stability, external fixation in the peri-injury period allows the patient to reduce dependency on opiate analgesia, facilitating pulmonary status and mobilization. External fixation is not used for definitive fixation because of its inability to maintain an accurate reduction during fracture healing. Definitive fixation involves ORIF after the patient becomes hemodynamically stable and fresh, active bleeding has stopped.

36. What is the timing of external fixation in the hemodynamically unstable patient?

External fixation is best applied as soon as the diagnosis of a mechanically unstable pelvic disruption is made. In many trauma centers, it is performed in the operating suite before exploratory laparotomy. For the patient in extremis, external fixation should be performed immediately in the emergency department. Many of these protocols are modified to fit the particular "culture" of the trauma center. In many trauma centers, angiography is readily available at a moment's notice; in these centers, immediate angiography may be a better choice. In centers where angiography is not as accessible, external fixation should be used initially, and if hemodynamic stability is not achieved, angiography should be performed. Remember that angiography allows control of arterial bleeding but has little effect on venous bleeding or fracture site bleeding; external fixation can control the latter two but not the former.

37. What types of external fixation are available for the pelvis?
External fixation can be applied anteriorly and posteriorly. Two types of frame constructs have been described for anterior frames: the Slatis frame and the Pittsburgh frame. The Slatis frame is a simple frame that is easily applied. This frame mainly controls the anterior portion of a pelvic disruption while providing some control, albeit poor, of the posterior disruption.

The Pittsburgh frame design was an attempt to increase control of the posterior disruption with a more complex anterior frame design. There has been a push to develop and use a C-clamp–type frame that is applied directly to the posterior disruption to achieve better control. Although several studies have shown its effectiveness, its advantage over a simple anterior frame is not as clear. A learning curve is involved in the use of the C-clamp, and there is the risk of injuring neurovascular structures, including include the superior gluteal artery and sciatic nerve, near the greater sciatic notch.

38. When is external fixation not effective in pelvic disruptions?
External fixation is not effective in controlling retroperitoneal volume and fracture-site motion when there is a fracture of the iliac wing or a concomitant acetabular fracture. This is why it is preferable to examine a good-quality anteroposterior radiograph of the pelvis before applying an external fixator.

39. Describe what additional information is obtained with inlet and outlet views of a pelvis. How is this additional information important?
The pelvic inlet view, taken with the x-ray beam directed obliquely 45 degrees from cephalad to caudad and with a cassette placed under the supine patient, best demonstrates anteroposterior deformities, including symphysis pubis disruptions and sacroiliac joint dislocations. Anterior or posterior displacement of the injured hemipelvis is best seen on this view. The pelvic outlet view is taken with the x-ray beam directed obliquely 45 degrees from caudad to cephalad and best demonstrates vertical instability and sacral body fractures.

40. What is the significance of blood at the meatus?
Blood at the meatus is an indication of urethral injury. The absence of blood at the meatus, however, does not rule out urethral injury, especially if the patient is being examined within 1 hour of the injury.

41. What is the significance of a high-riding prostate in a patient with a pelvic fracture?
A high-riding prostate in a patient with a pelvic fracture is pathognomonic of a urethral injury. However, the absence of this condition does not rule out urethral injury.

42. What determines mechanical stability in the pelvis?
The pelvis ring consists of two innominate bones joined posteriorly by the sacrum. These bones are not inherently stable; stability of the construct depends entirely on ligamentous structures. Anteriorly, the pubic portion of the innominate bones is joined by the pubic symphysis. Posteriorly, very strong posterior and anterior sacroiliac ligaments provide stability. There are also ligaments from the sacrum to the ischium of the innominate bone, known as the sacrotuberous ligaments and the sacrospinous ligaments. In the absence of bony discontinuity due to fracture,

injury to these ligamentous structures produces a mechanically unstable pelvis. Because ligamentous structures are not seen on radiographic views, it is possible to have a grossly unstable
pelvis with normal-appearing films, emphasizing the importance of clinical examination.

43. Describe the posterior lesions that can occur in an unstable pelvic fracture.

When an unstable pelvic disruption occurs, the presence of an anterior lesion, such as a
widened pubic symphysis or a pubic rami fracture, implies a concomitant posterior lesion. The
posterior lesions that may form lateral to the midline are fracture of the ilium, fracture dislocation
of the sacroiliac joint, pure dislocation of the sacroiliac joint, and sacral body fracture. Fractures
of the sacral body are further classified as those that are lateral to the sacral foramina, through the
foramina, and medial to the foramina. Injuries to the sacral nerve roots are common in fractures
that occur through the sacral foramina.

44. What are the considerations about the trauma patient who has an acetabular fracture that may require ORIF for a best functional outcome?

Although the acute care and evaluation of acetabular fractures are similar to those for pelvic
fractures, there are some differences and special considerations. Radiographically, 45-degree
oblique views of the pelvis are more useful than inlet and outlet views. For pelvic and acetabular
fractures, fine-cut computed tomography (CT) with bony windows is helpful in reconstructive
planning. Suprapubic catheters and colostomies may compromise the ability to perform anterior
approaches to the acetabulum. If a suprapubic catheter is necessary to treat a urologic injury, it is
best to tunnel the catheter from just below the umbilicus to keep it out of the potential acetabular
surgical field. Injury to and embolization of the superior gluteal artery may also prohibit the use of
an extended iliofemoral approach, because the flap may not have adequate collateral circulation
without the superior gluteal artery. Acetabular fractures usually are not emergent surgical problems, and skeletal traction can be used to temporarily stabilize the fracture until definitive fixation.

BIBLIOGRAPHY

1. Bone LB, Johnson KD, Weigelt J, Scheinberg R: Early versus delayed stabilization of femoral fractures:
   A prospective randomized study. J Bone Joint Surg Am 71:336–340, 1989.
2. Bosse MJ, MacKenzie EJ, Riemer BL, et al: Adult respiratory distress syndrome, pneumonia, and mortality following thoracic injury and a femoral fracture treated either with intramedullary nailing with
   reaming or with a plate. J Bone Joint Surg am 79:799–809, 1997.
3. Browner BD, Jupiter JB, Levine AM, Trafton PG (eds): Skeletal Trauma. Philadelphia, WB Saunders,
   1992.
4. Heppenstall RB, Scott R, Sapiga A, et al: A comparative study of the tolerance of skeletal muscle to ischemia. J Bone Joint Surg Am 68:820–827, 1986.
5. Kasser JR (ed): Orthopaedic Knowledge Update 5. Rosemont, IL, American Academy of Orthopaedic Surgeons, 1996.
6. Mayer T, Walker ML, Clark P. Further experience with the modified abbreviated injury severity scale. J
   Trauma 1984; 24:31–34.
7. Rockwood CA, Green DP, Bucholz RW, et al (eds): Fractures, 4th ed. Philadelphia, Lippincott-Raven,
   1996.
8. van Noort A, te Slaa RL, Marti RK, van der Werken C: The floating shoulder a multi-centre study. J Bone
   Joint Surg Br 83:795–798.

VIII. Vascular Trauma

27. VASCULAR TRAUMA

Carlos E. Donayre, M.D.

1. What are the most common mechanisms by which arterial injuries occur?

Because of the high incidence of urban trauma in the United States, penetrating injuries from gunshot wounds are the most common cause of arterial injuries. They are followed by stab wounds, which in turn predominate over blunt injuries. Blunt injuries tend to arise from motor vehicle accidents, falls, or recreational activities. Joint dislocations or fractures produce compression, torsion, and shearing forces that can lead to intimal or transmural injuries. Lower extremity vessels are the most frequently injured vessels owing to their long length, relatively superficial location, and close proximity to long bones.

Recently, rapid advances in cardiology and interventional radiology have increased the number of invasive procedures performed, and these procedures have been associated with femoral, axillary, and brachial arterial injuries. These iatrogenic complications are directly related to catheter diameter, length, and amount of time the catheter remains in position. (Trivia: Catheter diameters are reported in French [Fr] sizes: French size/3 = diameter in mm. For example, a 9 Fr catheter is 3 mm in diameter.) Female gender, diabetes, and pre-existing peripheral vascular disease are associated with an increased incidence of iatrogenic vascular injuries.

2. What are the most common presenting symptoms of a peripheral vascular injury?

The "hard" signs include pulsatile bleeding, expanding hematoma, palpable thrill, audible bruit, and regional ischemia as evidenced by the "6 P's": **p**ain, **p**aresthesia, **p**allor, **p**aralysis, **p**oikilothermia (cold-blooded), and absent **p**ulses. "Soft" signs include a history of moderate hemorrhage, injury close to a major artery (proximity), decreased but palpable pulses (ankle–brachial index < 0.9), or peripheral nerve deficit.

3. What is the ankle–brachial index or ratio (ABI)?

The ankle–brachial index (ABI) is the measurement of the systolic ankle pressure compared with the measured systolic brachial pressure using a Doppler probe and appropriately sized blood pressure cuff. The systolic Doppler pressure is the millimeter of mercury (mmHg) at which arterial flow can be detected by the Doppler probe. The normal ABI for the average person is between 0.9 and 1.1. Pressures must be obtained and compared for both posterior tibial arteries (PTA) and dorsalis pedis arteries (DPA) to avoid missing an injury. (Trivia: The anterior tibial artery gives rise to the DPA but is congenitally absent in 2% of the population. It is the predominant artery of the foot. In 7% of individuals the peroneal artery is the major source of blood to the foot. The PTA is absent in 5% of the population.)

Warning: The ABI will be decreased in older persons with pre-existing peripheral vascular disease and will be normal in patients sustaining an isolated injury to the profunda artery (main blood supply of the thigh musculature, not in direct continuity with the popliteal artery). ABIs are not as reliable in the upper extremity owing to the great number of collateral vessels in the shoulder and elbow region.

4. What types of vessel injuries occur commonly?

Laceration is the most frequent injury sustained by arteries and veins. Transection is associated with distal limb ischemia from either interruption of blood flow due to loss of vessel continuity or proximal and distal thrombosis due to retraction of the injured vessel ends. High-velocity weapons (muzzle velocity > 1,500 ft/sec) create a temporary cavity that fragments and disrupts the media and endothelium of adjacent vessels. This blast effect results in vessel contusions and associated segmental spasm or thrombosis. Pseudoaneurysms (false aneurysms) arise when vessel continuity is maintained by at least one of the layers of the vessel wall, usually the adventia. Arteriovenous fistulas result when a closely adherent artery and vein sustain an injury that creates an abnormal communication between them.

5. Is proximity of injury to a major vessel an indication for arteriography or operative exploration?

Those patients with the hard signs for vascular injury as outlined in question 2 generally can be taken directly to the operating room for operative intervention, though circumstances vary. In the hemodynamically stable patient with hard signs of arterial injury, angiography may be performed to delineate the injury and formulate an appropriate plan for its management (choice of incision and exposure). The diagnostic work-up in the patient with the soft signs of arterial injury is varied and not as straightforward as above. Patients with penetrating injuries in "proximity" to major vessels with pulses but with abnormal ABIs should undergo arteriography. If the ABI is >.9, the patient either can undergo serial clinical examinations for a defined period of time or must undergo a noninvasive study (duplex scan) to exclude arterial or venous injuries.

6. What is the preferred conduit for arterial reconstruction in peripheral vascular injuries?

The greater saphenous vein (GSV), the longest vein of the body, is the preferred conduit for peripheral vascular reconstruction in the trauma patient. It is usually harvested from the contralateral extremity. Removal of intact GSV from the injured extremity is usually avoided in case the major veins of the deep venous system have sustained an unrecognized injury. Furthermore, trauma patients requiring prolonged bed rest or immobilization are prone to develop deep venous thrombosis. Removal of the GSV in a patient with an injured or thrombosed deep venous system can result in debilitating lower extremity swelling and the development of chronic venous ulcers. (Trivia: The superficial femoral vein is part of the deep venous system of the thigh. It is called superficial because it accompanies the superficial femoral artery.)

7. What is a compartment syndrome? Can you define its etiology and pathogenesis?

Acute compartment syndrome is defined as increased pressure within a limited space, which compromises capillary blood perfusion and threatens tissue viability. Causes of increased compartment pressure include: (1) accumulation of blood due to bleeding from fractures, bleeding disorders (hemophilia), anticoagulation, or vascular injury and (2) edema formation after trauma (bony and soft tissue injury), thermal injury, surgery, crush injury, ischemia, or strenuous exercise. Edema formation is central to the pathogenesis of compartment syndrome. When the intracompartmental pressure exceeds 30 mmHg, lymphatic outflow is blocked, capillaries suffer damage, and their permeability is increased. The resultant protein leakage leads to increased oncotic pressure and decreased fluid resorption with a further increase in compartment pressure and decreased tissue perfusion. This vicious cycle of increased tissue pressure leading to ischemia and edema formation causes further increases in tissue pressure with inadequate tissue perfusion, anoxia, and ultimate tissue necrosis. Disabling contractures can result from muscle necrosis if compartment syndromes are not recognized and treated promptly.

8. Describe the signs and symptoms of acute lower extremity compartment syndrome.

Acute compartment syndrome is suggested by the following physical signs and symptoms:
1. Peripheral nerve deficits

2. Pain, often out of proportion to the clinical presentation and that worsens with passive motion of the affected muscle groups

3. Motor weakness

4. Palpable tenseness of the involved compartment

5. Loss of pulses in the very last stages, which often signals irreversible neural and muscle injury

Nerve function is more sensitive to ischemia than skeletal muscle function. Thus, the earliest sign of increased compartment pressure is the loss of two-point discrimination. (Trivia: Fast conductive nerve fibers are the first to cease functioning with increasing compartment pressures.)

9. What are the contents of the four fascial compartments of the lower extremity?

The four compartments of the lower extremity in which compartment syndrome is most common are the anterior, lateral, deep posterior, and superficial posterior (see Figure below).

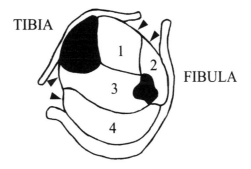

The anterior compartment is the most susceptible to the development of acute compartment syndrome and frequently occurs alone. The muscles of the anterior compartment (Trivia: The foot and toe dorsiflexors are the tibialis anterior, extensor digitorium brevis, extensor hallucis longus, and peroneus tertious.) are innervated by the deep peroneal nerve, which provides sensation to the first web space. The anterior tibial artery provides the vascular supply to this compartment.

The lateral (peroneal) compartment is the second most frequently involved compartment of the lower leg. The only two muscles occupying the lateral compartment are innervated by the superficial peroneal nerve, which provides sensation to the mid-dorsum of the foot. There are no major vessels in this compartment. (Trivia: Peroneus longus and brevis are responsible for foot eversion.)

Of the two remaining compartments, the deep posterior is more frequently involved in compartment syndrome. The muscles of the deep posterior compartment are innervated by the tibial nerve, which provides sensation to the sole of the foot. (Trivia: The muscles occupying the deep compartment are the tibialis posterior, flexor digitorium longus, and flexor hallucis longus and control toe plantar flexion. Ischemic muscular necrosis results in the claw toe appearance.) The posterior tibial artery travels in this compartment.

The superficial posterior compartment is least frequently involved in compartment syndrome. A deep posterior compartment syndrome must always be suspected with superficial compartment involvement. The muscles of the superficial posterior compartment are innervated by the tibial nerve, which travels outside this compartment. (Trivia: The muscles occupying the superficial compartment are the gastrocnemius, soleus, and plantaris, which control ankle plantar flexion. Ischemic muscular necrosis of this compartment also results in the claw toe appearance in addition to equinovarus ankle deformity.) The only nerve within this compartment is the sural, which provides sensation to the lateral dorsum of the foot and lateral malleolar region. The branches of the posterior tibial and peroneal arteries provide the vascular supply to this compartment.

10. What are the indications for performing a fasciotomy?

Lower extremity fasciotomies are indicated to prevent or treat compartment syndromes. Classic teaching dictates that after 6 hours of acute ischemia, compartment decompression must be performed to relieve or prevent intracompartmental hypertension. Combined peripheral arterial-venous injuries, ligation of major vessel without vascular reconstruction, presence of sustained or prolonged shock, crush injuries, and extensive soft tissue injury or swelling mandate the performance of fasciotomies. Objective data can be obtained by direct measurement of compartment pressures with needle-based manometers, Wick catheters, or solid state transducer-based catheters. Values over 40 mmHg indicate the need for fasciotomy.

11. How are lower extremities fasciotomies performed?

Fasciotomy refers to the surgical incision of a fascial compartment in order to relieve excessive pressure that has built up due to extremity injury. Fascial compartments contain neurovascular structures that are susceptible to injury when excessive and sustained high compartmental pressures develop (see question 7). The four compartments of the lower extremity can be decompressed using single or double incisions or by fibular excision also accompanied by a single incision. Regardless of the technique used, all the compartments must be decompressed. The double-incision fasciotomy is the most commonly used approach owing to its simplicity and the rapidity by which it can be performed. An anterolateral incision is made halfway between the tibia and fibula, but care must be taken to avoid injury to the superficial peroneal nerve in the lateral compartment. A second posteromedial incision is made 2 cm posterior to the medial border of the tibia to avoid injury to the saphenous nerve and vein (see Figure in question 9).

12. In a patient with a peripheral injury that includes bone, artery, vein, and soft tissue, what is the order of repair?

Typically, bony injuries are repaired first to return the limb to normal length. The vein is repaired next if a complex reconstruction is not required, followed by the arterial repair. Soft tissue injuries are repaired last after vascular supply to the affected extremity is re-established. In the face of prolonged ischemia, the artery should be repaired first, then the vein, followed by bone and soft tissue. Do not forget that fasciotomies should be performed prior to complex arterial repairs, shotgun wounds, or crush injuries to protect the collateral circulation and avoid prolonged ischemia to the affected extremity. Complicated bone injuries that require significant manipulation can sometimes be managed by placing an arterial shunt to provide circulation during the bone repair. This reduces the possibility of inadvertent disruption or compromise of the arterial repair, which can be safely performed after the bone is stabilized. However, the use of an arterial shunt requires anticoagulation, which may complicate the management of associated injuries. Sound clinical judgment and an open communication between the multiple caretakers involved in these complex repairs is required to avoid loss of limb or even life.

13. When should limb salvage be attempted when dealing with a mangled extremity?

The assessment of an extremity injury involves the evaluation of skin and subcutaneous tissue, muscles and tendons, bones, joints, arteries, veins, and peripheral nerves. In order to successfully restore the best possible limb function, an experienced surgeon should perform a careful and complete assessment in the operating room, after which the appropriate priority can be given to each component of the injury. The Mangled Extremity Severity Score (MESS) assigns points in the following four categories: skeletal and soft tissue, shock, ischemia, and age (see Table below). Based on the combined score obtained, management principles for attempted salvage can be undertaken, and a prognosis of limb salvage and favorable function can be made. A total MESS of 7 or more suggests the need for primary amputation. Primary amputation is also recommended if the extremity is completely insensate, because these patients do better with prosthetic limbs.

Mangled Extremity Severity Score

	POINTS	CHARACTERISTICS
Skeletal and Soft Tissue	1	Low energy
	2	Medium energy
	3	High energy
	4	Massive crush
Shock	0	Normotensive (systolic BP > 90)
	1	Transient hypotension
	2	Prolonged hypotension (> 30 minutes)
Ischemia	0	None
	1	Mild
	2	Moderate
	3	Advanced
Age	0	< 30 years
	1	30–50 years
	2	> 50 years

14. Should venous injuries be repaired?

Many vascular surgeons prefer venous repair over ligation for traumatic injury to prevent embolus from the ligated vein and provide venous drainage, even if only temporary. However, no solid evidence indicates that this is true. In fact, at initial follow-up, 50% of complex venous repairs will be thrombosed, though proponents of vein repair would argue that recanalization can occur. In certain situations, such as when dealing with a young, hemodynamically stable patient, venous repair is highly desirable because restoration of adequate venous drainage augments arterial inflow. Thus, popliteal veins, as well as combined arterial-venous injuries, should be repaired whenever possible.

15. What is the optimal exposure for an injury to the subclavian artery?

In general, to obtain proximal control of the right subclavian artery, a median sternotomy is indicated. The median sternotomy (see *A* in Figure) is the most versatile and most commonly employed incision for the control and repair of the aortic arch vessels. Proximal control of the left subclavian artery (L-SCA) is not as simple. The posterior and lateral course of the aortic arch displaces the origin of the L-SCA out of view if a median sternotomy incision is used. An anterolateral fourth intercostal thoracotomy provides the quickest control of the origin of this vessel from the chest (see *B* in Figure). Additional exposure of the L-SCA can be gained by a second incision along or above the clavicle, which, if combined with a median sternotomy, can be used to create a "trapdoor" (see *A, B,* and *D* in Figure). Transection of the clavicle or medial excision of the clavicle is necessary

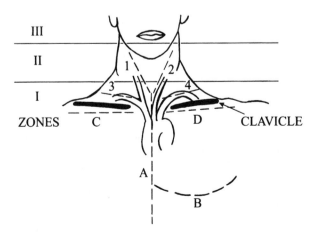

to allow the trapdoor to hinge out of the way, increasing access to the left subclavian vessels. If proximal clavicle resection is necessary, this should be done in a subperiosteal fashion to avoid injury to the underlying neurovascular bundle. Extension of the median sternotomy incision in a cephalad direction along the anterior border of the sternocleidomastoid muscle provides excellent exposure of the common carotid artery and internal jugular vein (see *1* and *2* in Figure).

For the control of distal subclavian artery injuries, a supraclavicular incision can be performed (see *3* and *4* in Figure). This requires division of the lateral head of the sternocleidomastoid and anterior scalene muscles. Care must be taken not to injure the phrenic, recurrent laryngeal, and vagus nerves. (Trivia: The phrenic nerve lies on the ventral surface of the anterior scalene muscle. The recurrent laryngeal nerves loop around the subclavian artery on the right and around the aortic arch and ligamentum arteriosum on the left.)

16. What are the defining borders of the axillary artery?
The lateral border of the first rib defines the origin of the axillary artery, which gives rise to the brachial artery upon crossing the lateral border of the teres major. The axillary artery is divided into three anatomic parts by the pectoralis minor muscle (see figure). The first (proximal) part is medial to pectoralis minor and is relatively fixed and anterior to the brachial plexus. The second (mid) portion courses beneath the pectoralis minor, and the third (distal) part extends from the lateral border of the pectoralis minor to the lateral border of the teres major. (Trivia: The first part of the axillary artery has one branch, the supreme thoracic artery. The second has two, the thoracoacromial and lateral thoracic artery. Finally, the third part has three branches, the subscapular and medial and lateral circumflex arteries.) A generous infraclavicular incision and transection of the pectoralis muscle can be used to achieve control and exposure of the proximal axillary artery (see *C* and *D* in question 15). Extension of this incision laterally is required for greater access to the distal axillary and proximal brachial arteries, or a separate incision along the lateral border of the pectoralis major can also be used. It should be pointed out that the long-term morbidity of injuries to the root of the neck and shoulder region is related to the frequent incidence of concomitant brachial plexus injuries and not ischemia. Control and exposure of the distal subclavian and proximal axillary vessels can be difficult and labor intensive in a young, muscular trauma victim. In this type of patient (if hemodynamically stable and not actively bleeding) placement of endoluminal balloons at the time of diagnostic angiography can greatly facilitate the management of these challenging injuries.

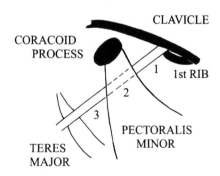

17. What are the zones of the neck?
In trauma, the neck is generally divided into three anatomic areas. Zone I (thoracic outlet) extends from the cricoid cartilage to the clavicles. This is considered to be a crowded, "high-rent district" because it houses the proximal carotid arteries, subclavian vessels, aortic arch and branches, lung apices, upper mediastinum, thyroid, trachea, esophagus, and thoracic duct! Zone II extends from the cricoid cartilage to the angle of the mandible. Zone III extends above the angle of the mandible to the base of the skull (see Figure in question 15).

18. What layer of the neck must be violated to consider an injury "penetrating"?

The platysma muscle must be violated to classify a neck injury as penetrating. Because no vital structures are above the platysma muscle, lack of platysma penetration obviates the need for further evaluation. (Trivia: The platysma is the only muscle that does not originate or terminate on a bone.) However, penetrating injuries to the neck should not be probed, cannulated, or "locally" explored in the emergency room to rule-out violation of the platysma. These maneuvers may dislodge clot and result in uncontrollable and life-threatening bleeding.

19. What is the appropriate work-up for a penetrating injury to zone IIof the neck without significant hematoma, bleeding, or neurologic deficit?

Two basic approaches have been proposed to evaluate the above-described injury in a hemodynamically stable patient lacking the hard signs of vascular aerodigestive injuries (presence of subcutaneous air, asphyxia, massive air leak). Nonoperative evaluation relies on angiography of the great vessels, esophagogram (first with Gastrografin, and if negative, then with barium) combined with rigid esophagoscopy and bronchoscopy. This selective approach gives approximately a 95% confidence that there is no operative lesion. An alternate, and perhaps less costly, algorithm relies on the direct exploration of zone IIof the neck, with supplemental rigid esophagoscopy and bronchoscopy if necessary. Proponents of this approach argue that this zone is the easiest to expose and evaluate in the operating room, and they add that cost can be further reduced if the exploration is done on an outpatient basis.

Initial arteriography of zones I and III is recommended in the hemodynamically stable patient. Exposure and assessment of potential vascular injuries in these regions is usually difficult and treacherous. High-quality angiography can prevent an unnecessary exploration and can help in the selection of the proper incision to adequately expose and repair the injury. In the patients with blunt neck injuries, indications for operative exploration are less clear because blunt injury to the carotid vessels is relatively uncommon. Thus, arteriography is recommended in selected patients with blunt neck trauma to rule out carotid injury that can result in transient or fixed neurologic deficits.

20. What is the incidence of abdominal vascular injuries in patients receiving treatment in urban trauma centers? What is the most common etiology of major abdominal vascular injury?

The incidence of abdominal vascular injury in military conflicts is only 2–3%. In the civilian arena, the incidence of abdominal vascular injuries is increased tenfold to 25–35%. Military injuries to the abdominal vessels are usually lethal owing to the potent firepower that is used in the field. Delays in transport to appropriate surgical facilities also have a negative impact on this type of injury.

The incidence of injury to major abdominal vessels in patients with blunt trauma is 5–10%. Patients with penetrating stab wounds to the abdomen also have a similar incidence of vascular injuries, at 10%. Not surprisingly, abdominal gunshot wounds account for 25% of all abdominal vascular injuries.

21. What types of vascular injuries are produced by blunt abdominal trauma?

Blunt abdominal trauma from motor vehicle accidents is associated with decelerating injuries. Rapid deceleration can result in avulsion of small arterial branches or intimal tearing in larger arteries because the aorta and its major branches are relatively fixed in the retroperitoneum. The freely moving small bowel and colon readily avulse branches from the relatively fixed superior mesenteric artery. Forward and rapid movement of decelerating kidneys can produce intimal tears and thrombosis of renal vessels. Another pattern of vascular injury in abdominal blunt trauma is the so-called seat belt aorta. This type of injury occurs when the seat belt crushes the aorta against the spine, resulting in a large intimal tear or flap with subsequent thrombosis

22. What are the major branches of the abdominal aorta, and what is their approximate level of branching?

Major Branches of the Abdominal Aorta

BRANCH	APPROXIMATE LEVEL OF BRANCH
Celiac axis	T12
Superior mesenteric artery	L1
Left and right renal arteries	L2
Inferior mesenteric artery	between L3 and L4
Aortic bifurcation	lower border of L4

23. Should all retroperitoneal hematomas be routinely explored?

No. In blunt trauma, nonexpanding hematomas of the retroperitoneum need not be explored. In fact, kidney salvage is more successful in those situations where the hematoma is not surgically violated. This algorithm of management does not hold true for penetrating trauma, however. In general, where the bullet (or knife) goes, you go.

Exposure of the supraceliac aorta is necessary when a central hematoma in that region is identified. Proximal control of the aorta can be obtained at the diaphragmatic hiatus or, occasionally, in the chest through a separate thoracotomy incision. Exposure of the aorta is then achieved by performing a medial visceral rotation of the left colon, spleen, pancreas, and stomach to the midline. The left kidney also may be rotated simultaneously (colloquially known as the Mattox maneuver) to allow further visualization of the abdominal aorta. Dissection is initiated by taking down the "white line of Toldt" followed by division of the ligament of Treitz and mobilization of the fourth part of the duodenum. Blunt retroperitoneal dissection is then performed to allow rotation of the viscera medially (frequently, the existing hematoma aids with this maneuver). This approach provides exposure of the aorta from the level of the diaphragm to the bifurcation and can be performed rapidly, with little risk of complication if done properly.

24. Is the management of pelvic hematomas arising from blunt trauma different than for those arising from penetrating injuries?

Yes, some of the most lethal injuries encountered are gunshot wounds to the pelvic region. Pelvic hematomas seen in blunt trauma arise from fractures and tend to be venous in nature. Retroperitoneal hematomas from gunshot wounds are usually not intact and cannot tamponade venous bleeding. Furthermore, hemorrhage may be brisk from associated arterial injuries. Injury to the common and external iliac arteries should be repaired to lower the risk of amputation if ligation is undertaken (40–50% risk of limb loss if accompanied by prolonged hypotension). Injured internal iliac arteries can be ligated with impunity, and even bilateral ligation can be performed to control ongoing bleeding.

The complex venous anatomy in the pelvis does not lend itself to straightforward repairs, and, in the face of exsanguination from a penetrating injury to an iliac vein, transection of the iliac artery may be warranted in order to achieve rapid and adequate control of the ongoing hemorrhage. After the venous injury has been repaired, the iliac artery can be reanastomosed. If, after control of arterial hemorrhage, venous bleeding still continues, the pelvis may have to be packed with laparotomy pads and the iliac veins ligated.

25. How are aortic injuries repaired?

Aortic injuries can be repaired directly (a 50% reduction in aortic diameter is readily tolerated), resected and repaired with an end-to-end reanastomosis, patched with autologous or prosthetic material, or replaced with a prosthetic graft. Aortic replacement with prosthetic material can be done even if enteric contamination from associated bowel injuries occurs. Adjunctive maneuvers such as copious irrigation with saline, coverage of the prosthetic graft with omentum, and long-term antibiotic therapy must be undertaken. The postoperative course in these patients can be complicated by ongoing sepsis, pseudoaneurysm formation, and aortic blow-out.

26. Can the portal vein be ligated?

Yes, ligation of the portal vein is compatible with survival. However, if this is done, aggressive and massive fluid resuscitation must be undertaken to reverse the transient peripheral hypovolemia, which results from splanchnic hypervolemia. Another alternative when faced with portal veins that cannot be repaired is to perform a portocaval shunt.

27. At what angle from a vessel is the Doppler probe designed to be held?

The basis for the use of Doppler devices is the detection of frequency shifts that occur when ultrasound encounters moving blood. This relationship and effect on the transmitted frequency is expressed by the Doppler equation:

$$\text{Frequency Shift} = \frac{2F \times V \times \cos \Theta}{C}$$

where 2 = round-trip of the ultrasound; C/F = wavelength of ultrasound; and V cos Θ = closing speed between the erythrocytes and the Doppler probe.

In order to maximize the above frequency shift, the Doppler probe must be held at a 60° angle, because the cosine of 60° = 1.

28. What was Doppler's occupation?

Christian Doppler (1803–1853) was an Austrian mathematician and physicist who originally described the change in pitch that results from a shift in the frequency of sound waves. Electromagnetic radiation emitted by a moving object also exhibits this Doppler effect. The radiation emitted by an object moving toward an observer is squeezed, and its frequency appears to increase and is therefore said to be *blueshifted*. In contrast, the radiation emitted by an object moving away is stretched, or *redshifted*. Cosmologic redshift results from the expansion of space. Despite the fact that Doppler first noted this effect by observing passing trains, there is no evidence that Doppler was ever employed as a railroad conductor or engineer!

BIBLIOGRAPHY

1. Bongard FS, Wilson SE, Perry OM (eds): Vascular Injuries in Surgical Practice. Norwalk, CT, Appleton & Lange, 1991.
2. Feliciano DV, Moore EE, Mattox KL (eds): Trauma, 3rd ed. Stamford, CT, Appleton & Lange, 1996.
3. Ivatury R, Cayten CG (eds): The Textbook of Penetrating Trauma. Baltimore, Williams & Wilkins, 1996.

28. CERVICAL VASCULAR INJURIES

Christian de Virgilio, M.D.

GENERAL INFORMATION

1. To identify the location of penetrating injuries, the neck is divided into what three zones?

Zone I extends from 1 cm above the clavicle inferiorly and includes the base of the neck and the thoracic inlet. Zone II extends from 1 cm above the clavicle to the angle of the mandible. Zone III extends from the angle of the mandible to the base of the skull.

2. Why is it important to identify which zone of the neck is penetrated by the injury?

Penetrating trauma to zones I and III of the neck may injure major vessels that are surgically inaccessible through a standard cervical incision (e.g., innominate or subclavian artery for zone I; intracranial carotid artery for zone III injuries). In addition, major injury to vessels in these areas may not be readily apparent by clinical examination. Thus, preoperative arteriography is usually recommended for zone I and III penetrating injuries in hemodynamically stable patients.

3. What are the structures most commonly injured with penetrating cervical trauma?

The common carotid artery is most commonly injured. Associated venous injuries occur in 27% of patients with penetrating cervical trauma. Twelve percent have vertebral, subclavian, and innominate artery injuries. Tracheal and laryngeal injuries occur in 9% of patients. Esophageal and pharyngeal injuries occur in 4% and spinal cord and brachial plexus injuries in 2% of patients.

ETIOLOGY

4. What is the most common mechanism of blunt common carotid injury?

Hyperextension of the neck with contralateral rotation of the head causing compression of the artery against the transverse process of the cervical spine.

5. Name other described mechanisms of blunt carotid injury.

Direct blows to the neck, blunt intraoral trauma, basilar skull fractures, therapeutic and diagnostic carotid massage, and attempted strangulation.

6. What is the most common mechanism of vertebral artery trauma?

Ninety-five percent of traumatic vertebral artery injuries are the result of penetrating trauma.

DIAGNOSIS

7. What neurologic findings are commonly associated with carotid artery trauma?

Hemiparesis, hemiplegia, ipsilateral Horner's syndrome, cranial nerve dysfunction (IX, X, XI, XII), and coma.

8. What are considered *unequivocal* signs of carotid arterial injury?

Pulsatile or expanding hematoma, signs of definite arterial bleeding, and hemiparesis or hemiplegia.

9. What are considered *equivocal* signs of carotid artery injury?

Stable hematoma, adjacent nerve injury (cranial nerves IX, X, XI, XII), proximity of the injury to the carotid artery, presence of shock, and history of arterial bleeding.

10. Why is there often a delay in the diagnosis of blunt carotid injury?

Patients with blunt carotid injury may not develop symptoms for hours or days following the injury. This is because blunt trauma often causes an intimal injury instead of hemorrhage. The intimal injury may cause immediate or delayed thrombosis. Furthermore, patients with blunt carotid injury frequently have associated head trauma, making neurologic assessment difficult. In addition, neurologic abnormalities may be incorrectly attributed to the head injury. One must remember that the finding of hemiplegia in an awake trauma patient should raise the suspicion of blunt carotid injury.

11. Is it common for patients with isolated vertebral artery trauma to have neurologic symptoms?

No. The posterior circulation of the brain is supplied by paired vertebral arteries that form the basilar artery. Thus, occlusion of a single vertebral artery would only cause symptoms in the rare case of atresia of the contralateral vertebral artery.

INITIAL MANAGEMENT AND ASSESSMENT

12. What is the initial management of cervical vascular injury?

Initial management should address the ABCs: airways, breathing, and circulation. With obvious vascular injury, control of the airway should be achieved by suctioning and endotracheal intubation. Rarely, control of the airway may require cricothyroidotomy or tracheostomy, but care must be taken to avoid entering the neck hematoma because this may lead to exsanguination.

13. What is the next step in the management?

The next step is control of hypovolemia by direct digital pressure if there is active external bleeding and placement of two large-bore IVs. One IV should be placed in the lower extremity if there is a zone I injury (in the event of a major upper extremity venous injury, this will avoid infusing fluid into the extravascular space). Blood should be sent for typing and crossmatching, complete blood count, prothrombin time, partial thromboplastin time, and electrolytes.

14. Patients with presumed vascular injuries can be triaged into what three groups?

Group I patients have obvious life-threatening vascular injury that requires immediate operation. Group II have obvious non–life-threatening vascular injury in whom there is time for a thorough evaluation. Group III have wounds in proximity to the carotid vessels but without obvious signs of vascular injury.

PREOPERATIVE IMAGING

15. What radiographs are recommended?

A radiograph of the chest is recommended to rule out hemothorax, pneumothorax, and widened mediastinum. A radiograph of the neck is obtained to look for evidence of vertebral fracture and for subcutaneous air, which is suggestive of tracheal or esophageal injury. Skull x-rays may show the track of the bullet by demonstrating intracranial bullet fragments or a skull fracture. In patients with suspected blunt carotid injury, computed tomography (CT) scan of the head should be obtained to rule out an intracranial bleed.

16. What is the rationale for obtaining preoperative arteriography?

Preoperative arteriography should be used only in hemodynamically stable patients without active bleeding or expanding hematomas. Arteriography helps identify the injury and unsuspected injuries, plan the type of surgical incision, and sometimes may allow for nonoperative management if there is no injury or minimal injury. It is particularly useful in penetrating injuries to zone I and zone III of the neck. Zone I injuries may injure the great vessels in the mediastinum. The surgical approach to such an injury usually requires a median sternotomy incision for proximal control of the innominate, right, and left common carotid arteries and a left anterolateral thoracotomy for control of the left subclavian artery. Zone III injuries may injure the intracranial carotid artery, which is considered surgically inaccessible. In these instances, percutaneous embolization may be necessary.

17. Is there a role for preoperative arteriography for penetrating zone II injuries?

Yes. Zone II injuries that penetrated the platysma were historically managed by mandatory operative exploration to rule out carotid and aerodigestive tract injuries (esophagus, trachea). However, more recently, a nonoperative approach has been advocated because of the high incidence of negative neck explorations. In order to rule out these injuries, a combination of arteriography, endoscopy, or Gastrografin swallow is recommended. If these are negative, operative exploration can be avoided.

MANAGEMENT

18. What are the therapeutic alternatives in the management of carotid injury?

Observation with or without anticoagulation, ligation of the carotid artery, and arterial reconstruction.

19. What factor(s) influence which of these alternatives is chosen?

Several factors influence the management decision including the presence of active arterial bleeding, the mechanism of injury (blunt vs. penetrating), the location of the carotid injury (intracranial vs. extracranial), the presence and degree of neurologic deficit (i.e., mild paresis, paralysis, or coma), and the time interval between injury and recognition of the injury. Patients with active arterial bleeding require immediate operative exploration.

20. How does the mechanism of injury alter the management approach?

Penetrating injuries to the carotid in general should be repaired surgically because of the risk of bleeding. An exception would be an intracranial carotid injury that is surgically inaccessible. On rare occasions, minimal injuries (such as a small, nonoccluding intimal flap) can be managed with observation. Blunt injuries tend to be managed nonoperatively because most are recognized in a delayed fashion. The injury often results in a dissection and thrombosis of the artery which may extend up into the inaccessible intracranial portion of the carotid. If there is no contraindication, heparin is usually recommended for blunt carotid injury.

21. How does the presence of a neurologic deficit influence management?

Controversy exists as to whether the injured carotid artery should be ligated or repaired in the presence of a neurologic deficit, for fear of converting an ischemic infarct into a hemorrhagic one. This concern is heightened when there is a long delay (greater than 6 hours) between onset of neurologic deficit and attempt at repair. Most surgeons advocate an attempt at repair of the injured carotid artery provided that the injury is surgically accessible (i.e., does not originate or extend into the intracranial carotid), the neurologic deficit is mild or moderate (i.e., the patient is not comatose), and there has not been an inordinate delay from injury to surgery (less than 6 hours).

22. What techniques are used to repair the carotid artery?

Repair of the carotid artery can be achieved either by lateral arteriorrhaphy or by resection followed by primary anastomosis or interposition reverse saphenous vein graft. Prosthetic grafts are generally not recommended for fear of graft infection. External carotid artery injuries can be treated with ligation.

23. What is the recommended management for vertebral artery injury?

Vertebral artery injuries can be managed either by embolization or by operative ligation. Embolization can be achieved by metal coils, Gelfoam, or detachable balloons. Surgical ligation requires proximal and distal ligation of the artery through a cervical incision. Distal ligation of the vertebral artery is technically more demanding because the artery courses through the foramina of the cervical vertebrae from C6 to C1.

BIBLIOGRAPHY

1. Clark G: Penetrating and blunt extracranial carotid injuries. In Ernst C, Stanley J (eds): Current Therapy in Vascular Surgery. Philadelphia, Mosby, 1991, pp 609–612.
2. Fry R: Penetrating and blunt vertebral artery trauma. In Ernst C, Stanley J (eds): Current Therapy in Vascular Surgery. Philadelphia, Mosby, 1991, pp 613–616.
3. Liekweg W, Greenfield L: Management of penetrating carotid arterial injury. Ann Surg 188:587–592, 1978.
4. Martin R, Eldrup-Jorgensen J, Clark D, Bredenberg C: Blunt trauma to the carotid arteries. J Vasc Surg 14:789–795, 1991.
5. Parikh A, Luchette F, Valente J, et al: Blunt carotid artery injuries. J Am Coll Surg 185:80–85, 1997.
6. Perry M: Injuries of the brachiocephalic vessels. In Rutherford R (ed): Vascular Surgery. Philadelphia, W.B. Saunders, 1989, pp 604–612.
7. Perry M: Carotid artery trauma. Semin Vasc Surg 4:147–152, 1991.
8. Reid J, Weigelt J: Forty-three cases of vertebral artery trauma. J Trauma 28:1007–1012, 1988.
9. Towne J, Neis D, Smith J: Thrombosis of the internal carotid artery following blunt cervical trauma. Arch Surg 104:565–568, 1972.
10. Unger S, Tucker S, Mrdeza M, et al: Carotid arterial trauma. Surgery 87:477–487, 1980.

29. DEEP VENOUS THROMBOSIS

Frederic S. Bongard, M.D., and Mary-Anne Purtill, M.D.

1. What is deep venous thrombosis (DVT), and what are common locations?

A DVT is a blood clot (thrombus) in the deep system veins. DVT develops most frequently in the posterior tibial veins, in the popliteal vein just above the knee, in the common femoral vein, and in the pelvic veins. Despite previous beliefs, significant thrombi form in the upper extremity veins, as well as in the axillo-subclavian system.

2. What is Virchow's triad?

Virchow described three factors that contribute to the formation of venous thrombi:
1. altered vessel wall integrity
2. hypercoagulable state
3. stasis of flowing blood

Of interest, Rudolf Virchow was a pathologist who died of Laennec's cirrhosis.

3. Are trauma patients at increased risk of developing a DVT?

Yes. Although the risk of venous thromboembolism is increased after trauma, the true incidence is unknown.

4. What is the incidence of DVT in trauma patients?

The incidence of DVT in injured patients is not known accurately because not all trauma patients undergo screening tests routinely. A reasonable estimate of the incidence is about 10%. The autopsy incidence is between 4% and 20%.

5. What are some of the risk factors that predispose trauma patients to developing DVT?

Risk for DVT increases as more days are spent in the hospital immobilized and as more transfusions are received. Patients who are older (> 45 years), or have clotting abnormalities on admission as demonstrated by a prolonged partial thromboplastin time (PTT) are also at greater risk.

Other studies have identified blunt trauma, spinal fractures with or without a neurologic deficit, subluxations, head injuries (Glasgow Coma Score < 7), pelvic fractures, and major venous injuries as risk factors.

6. What effect does mild to moderate trauma have on the prothrombin time (PT) and PTT?

In minimally injured patients, both the PT and the PTT remain essentially normal. In more severely injured patients, these studies are elevated early and then usually return to normal within 4–6 hours.

7. What effect does hypothermia have on the clotting cascade?

Because the clotting cascade is a temperature-dependent series of enzymatic steps, hypothermia decreases the rate at which these steps occur and increases the time required for blood to clot.

8. What is the most common coagulation abnormality in patients who die after trauma?

Up to 97% of such patients have abnormal PTs, while 72% have abnormal platelet counts, and 70% have abnormal PTTs.

9. What type of injury causes the most significant derangement in the clotting cascade?

Head injury.

10. What are the risk factors for developing a pulmonary embolism (PE) after trauma?

Patients who develop a PE are more likely to have had blunt injury, a GCS score < 8, shock on admission, or fractures of the pelvis or lower extremity. They also tend to have an Injury Severity Score of 16 or greater and the presence of an extremity or pelvic injury.

11. Is physical examination accurate in the diagnosis of DVT?

Physical examination findings are falsely negative in 50% of patients with DVT, and they are falsely positive in patients with symptoms related to conditions other than DVT.

12. What percentage of patients who died from PE had the diagnosis of DVT at the time of their death?

Less than 20%.

13. What are some commonly used methods for diagnosing DVT in trauma patients?

Radionuclide phlebography, duplex ultrasound, and venography.

14. How is radionuclide-labeled fibrinogen used in the diagnosis of DVT?

Radionuclide-labeled (125I) fibrinogen circulating in the bloodstream is incorporated into developing thrombi. Although the method is useful for the detection of calf thrombi, it is poor at detecting pelvic thrombi and already established clots. The method requires 18–72 hours before a diagnosis can be made and has a significant number of false positives. Because of the risk of blood-borne infection, radio-labeled fibrinogen is no longer available in the United States.

15. What is radionuclide phlebography?

Radionuclide phlebography uses technetium-99m-labeled microaggregated albumin injected into a dorsal vein of both feet. Tourniquets are applied to the ankles, forcing the substance into the deep venous system, where its course up the leg is tracked by a special gamma camera. The popliteal, femoral, and iliac veins are seen as well-defined columns of radioactivity. The iliac veins are seen less well than the extremity veins because of venous admixture from the pelvis. Venous obstruction is indicated by nonfilling, visualization of collateral channels, slow ascent of the isotope, and residual areas of increased activity. Appearance of the tracer in superficial veins is suggestive of deep venous occlusion. Although the accuracy of the technique varies among authors, its overall correlation with conventional venous phlebography has been reported to be as high as 89–96%.

16. What is the accuracy of duplex imaging for diagnosing *asymptomatic* deep venous thrombosis in postoperative surveillance studies?

By site, the accuracy in reported studies is:
- Total limb: 81–97%
- Above knee: 93–100%
- Below knee: 83–97%

17. What are the most commonly used prophylactic measures to prevent DVT in trauma patients? Are they effective?

Low-dose subcutaneous heparin, sequential compression devices, and antiembolism stockings are all used, although none of them has been shown to be effective in patients following trauma.

An interesting study by Ruiz (reported in 1985) randomized 100 consecutive trauma patients with an Injury Severity Score greater than 10 to no treatment (control) or subcutaneous heparin prophylaxis for deep venous thrombosis. Twenty-eight percent of those who received heparin developed a DVT, while only 2% of the nontreated controls developed DVT! The lack of efficacy may be explained by the fact that treatment is usually started well after injury, thereby allowing the clot to develop.

18. Is there a group of patients in whom these measures might be effective?

A recent study by Knudson et al. randomized 400 patients to receive either subcutaneous heparin or sequential compression boots. A control group was also included that received no prophylaxis. Neither of the experimental groups had a significant reduction in the incidence of DVT except for the subgroup of head-injured patients (who could not receive heparin) in whom sequential venous compression devices were more effective than no treatment in preventing DVT.

19. Are vena cava filters useful in PE prophylaxis among trauma patients?

The lack of efficacy of standard measures has prompted some clinicians to try vena cava filters. A recent study reported 63 high-risk patients in whom prophylactic filters were inserted. Thirty percent developed DVT and 1% sustained a PE. Follow-up examination with abdominal duplex ultrasound found the 30 day patency rate of the filters to be 100% and the 2-year patency rate to be 96%.

20. What is the mortality rate among trauma patients who sustain a PE?

About 25%.

21. What is the mechanism of action of heparin?

Heparin binds with antithrombin III to prevent the conversion of prothrombin to thrombin. The postulated mechanism of action of low dose heparin therapy is enhancement of antithrombin III. Heparin does *not* dissolve established clots.

22. What is low–molecular-weight heparin (LMWH)?

LMWH is prepared from standard (unfractionated) heparin. LMWH does not prolong the activated PPT but retains its ability to inhibit activated factor X.

23. What are some advantages of LMWH over unfractionated heparin?

LMWH seems to have fewer bleeding complications, to produce less thrombocytopenia, and to have a more predictable half-life than unfractionated heparin.

24. Is LMWH effective in trauma patients?

A study from Canada compared (using venography) 344 randomized patients who received either low-dose unfractionated heparin or LMWH (enoxaparin). Forty-four percent of those receiving low-dose heparin developed a DVT, while 31% of those receiving enoxaparin developed DVT. The rates of proximal vein thrombosis were 15% and 6%, respectively. The risk reduction with enoxaparin compared with standard low-dose heparin was 30% for all DVT and 58% for proximal vein thrombosis. A nonsignificant increase in major bleeding was noted in the group that received enoxaparin.

LMWH has also been used with encouraging results in spinal cord–injured patients and in those sustaining orthopedic trauma.

25. Are thrombolytics useful in the management of trauma patients with DVT and PE?

Thrombolytic agents include streptokinase, urokinase, and tissue plasminogen activator (TPA). These agents, unlike heparin, actually dissolve established clots. However, a systemic lytic state may occur that will dissolve clots anywhere in the body. Therefore, these agents have not been used routinely in trauma patients. They are specifically contraindicated in patients with intracranial hemorrhage.

26. How do sequential compression devices work?

Sequential compression devices are thought to have two effects that prevent DVT. First, they compress the legs to increase venous velocity and empty stagnant blood from the venous reservoirs. In this regard they simulate the normal muscle pumping activity. Second, and perhaps of greater importance, compression of the veins causes release of plasminogen activator, which increases fibrinolytic activity. Theoretically, this fibrinolytic effect can be produced by placing a compression garment around an arm.

27. What is the most common site of origin of clinically significant PEs?
The veins of the pelvis and thigh (iliofemoral system).

28. Is Coumadin (warfarin) useful in trauma patients for the prevention of DVT and PEs?
No. Coumadin's action decreases synthesis of vitamin K–dependent clotting factors. Therefore, Coumadin takes about 48 hours to have an effect—long after clots begin to form in the veins of immobilized trauma patients.

29. How does low–molecular-weight dextran prevent DVT?
The effect is probably multifaceted. Dextran 40 coats platelet surfaces to reduce adhesion. This prevents the build-up of platelets on vessels whose endothelium has been damaged as well as on the cusps of venous valves. It also increases plasma volume and decreases blood viscosity.

30. How did warfarin get its name?
A research effort to determine the cause of fatal livestock hemorrhage was funded by the University of **W**isconsin **A**lumni **R**esearch **F**oundation. When the compound was identified in the diet of the animals, it was named W**ARF**-arin.

31. Is there any value in trying to remove deep venous thrombi surgically?
Yes. New devices that break up the clot and infuse thrombolytics have been developed. When the clot has been liquefied, it is suctioned away. The device has an inflated balloon proximally to prevent embolization. These procedures prevent the development of a post-phlebitic limb.

BIBLIOGRAPHY

1. Dennis JW, Menawat S, Von Thron J, et al: Efficacy of deep venous thrombosis prophylaxis in trauma patients and identification of high-risk groups. J Trauma 35:132–138, 1993.
2. Geerts WH, Jay RM, Code KI, et al: A comparison of low-dose heparin with low–molecular-weight heparin as prophylaxis against venous thromboembolism after major trauma. N Engl J Med 335: 701–707, 1996.
3. Hoyt DB, Simons RK, Winchell RJ, et al: A risk analysis of pulmonary complications following major trauma. J Trauma 35:524–531, 1993.
4. Knudson MM, Lewis FR, Clinton A, et al: Prevention of venous thromboembolism in trauma patients. J Trauma 37:480–487, 1994.
5. Rogers FB: Venous thromboembolism in trauma patients. Surg Clin North Am 75:279–291, 1995.
6. Rogers FB, Shackford SR, Ricci MA, et al: Routine prophylactic vena cava filter insertion in severely injured trauma patients decreases the incidence of pulmonary embolism. J Am Coll Surg 180:641–647, 1995.
7. Ruiz AJ, Hill SL, Berry RE: Heparin, deep venous thrombosis, and trauma patients. Am J Surg 162: 159–162, 1991.
8. Wilmore, Cheung, Harkin, et al: ACS Surgery: Principles and Practice. New York, 2002.

IX. Endocrinology

30. ENDOCRINE PROBLEMS IN TRAUMA

Elizabeth Beale, M.B.B.Ch., M.Med.

DIABETES MELLITUS AND HYPOGLYCEMIA

1. How may diabetes mellitus complicate the management of the trauma patient?

Acute metabolic problems precipitated by the trauma

Diabetic ketoacidosis

Hyperosmolar hyperglycemic nonketotic coma

Hyperglycemia causing, for example, volume depletion with hemodynamic deterioration or gastroparesis

Electrolyte imbalance (e.g., hyperkalemia, hypokalemia, hypernatremia, hyponatremia, hypophosphatemia)

Hypoglycemia

Increased protein breakdown

New onset of diabetes

Chronic organ changes

Nephropathy and impaired renal function

Cardiovascular disease with greatly increased risk of ischemic heart disease and compromised peripheral vasculature

Peripheral and autonomic neuropathy leading to complications such as postural hypotension

Diabetic eye disease, including cataracts or retinopathy, that impairs mobility

Increased infections

The most common postoperative infection in diabetics is urinary tract infection.

Foot infection causes the greatest overall morbidity in diabetics.

Hyperglycemia impairs neutrophil phagocytic function and other host defense mechanisms.

Poor wound healing

Increased catabolism with poor diabetic control

Impaired fibroblast function with uncontrolled hyperglycemia

Macrovascular and microvascular disease

Associated medical problems

Obesity in non–insulin-dependent diabetes mellitus (NIDDM)

Hypertension in NIDDM

Medication-related problems

Insulin dose needs to be adjusted frequently as patient's status changes.

Oral agents frequently need to be changed to insulin.

Drug interactions may occur; alcohol may cause severe hypoglycemia with oral hypoglycemic agents.

2. What are the principles in the management of the critically ill diabetic?

- Glucose should be maintained in the range of 90 to 180 mg/dL range.
- Regular insulin by continuous intravenous infusion is the treatment of choice.

- Capillary blood glucose should be monitored hourly and accurately at the bedside and checked intermittently at the laboratory.
- When the glucose level is less than 250 mg/dL, glucose-containing solutions should be infused with the insulin. Insulin infusion must be continued to prevent ketoacidosis. A commonly used maintenance fluid is 5% dextrose at 100 mL/hour.
- Serum potassium levels and fluid balance should be monitored frequently and adjusted appropriately.
- Factors that may precipitate an acute metabolic crisis, such as infection or myocardial infarction, should be prevented or treated promptly.
- Be alert for complications such as diabetic ketoacidosis, hyperosmolar nonketotic coma, and hypoglycemia.

3. Give an example of an insulin infusion regimen suitable for the management of a critically ill diabetic trauma patient in the intensive care unit (ICU) and perioperatively.

1. Put 25 units of regular insulin in 250 mL of normal saline (1 U/10 mL).
2. Flush tubing with 50 mL of solution.
3. Monitor the blood glucose level hourly at the bedside and every 6 hours at the laboratory.
4. Give maintenance and replacement fluids as required, including dextrose-containing solutions when the glucose level is less than 250 mg/dL.
5. Administer insulin intravenously by continuous infusion.

Blood glucose (mg/dL)	Insulin Dosage	
	U/hr	mL/hr
< 80	0.0	0.0
81–100	0.5	5.0
101–140	1.0	10
141–180	1.5	15
181–220	2.0	20
221–260	2.5	25
261–300	3.0	30
301–340	4.0	40
> 341	5.0	50

6. If the blood glucose level is less than 80 mg/dL, stop intravenous insulin administration, and give 25 mL of 50% dextrose in water. When the glucose level is more than 80 mg/dL, insulin infusion can be restarted.
7. A patient with diabetic ketoacidosis requires higher doses, usually about 0.1 U/kg/hr. A patient with sepsis or other significant physical stress or obesity or who is on steroids may also require higher doses.
8. Lower doses may be adequate in patients normally treated with diet or oral agents only or with less than 50 U of insulin each day.

4. Outline a regimen that may be used perioperatively in a diabetic on oral hypoglycemic agents.

1. As a general rule, all diabetics are put on insulin perioperatively.
2. The usual oral medication is given the night before the surgery.
3. Surgery is scheduled for early in the day.
4. Intravenous insulin and dextrose infusions as outlined in Question 3 are started at least 2 to 3 hours before the operation to obtain a glucose level in the range of 90 to 180 mg/dL preoperatively.
5. Intravenous insulin and dextrose infusions are continued postoperatively until food is well tolerated.
6. It may be necessary to give multiple-dose insulin regimens for several days before restarting oral agents.

5. The general rule is that all diabetics should be on insulin perioperatively. When may an exception be made?

An exception may sometimes be made in the case of NIDDM patients who are well controlled (fasting blood glucose [FBG] <180 mg/dL, glycosylated hemoglobin [HbA$_1$c] <10%) on diet or oral agents, who are undergoing surgery of less than 2 hours, when the body cavity is not penetrated, and when food intake will be resumed within a few hours after the operation.

6. Calculate an approximate daily insulin dose for a 70-kg diabetic man receiving a standard total parenteral nutrition (TPN) infusion of 25% dextrose at 100 mL/hr.

- A starting basal rate for insulin is 1 U/hr.
- The usual additional insulin with TPN is 2 to 3 U/100 mL of 25% dextrose (i.e., 2 to 3 U/hr).
- The total daily dose is therefore 3 to 4 U/hr of regular insulin given as a continuous intravenous infusion (i.e., 72 to 96 U/day).
- A stressed or septic patient usually requires additional insulin.

7. What are some causes for abdominal pain in a diabetic patient?

Gastrointestinal causes
    Acute gastric dilatation with ketoacidosis
    Mesenteric infarction
    Ileus due to electrolyte disturbance
Pancreatic causes
    Chronic pancreatitis
    Pancreatitis with type IV hyperlipidemia (hypertriglyceridemia). *Note:* Elevated serum
       amylase is found in 75% of cases of diabetic ketoacidosis.
Hepatobiliary causes
    Cholecystitis
    Hepatic capsular distension owing to fatty infiltration in poorly controlled diabetics
Urogenital causes
    Urinary tract infection
    Bladder distention
Referred pain, such as myocardial infarction
Thoracolumbar neuropathy
Acute "surgical" abdomen, particularly in patients older than 40 years

8. Why should special care be paid to the feet of diabetic patients?

Diabetic foot ulcers occur in 15% of diabetics, and 15% to 20% of these patients will undergo amputation. Diabetic ulcers are usually caused by infection in a minor lesion caused by trauma to a neuropathic foot. An estimated 50% of amputations for diabetic foot ulcers and their sequelae could be prevented with careful management.

9. Why may infection be difficult to diagnose in a diabetic patient?

- A high white blood cell count may occur with diabetic ketoacidosis and does not necessarily indicate an infection. A band count of greater than 10 has been reported to indicate infection.
- Temperature may not be elevated in cases of infection.
- A confused or comatose diabetic patient is unable to describe symptoms or help in localizing the infection.

10. Does normalization of hyperglycemia improve prognosis in critically ill patients?

According to a study by Van den Berghe et al., normalization of blood glucose levels (i.e., maintenance of blood glucose levels at 80 to 110 mg/dL) reduces morbidity and mortality even in patients without prior diabetes. This single-center trial suggested that intensive treatment of modest hyperglycemia using intensive insulin therapy significantly decreased multiple-organ failure due to sepsis and acute renal failure and substantially improved the prognosis of critically ill patients.

11. When should hypoglycemia be suspected in a trauma patient?
Although hypoglycemia is uncommon in trauma patients, it should be sought in all patients with an altered mental state, especially in patients taking insulin or oral hypoglycemic agents in the following settings:
- Interruption of normal caloric intake
- Alcohol use
- Elderly patients
- Renal insufficiency

THYROID

12. What is the most common cause of thyroid hormone abnormalities in the critically ill patient?
The euthyroid sick syndrome is the most common cause.

13. What is the euthyroid sick syndrome?
It is an abnormality of thyroid function tests that occurs with nonthyroidal illness in critically ill patients. The most common finding is a low triiodothyronine (T_3) level. A low thyroxine (T_4) level may also be found, and thyroid-stimulating hormone (TSH) levels are normal, slightly suppressed, or slightly elevated. In a stressed individual (e.g., critically ill trauma patient), there is decreased conversion of T_4 to T_3 in the periphery, and there is decreased binding of thyroid hormone to thyroxine-binding globulin.

14. Should critically ill patients with changes in thyroid function tests consistent with the euthyroid sick syndrome be treated with thyroid hormone?
Despite many studies of the subject, it is unclear whether treating critically ill patients with thyroid hormone is beneficial or harmful. In general, authorities advise giving thyroid hormone therapy to critically ill patients only if there is clear clinical or laboratory evidence for hypothyroidism.

15. How can hypothyroidism be distinguished from the euthyroid sick syndrome?
The hypothyroid patient may have a history of thyroid illness, including thyrotoxicosis, radioiodine ablation of the thyroid, or thyroid surgery. Antimicrosomal antibodies are frequently present with hypothyroidism due to Hashimoto's thyroiditis. In hypothyroidism, T_4 is reduced proportionately more than T_3, and the TSH level may be very high. In the euthyroid sick syndrome, T_3 is decreased proportionately more than T_4, and the TSH level is normal or only slightly abnormal. The T_3-resin uptake is decreased in primary hypothyroidism but increased in the euthyroid sick syndrome.

16. What causes thyroid storm?
A thyroid storm is caused by inadequate treatment of thyrotoxicosis in association with a superimposed stress such as trauma, infection, or thyroid or nonthyroid surgery.

17. How does thyroid storm manifest?
There are marked features of thyrotoxicosis as well as fever, tachycardia out of proportion to the fever, and central nervous system (CNS) dysfunction, which may include agitation, seizures, or coma. There may be features of Graves' disease, a goiter, or heart failure.

18. What is the prognosis of thyroid storm?
Untreated, the mortality rate is almost 100%, but with aggressive treatment, it is about 20%.

19. Outline the management of thyroid storm.

Specific measures

1. Antithyroid drugs to prevent formation of more thyroid hormone (e.g., propylthiouracil [PTU], 1000 mg orally or by nasogastric tube as soon as possible and then 300 to 400 mg every 6 to 8 hours, or methimazole, 30 to 40 mg orally or per rectum every 6 to 8 hours).

2. Sodium iodide, 1 to 2 g every 24 hours by continuous intravenous infusion or saturated solution of potassium iodide (SSKI); 5 drops orally every 6 hours starting 1 hour after the antithyroid drugs to prevent release of preformed thyroid hormone.

3. Dexamethasone, 2 mg intravenously every 6 hours to prevent peripheral conversion of T_4 to T_3.

4. Propranolol is given intravenously to achieve a pulse of about 100 beats per minute. Caution should be used in cases of congestive heart failure, because it may be aggravated by beta-blocker therapy. However, if the failure is caused by tachycardia, beta-blockade may be an effective treatment. A typical dose is 40 to 80 mg orally or 1 to 2 mg intravenously every 6 to 8 hours.

Supportive measures

1. Treat the precipitating cause.

2. Apply external cooling.

3. Administer nonaspirin antipyretics. Aspirin displaces T_4 from binding proteins and may raise the circulating free T_4 level.

4. Give fluids.

5. Glucose, phenobarbital, and B vitamins have also been recommended by some authorities.

20. When may myxedema coma occur in a trauma patient?

Myxedema coma usually occurs in an elderly individual with compensated hypothyroidism (i.e., an individual with a high TSH but normal T_4) who undergoes a severe stress, such as trauma, prolonged cold exposure, infection, surgery, or administration of CNS depressants.

21. Summarize the management of myxedema coma.

1. Draw blood for TSH and thyroid hormone testing, but do not delay treatment while tests are obtained.

2. Give T_4, 0.3 to 0.5 mg intravenously and then 0.025 to 0.05 mg/day until awake, after which administer 0.05 to 0.1 mg/day of the oral replacement.

3. Administer hydrocortisone, 75 mg intravenously every 6 hours, for possible coexistent adrenal insufficiency.

4. Offer supportive measures:

Begin slow rewarming.

If necessary, support respiration and circulation.

Treat underlying precipitating cause.

5. Be alert for myocardial ischemia caused by a rapid increase in myocardial oxygen use.

22. What drugs commonly used in the critically ill patient may cause suppression of TSH?

Dopamine (profound suppression that can lead to a fall in T_4 and T_3)

Glucocorticoids

Phenytoin

Amiodarone (more commonly causes TSH elevation)

23. How may dopamine and furosemide interact to cause significant hypothyroxinemia?

Dopamine suppresses TSH release, leading to low T_4 levels. Furosemide inhibits T_4 serum protein binding, leading to increased clearance.

ADRENAL

24. What is the incidence of adrenal insufficiency in ICU trauma patients?

A wide range (<1% to >30%) has been reported for the incidence of adrenal insufficiency; the rate depends on the population studied and the tests used. Two studies in surgical ICU patients found an incidence of 0.7%. The incidence increased to 6% for patients with an ICU stay longer than 14 days and to 11% for patients with an ICU stay longer than 14 days who were older than 55 years of age. Barquist et al. found that the incidence of adrenal insufficiency after adrenocorticotropic hormone (ACTH, Cortrosyn) testing was lower in trauma patients than in general surgical ICU patients. They consider that this finding may have reflected the overall better state of health of the trauma patients before hospitalization.

25. Why is it important to diagnose and treat adrenal insufficiency?

Untreated, the mortality is 100%. Treatment is simple and effective.

26. When should adrenal insufficiency be suspected in an ICU patient?

The clinician should have a high index of suspicion because the signs and symptoms are often nonspecific. The typical ICU presentation is with hypotension that is unresponsive to fluids and inotropes. There is often a high cardiac output with low systemic vascular resistance. Other presenting signs and symptoms include fever, abdominal pain, anorexia, nausea, vomiting, diarrhea, fatigue, weakness, altered mental state, and eosinophilia. The presentation may be similar to septic shock.

27. How may the presentation of adrenal insufficiency in the critically ill trauma patient differ from that in the general population?

* Fluid and electrolyte changes may be masked by therapy given in the intensive care.
* The patient may be unconscious or sedated and therefore is "asymptomatic."
* The presentation may be masked by other medical problems such as septic shock.

28. How is the diagnosis of adrenal insufficiency made in the critically injured ICU patient?

In the standard test, 250 μg of ACTH (Cortrosyn) is given intravenously after drawing a baseline cortisol level. Cortisol is rechecked at 30 minutes and 60 minutes.

The normal reference range for cortisol, basal and stimulated, in the ICU is controversial. In general a baseline value of less than 3 μg/dL or a stimulated level of less than 20 μg/dL is considered diagnostic of adrenal insufficiency. Other practitioners have considered a basal level less than 15 μg/dL and a stimulated level less than 25 μg/dL as being diagnostic of adrenal insufficiency in the ICU.

29. What is the treatment of adrenal crisis?

1. Draw blood for cortisol and ACTH determinations. Treatment should be given on clinical suspicion of adrenal insufficiency in a critically ill patient without waiting for test results.

2. Steroid replacement consists of hydrocortisone, 100 mg given intravenously every 6 to 8 hours, or 2 mg of dexamethasone given intravenously every 6 to 8 hours. Because dexamethasone does not cross-react with endogenous cortisol, it can be used before performing diagnostic tests.

3. Fluids and electrolytes should be monitored. Patients with hypovolemia and hyponatremia should be given normal saline intravenously.

4. Glucose is usually given as 5% dextrose with the replacement normal saline.

5. Treat the precipitating cause.

30. What are some controversies in the diagnosis of adrenal insufficiency in the critically ill patient?

The value of serum cortisol above which adrenal insufficiency can safely be excluded is uncertain. When in doubt, the patient should be treated on the basis of clinical suspicion.

The standard cosyntropin test result may be falsely normal for several months after the onset of secondary adrenal insufficiency. The cause of adrenal insufficiency in the ICU is not clear but appears to include some cases with secondary adrenal insufficiency. The low-dose (1-μg) ACTH test may detect these cases.

31. How may trauma precipitate an adrenal crisis?

A patient with preexisting adrenal insufficiency may develop a crisis due to the stress of trauma itself, a diagnostic procedure, surgery, or an infection. An individual who is taking or was recently taking exogenous corticosteroids may develop an adrenal crisis if these drugs are not administered regularly or are tapered too rapidly.

32. If a patient is taking exogenous glucocorticoids, can the risk for hypothalamic-pituitary-adrenal (HPA) suppression be predicted from the amount of corticosteroids a patient has used or from the duration of use?

No. It has been reported that in patients receiving more than the equivalent of 10 mg/day of prednisone, suppression of the HPA cannot be predicted from the total dose, the highest dose, nor the duration of treatment.

33. How long does the HPA take to recover from suppression by exogenous glucocorticoids?

The time to HPA recovery after stopping glucocorticoids varies from 2 days up to a year.

34. What perioperative hydrocortisone dosages are recommended for patients on long-term glucocorticoid therapy?

Type of Surgery	Dose of Hydrocortisone	Duration of Therapy (in the absence of complications)
Minor	25 mg/day	1 day
Moderate	50–75 mg/day	1–2 days
Major	100–150 mg/day	2–3 days

35. What complications may occur in the trauma patient who is taking long-term, high-dose glucocorticoids?

- Exacerbation of the condition (e.g., asthma) for which the glucocorticoids were initially prescribed
- Adrenal crisis due to inadvertent, rapid withdrawal of glucocorticoids
- Increased risk of infection
- Slow healing of wounds
- Osteoporotic fractures
- Glucose intolerance or even diabetes mellitus
- Muscular weakness
- Thinning of the skin
- Easy bruising
- Mental changes

36. What are adrenal incidentalomas, and what is their significance?

Adrenal incidentalomas are lesions found unexpectedly on 0.3% to 5.0% of abdominal computed tomography (CT) scans. They are usually benign, nonfunctioning adrenocortical adenomas. Malignant adrenocortical adenocarcinomas are rare and found in only 0.6 to 1.7 persons per million people. The adrenal glands are common sites for metastases from the lung, breast, stomach, and kidney.

37. Outline an approach to the management of an adrenal incidentaloma.

1. Take a history and examine the patient, looking especially for features of malignancy (e.g., weight loss), pheochromocytoma (e.g., hypertension, sweating, anxiety), Cushing's syndrome (e.g., hypertension, striae, central obesity), and virilization.

2. Check serum potassium; obtain a 24-hour urine collection for vanillylmandelic acid (VMA), metanephrines, and catecholamines for pheochromocytoma; and determine 17-hydroxy-corticosteroid (17-OH) and 17-ketosteroid levels for Cushing's syndrome.

3. Resect the incidentaloma if it is biochemically active.

4. If the lesion is larger than 6 cm in diameter, it is usually resected, because it is likely to be malignant.

5. A lesion between 3 and 6 cm in diameter is usually resected if it is solid and has suspicious features on CT or if it is a thick-walled cyst with positive cytology results for the aspirate. Otherwise, such lesions are followed with three monthly CT scans for 1 year and then annual scans.

6. Lesions less than 3 cm in diameter that are not suspicious on CT scan may be followed with three monthly CT scans for 1 year and then annual scans.

7. Repeat a 24-hour urine collection for VMA, metanephrines, and catecholamines for pheochromocytoma at 3 months, and obtain serum potassium levels and 17-OH corticosteroid and 17-ketosteroid levels for Cushing's syndrome annually.

8. Resect the lesion if it increases in size or becomes biochemically active.

PITUITARY

38. Describe the clinical features of posttraumatic hypopituitarism.

Benvenga et al. reported the following features of hypopituitarism occurring after head trauma:
Male to female ratio of 5:1
Age at trauma: 35% of cases in the third decade of life
Time from trauma to diagnosis: days to more than 40 years; 71.0% were less than 1 year from trauma
Most frequent type of trauma: road accident (74.1%)
Occurrence of skull fracture (55%)
Occurrence of coma or unconsciousness (93%)
Most frequent type of anatomic lesions (CT or MRI): hemorrhage of the hypothalamus (29.0%) and hemorrhage of the pituitary posterior lobe (26.3%)
Occurrence of diabetes insipidus (30%)

39. Name some causes of polyuria in a trauma patient.

- Overhydration
- Osmotic diuresis after rhabdomyolysis
- Diabetes insipidus
- Recovery from renal failure

40. What type of head trauma is most commonly associated with diabetes insipidus?

The usual cause of posttraumatic diabetes insipidus is an automobile accident causing injuries to the lateral skull. Injuries result from a shearing action on the pituitary stalk or hemorrhagic ischemia of the posterior pituitary and hypothalamus. One of six patients has associated anterior pituitary damage.

41. How is diabetes insipidus diagnosed?

- Exclude osmotic or water diuresis.
- Cautiously reduce intravenous fluid administration while following the serum sodium, hourly urine output, and urine osmolality.
- Diabetes insipidus is diagnosed by the finding of a serum sodium greater than 145 mEq/L,

serum osmolality greater than 290 mOsm/L, and urine specific gravity less than 1.0003 or urine osmolality less than 150 mOsm/kg. Urine output is often greater than 300 mL/hr.

42. Outline the management of diabetes insipidus.

1. The conscious subject usually spontaneously increases his or her oral fluid intake until the condition resolves.

2. The critically ill or unconscious patient should be given 1-deamino-8-D-arginine vasopressin (DDAVP), with a starting dose of 1 mg given intravenously.

3. Hourly urine output and urine osmolality are measured.

4. When dilute polyuria restarts, the next dose of DDAVP is administered.

5. Maintenance hypotonic fluids are given intravenously until the patient is alert enough to sense thirst and take adequate amounts of water orally.

6. Overtreating with fluids or DDAVP should be avoided because it produces fluid overload and hyponatremia.

7. Stress doses of hydrocortisone are given until anterior pituitary function has been evaluated.

43. What is triphasic diabetes insipidus?

It is a syndrome consisting of three phases that may occur after head trauma or surgery. Any one of the phases may not be clinically obvious.

Phase 1: Diabetes insipidus occurs hours to days after the injury and results from neuronal shock causing impaired release of vasopressin.

Phase 2: Inappropriate antidiuresis, often with hyponatremia, occurs 2 to 14 days after the head injury and results from leakage of vasopressin from damaged neurons.

Phase 3: Return of diabetes insipidus occurs 2 to 14 days after trauma as the intraneuronal vasopressin granules are depleted. This phase may be permanent, or it may resolve. Recovery has been seen 10 years after the injury.

MISCELLANEOUS ENDOCRINE PROBLEMS

44. What endocrine parameters predict outcome in intensive care patients?

Low concentrations of TSH and thyroxine and high concentrations of cortisol are associated with a poor prognosis.

An endocrine index derived from the admission levels of cortisol, thyroxine, and TSH was shown in one study to be a better predictor of patient outcome than the Acute Physiology and Chronic Health Evaluation (APACHE) II score.

45. What is immobilization hypercalcemia, and how can it be treated?

This is an uncommon cause of hypercalcemia overall but is an important cause of hypercalcemia in trauma patients. It is seen in patients immobilized, for example, with spinal cord injury, burns, or fracture of the femur. Untreated, it may lead to renal dysfunction, renal stones, and osteoporosis. It has most often occurred in adolescent males, probably because of their high rates of skeletal growth. The cause of immobilization hypercalcemia is not clear, but it is associated with normal levels of parathyroid hormone (PTH), which appear to act with increased activity on the immobilized bone. In one study, a single dose of 60 mg of pamidronate resolved the hypercalcemia or its symptoms in 7 (78%) patients with immobilization hypercalcemia caused by spinal cord injury. Pamidronate is easy to administer, has a long duration of treatment, and eliminates the need for long-term intravenous saline or daily medications.

46. What is the prognosis after osteoporotic hip fracture?

Twenty percent risk of dying in the first year. Seventy-five percent of survivors have an impaired ability to perform activities of daily living.

BIBLIOGRAPHY

1. Angelis M, Yu M, Takanishi D, et al: Eosinophilia as a marker of adrenal insufficiency in the surgical intensive care unit. J Am Coll Surg 183:589–596, 1996.
2. Barquist E, Kirton O: Adrenal insufficiency in the surgical intensive care unit patient. J Trauma 42:27–31, 1997.
3. Benvenga S, Campenni A, Ruggeri RM, Trimarchi F: Clinical review 113: Hypopituitarism secondary to head trauma. J Clin Endocrinol Metab 85:1353–1361, 2000.
4. Boulanger BR, Gann DS: Management of the trauma victim with pre-existing endocrine disease. Crit Care Clin 10:537–554, 1994.
5. Brent GA, Hershman JM: Thyroxine therapy in patients with severe nonthyroidal illnesses and low serum thyroxine concentration. J Clin Endocrinol Metab 63:1–8, 1986.
6. Buonocore CM, Robinson AG: The diagnosis and management of diabetes insipidus during medical emergencies. Endocrinol Metab Clin North Am 22:411–422, 1993.
7. Gavin LA: Perioperative management of the diabetic patient. Endocrinol Metab Clin North Am 21: 457–475, 1992.
8. Karpati RM, Mak RH, Lemley KV: Hypercalcemia, hypertension, and acute renal insufficiency in an immobilized adolescent. Child Nephrol Urol 11:215–219, 1991.
9. McDermott MT: Thyroid disease in the critical care setting. In Parsons PE, Wiener-Kronish JP (eds): Critical Care Secrets. Philadelphia, Hanley & Belfus, 1992, pp 252–256.
10. Robinson GA, Verbalis JG: Diabetes insipidus. In Bardin CW (ed): Current Therapy in Endocrinology and Metabolism, 6th ed. St. Louis, Mosby, 1997, pp 1–7.
11. Rothwell PM, Lawler PG: Prediction of outcome in intensive care patients using endocrine parameters. Crit Care Med 23:78–83, 1995.
12. Sanders LJ: Diabetes mellitus: Prevention of amputation. J Am Podiatr Med Assoc 84:322–328, 1994.
13. Schneyer CR, Kerkvliet GJ: The critically ill diabetic. In Shoemaker WC, Ayres SM, Grenvik G, Holbrook PR (eds): Textbook of Critical Care. Philadelphia, WB Saunders, 1995, pp 1081–1093.
14. Staren ED, Prinz RA: Selection of patients with adrenal incidentalomas for operation. Surg Clin North Am 75:499–509, 1995.
15. Stathatos N, Levetan C, Burman KD, Wortofsky L: The controversy of the treatment of critically ill patients with thyroid hormone. Best Pract Res Clin Endocrinol Metab 15:465–478, 2001.
16. Stockigt JR: Serum thyrotropin and thyroid hormone measurements and assessment of thyroid hormone transport. In Braverman LE, Utiger RD (eds): Werner and Ingbars's the Thyroid: A Fundamental and Clinical Text, 7th ed. Philadelphia, Lippincott-Raven, 1996, pp 377–396.
17. Van den Berghe G, Wouters P, Weekers F, et al: Intensive insulin therapy in the surgical intensive care unit. N Engl J Med 345:1359–1367, 2001.

X. Surgical Issues

31. PLASTIC SURGERY

William R. Dougherty, M.D., and Thuan T. Nguyen, M.D.

WOUND HEALING AND LACERATION MANAGEMENT

1. Summarize the processes of normal wound healing.

Wound repair is an amalgam of two synergistic processes: biochemical and cellular. Their relative function and contribution change during the course of healing. The time line of healing is commonly broken down into overlapping phases, which, for didactic purposes, are named for the dominant features exhibited by each of the two processes: injury (hemostasis), inflammatory (fibroplasia), proliferative, and remodeling (see figure).

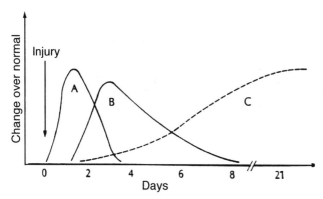

Schematic diagram of the phases of wound healing; injury and hemostasis; A = inflammatory phase; B = proliferative phase; C = maturation/remodeling phase (Reprinted from Mathes SJ, Abouljoud M: Wound healing. In Davis JH (ed): Clinical Surgery. St. Louis, Mosby, 1987; with permission.)

The Phases of Wound Healing

HEMOSTASIS: IMMEDIATE	INFLAMMATORY PHASE: FIRST 5 DAYS	PROLIFERATIVE PHASE: 5 DAYS–3 WEEKS	REMODELING PHASE: 3 WEEKS–1.5 YEARS
Disruption of normal anatomic structures	Rubor	Epithelial regeneration	Restoration of the normal ratio of
Division of blood vessels	Tumor	Contraction	type I and type III
Exposure of matrix molecules	Calor	Fibroplasia	collagen by
	Dolor	Wound contraction	degradation and
Clotting cascade	Functio delasa	PDGF from platelets—	resynthesis
Fibrinogen-fibrin plug	PMNs—first 48 hours	chemotactic and	Collagen realigned
Platelet trapping	release inflammatory	mitogenic for	Fibroblasts diminish
Release of growth	mediators	fibroblasts	Vessels constrict
factors PDGF,	Monocytes—	BFGF—angiogenesis	
TGF(B), FGF	macrophages	and synthesis of	
	Main role—debride	collagen matrix	
	ment—phagocytosis		

(continued)

The Phases of Wound Healing (Continued)

HEMOSTASIS: IMMEDIATE	INFLAMMATORY PHASE: FIRST 5 DAYS	PROLIFERATIVE PHASE: 5 DAYS–3 WEEKS	REMODELING PHASE: 3 WEEKS–1.5 YEARS
Complement cascade Cellular migration	Remain as long as wound is open Secrete BFGF Fibroblast ingrowth Formation of all connective tissue components Collagen, glycosaminoglycans, elastin Reepithelialization	TGFB—potent activator of extracellular matrix protein synthesis	

The biochemical processes include the coagulation cascade, the complement system cascade, arachidonic acid metabolism, histamine/kallikrein release, and collagen synthesis. The structural components of wound repair include collagen, glycosaminoglycans, and elastin. These biochemical events modulate cellular events such as the margination of leukocytes (PMNs, monocytes, and macrophages) and the migration of fibroblasts, angiogenesis, and reepithelialization (see figures).

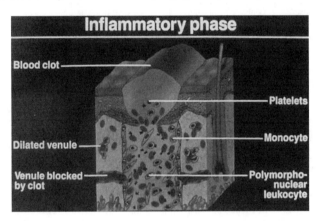

The inflammatory phase of wound healing. (Reprinted from Current Concepts in Wound Healing. C.R. Bard Home Healthcare Division, Covington, GA; with permission.)

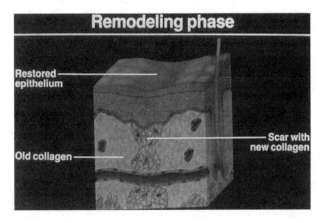

The remodeling phase of wound healing. (Reprinted from Current Concepts in Wound Healing. C.R. Bard Home Healthcare Division, Covington, GA; with permission.)

Wound closure involves the biomodal process of epithelial migration and contraction of the wound edges. Full epithelialization heralds the completion of the inflammatory phase. The longer the wound remains open, the more extensive the eventual scarring.

2. What differentiates the inflammatory phase of wound healing from acute infection?
The inflammatory phase usually lasts the first 5 days after injury but will continue until the wound has reepithelialized. The signs of inflammation are rubor (redness), tumor (swelling), calor (heat), dolor (pain), and functio laesa (reduced function). Unfortunately, these are the same symptoms seen in an acute infection and may cause initial confusion for the clinician. The timing of symptoms and systemic manifestations of infection help differentiate the two. There are only two common organisms that establish wound infection within the first 24–36 hours after surgery or injury, β-hemolytic streptococcus and *Clostridum perfringens*. These early infections have concomitant signs such as fever, rapidly advancing cellulitis, tenderness, fetid drainage, tissue crepitus, bullous formation, and tissue necrosis.

Humoral Events in the Inflammatory Phase

RUBOR	TUMOR	CALOR	DOLOR
Vasodilation; increased vascular permeability PGI(2)-Prostacyclin Also PGA, PGD, and PGE	Leakage of plasma proteins into extra-vascular space; PGE(2), PGF(2A) involve permeability. While PGI(2), PGE(2) enhance flow.	Local tissue temp. elevation due to increased local blood flow and increased metabolic activity	Pain brought on by arachidonic acid, PGI(2), PGE, and PGE(2)

The other common organisms usually require 5–7 days to establish an infection. Drainage, dehiscence, and signs of inflammation that appear to leave the zone of injury herald wound infection and cellulitis.

3. Compare acute and chronic wounds.
An acute wound is one that proceeds through an orderly and timely reparative process that results in sustained restoration of anatomic and functional integrity. The majority of acute civilian traumatic wounds can be closed primarily if adequately debrided. Chronic wounds do not proceed through an orderly and timely process and cannot be closed primarily. Some examples of chronic wounds are nonacute thermal burns, lacerations more than 24 hours old, traumatic wounds with large soft tissue defects, and vascular ulcers. A common ingredient to all chronic wounds is granulation tissue. Debridement and topical antimicrobials with good tissue penetration are the standard for treating chronic wounds. Systemic antibiotics are often not effective since they do not penetrate the fibrous bed of granulation tissue. Final closure is usually achieved by secondary intention or skin grafts.

4. What is the role of collagen in wound healing?
Collagen is the principle building block of connective tissue, accounting for one third of the total body protein content. Collagen is almost devoid of the sulfur-containing amino acids cysteine and tryptophan; instead, it is composed of hydroxyproline and hydroxylysine. Collagen has a very complex tertiary and quaternary molecular structure consisting of three polypeptide chains: Each chain is wound upon itself in a left-handed helix and the three chains together wind in a right-handed coil to form the basic collagen unit. The polypeptide chains are held in their relative configurations by covalent bonds. Each triple helical structure is a tropocollagen molecule. Tropocollagen units associate in a regular fashion to form collagen filaments; collagen filaments aggregate as collagen fibrils, and collagen fibrils unite to form collagen fibers, which are visible under the light microscope.

Normal connective tissue is in a state of dynamic equilibrium, balanced between ongoing synthesis and degradation of collagen. The process of collagen remodeling and collagenolysis offer the opportunity of therapeutic intervention in abnormal scarring.

5. Define tensile strength and breaking strength.
The tensile strength of a wound is a measurement of its load capacity per unit area. Breaking strength is defined as the force required to break a wound, regardless of its dimensions. Tensile strength is constant for wounds of similar size, whereas breaking strength can vary, depending solely on different skin thickness.

6. When is peak tensile strength achieved during wound healing?
All wounds gain strength at approximately the same rate during the first 14–21 days; thereafter, the curves may diverge significantly according to the tissue involved. In skin, the peak tensile strength is achieved at approximately 60 days after injury (see figure).

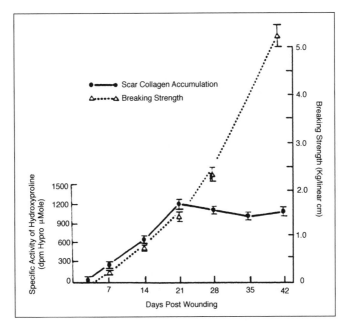

Scar collagen acumulation and breaking strength in rat skin wounds. (Reprinted from Madden JW, Peacock EE Jr: Studies on the biology of collagen during wound healing. Ann Surg 174:511–520, 1971; with permission.)

7. What are primary closure, delayed primary closure, and closure by secondary intention?
Traumatic wounds can be closed primarily, by delayed primary closure, or can be allowed to close by secondary intention. Several factors must be considered when a wound is evaluated for closure. Clean, incised wounds can be closed within 6 hours after injury by suture or skin graft (**primary closure**), providing all the contaminated and nonviable tissue is adequately debrided and there is sufficient soft tissue for a nontension closure. Wounds that are contaminated or are more than 6 hours old (facial wounds up to 24 hours) should not be closed primarily. These wounds are debrided and dressed and evaluated daily for closure over a period of 4–6 days, prior to granulation tissue formation (**delayed primary closure**). Wounds with large soft tissue defects, sinuses, fistulae, and severe gross contamination are best managed by serial dressing changes and allowed to close by contraction and epithelialization (**secondary intention**).

8. What is debridement, and who coined the term?

Debridement is the surgical removal of diseased or nonviable tissue from a wound. Ambroise Paré, a French surgeon (1517?–1590), coined the term. Paré reintroduced the ancient method of hemostasis by suture ligature and was also responsible for abandoning the use of boiling oil in the treatment of battle amputations.

9. What is the function of suture?

The function of suture is to bring tissue into apposition without compromising its vascularity. The judicious use of suture is key to the restoration of a normal anatomic relationship of severed structures while reducing the dead space. Dead space leads to accumulation of exudate, which is prone to infection and is replaced solely by scar tissue.

10. Describe the different types of suture material with respect to their tensile strength, tissue reaction, knot-holding ability, pliability, and capillary (or wick) action.

Sutures are generally considered to be absorbable (catgut, polyglycolic acid, polydioxanone) or nonabsorbable (nylon, Dacron, polypropylene, silk, cotton, stainless steel). Nonabsorbable sutures may be coated with a medical grade of silicone (on silk), Teflon (on braided Dacron), or other synthetic materials to make them smoother and less reactive.

Absorbable sutures made of collagen, polyglycolic acid, or polydioxanone are digested by body enzymes. They are frequently used to close subcutaneous tissues and to repair mucous membranes. They are also advantageous for children to avoid painful removal of skin sutures. Catgut is made from collagen of the submucosal layer of the small intestine of sheep or the serosal layer of the small intestine of cattle. Chromic catgut retains its tensile strength for 30 days, twice as long as plain catgut. Polyglycolic acid (Dexon) and polyglactin 910 (Vicryl) are made of a polymerized amino acid (glycolic acid), which is stretched and braided to form the suture. These sutures are stronger and have a greater knot-holding ability than catgut. Dexon and Vicryl lose their tensile strength in about 30 days.

Synthetic sutures (nylon, Dacron, stainless steel, or polypropylene) or stainless steel staples can be used to close the skin. These sutures are stronger and less reactive than absorbable sutures. Silk and cotton consistently produce more tissue reaction than the synthetic sutures. Multifilament sutures are more reactive than the same material in a monofilament suture and are more likely to develop a discharging sinus in the skin wound.

11. Compare and contrast the healing of skin, muscle, tendon, nerve, cartilage, and bone with respect to regeneration and scarring.

Skin. Epithelialization is a regenerative process that proceeds from the basal layer contrasted to dermal repair, which heals by scar formation and not regeneration. With epithelial regeneration, cells at the wound margin flatten then migrate into the open wound. Dermis heals by scar formation.

Muscle. Once injured, the myocyte degenerates, and the muscle heals with scar formation.

Tendon. Tendon healing progresses through the inflammatory, proliferative, and remodeling stages as seen with other connective tissues. Additionally, there is a requisite third phase of healing where the tendinous repair gains strength while the peritendinous adhesions degenerate. This is not a regenerative process as seen with the epithelium but another example of healing with scar formation.

Peripheral nerves. Peripheral nerves repair through regeneration of their sheaths and axons; the Schwann cell closest to the site of injury responds by repairing the axonal damage. Initially, this cell swells then proliferates primarily in the distal nerve stump. It becomes motile, forming dense cords along the former line of the axon. The Schwann cell phagocytizes the degenerating axon, fragments of myelin, and other debris. If the injury does not ultimately result in neuronal death, regeneration proceeds. Myelin sheaths first make their appearance on the regenerating axon in 6–7 days. Nodes of Ranvier appear some 2 weeks later. The process of myelination continues for nearly a year. This is a regenerative process as seen with the epithelium; however, scar formation in the form of neurilemomas develops from the sheath of the Schwann cell when axonal regeneration is inhibited.

Cartilage. Cartilage has a low metabolic rate and is relatively avascular with few cell populations. Once wounded, cartilage regenerates by neochondrogenesis. This process becomes less apparent with aging where connective tissue replacement (scar formation) becomes more prominent. In healing cartilage, the primary cell type is the chondrocyte. This cell produces collagen in addition to extracellular cartilage. The long-term success of cartilage graft survival depends on an adequate blood supply in addition to the chondrocyte maintaining the graft's bulk.

Bone. The three cell types present in bone are the osteoblast, the osteoclast, and the osteocyte. The osteoblast produces bone matrix, and the osteoclast absorbs bone material. The osteocyte constitutes the majority cell type in mature bone, and it has matrix-producing and resorptive capacities.

The healing of bone is divided into three phases. Initially, there is the inflammatory phase lasting approximately 5 days. It resembles the corresponding phase seen in soft tissue with PMNs and monocytes removing necrotic tissue and debris.

The proliferative phase is characterized by mineralization and the formation of a callus around the fracture with the transition to mature bone formation. As seen within the cells, there is an orderly progression of endochondral ossification of cartilage with woven trabecular bone bridging the fracture site.

The remodeling phase is the longest phase of bone healing. As the callus diminishes in size, angular deformities at the fracture site also decrease. This bone remodeling follows Wolff's law stating that bone adapts to functional forces acting on it.

Contrasting the different types of bone, cortical and endochondral bone provides weight-bearing functions and allows for locomotion. Membranous bone, on the other hand, serves to protect vital soft tissue structures from injury. Endochondral bone has a cartilaginous intermediate phase, whereas membranous bone lacks this cartilaginous stage. Also, endochondral bone has an epiphyseal plate while membranous bone has no identifiable epiphysis.

12. What are the differences between keloid and hypertrophic scarring and normal scar formation?

In humans, virtually all wounds heal by scar formation rather than regeneration. The degree of scarring between normal and keloid is a spectrum. Clinicians and pathologists still disagree about the exact definition of keloid versus hypertrophic scarring.

In general, keloid scars tend to grow beyond the wound margin. They are more common in certain parts of the body (sternum, neck, shoulders, pinna, and back), but it can be seen anywhere. There is striking racial predominance of keloid scarring in blacks and Asians. Keloid scarring is disproportionate to the degree of injury, for example, ear piercing that leads to baseball-sized scar mass. Excision of the keloid alone can lead to even worse scarring.

In contrast hypertrophic scars scale with the degree of injury. Circumstances that prolong the inflammatory phase, such as the loss of tissue, burns, presence of foreign body, ischemia, or ongoing trauma, often lead to hypertrophic scars. There are no specific common sites and no racial differences; however, children are more often affected. Hypertrophic scars are limited to the area of injury and usually stop growing after 6 months. Clinically, they are pink or red in color, which signifies that the inflammatory process is still active. Hypertrophic scars may be prevented with appropriate tissue handling to minimize scarring.

13. Is there a nonoperative treatment for hypertrophic and keloid scarring?

Because the etiology of hypertrophic and keloid scarring is not known, the treatment tends to be nonspecific and based on trial and error. Several available treatment modalities to decrease scar thickness are being assessed; positive-polarity electrotherapy ultrasound, pressure garments, topical and intralesional injection of steroids, topical application of silicone sheets, and laser techniques. The putative goal of the treatment is to modulate collagen deposition and turnover.

14. What is the operative treatment of hypertrophic and keloid scarring?

The mainstay of operative therapy is debulking the scar mass followed by topical pressure and intralesional steroid injection. Intralesional therapy involves injecting triamcinolone diacetate into the wound at the time of surgery and then every 3–4 weeks in an effort to manipulate collagen deposition. Injections are continued until the inflammatory phase has resolved. For keloid scars some clinicians add a short course x-ray therapy to the above regimen.

15. What are the factors that affect wound healing?

The goal of traumatic wound closure is to obtain a closed wound preventing infection, fibrosis, and secondary deformity. In order to achieve this goal, several local and systemic factors must be observed to prevent wound breakdown and dehiscence.

Systemic factors are anemia, systemic sepsis, malnutrition, vitamin deficiency, zinc deficiency, steroid use, chronic illness, renal or liver failure, diabetes, hypoproteinemia, atherosclerosis, and immunosuppressive therapy.

Local factors are excessive tension on wound edges leading to ischemia, hematoma, wound infection, irradiation, foreign body, obesity, malignancy, poor blood supply, fistulization, and eschar.

16. What inoculum of bacteria leads to wound infection and graft failure?

All traumatic wounds are contaminated to some degree. A wound can tolerate an inoculum of up to 100,000 (10^5) organisms per gram of tissue and still heal or be repaired. Contamination with greater than 10^5 organisms/gram tissue may lead to wound infection. β-hemolytic streptococcus can produce clinical wound infection regardless of the inoculum.

17. What is the reconstructive ladder?

The surgical techniques available to the clinician for the management of a wound problem are ranked from simple (low complication rate) to complex (higher complication rate) in a step fashion, like the rungs of a ladder. In general one chooses the simplest solution to solve the problem (see figure).

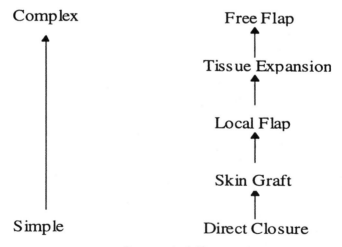

Reconstructive ladder.

18. Define Z-plasty and give indications for its use.

Z-plasty is simply a technique by which two triangular flaps are interchanged one for the other to achieve lengthening of the scar and to change its direction. The three limbs of the Z must always be of equal length. The length gained by Z-plasty of a contracted scar is based on the angle between its limbs. A Z-plasty can be designed with angles ranging from 30–90°, but the maximum length of the central axis will be obtained when using 60° angles. The length gained will be the difference between the long and short diagonals minus the 25–45% lost to skin elasticity. Z-plasty revisions are indicated for:

1. Anti–tension line scars of the eyelids, lips, nasolabial folds, and nonfacial areas
2. Scars on the forehead, temples, nose, cheeks, and chin running at less than 35° of inclination to the resting skin tension lines
3. Small linear scars not amenable to fusiform excision
4. All severe trapdoor and depressed scars
5. Most areas of multiple scarring

Scar revision by W-plasty is indicated for anti–tension line scars on the forehead, eyebrows, temples, cheeks, nose, and chin. It is also indicated for scars on the face whose long axes are at angles of 35° or more to the resting skin tension lines (see figure).

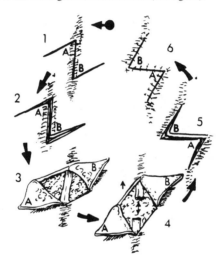

Z-plasty technique: Centra limb designed along the scar. Both limbs are equal in length. *1*, angles A and B are 60°. *2* and *3*, flaps are incised and elevated. *4*, release of deeper portion of the scar. *5*, transposition of triangular flaps. *6*, wounds are approximated. Note lengthening and new direction of scar. (Reprinted from McCarthy JG: Plastic Surgery: General Principles. Vol. 1. Philadelphia, W.B. Saunders, 1990, p 56; with permission.)

19. What are the fundamentals of wound closure that will produce a fine line scar that compromises neither function nor appearance?

Optimal healing is the product of appropriate scar orientation, satisfactory wound closure, and minimal inflammation. An elective incision should be placed in Kraissel's lines of minimal tension as opposed to Langer's lines of tension. Kraissel's lines are those lines perpendicular to the underlying muscular pull. Thus, they minimize the tension in the incision even when the muscle contracts; this prevents hypertrophic scar formation. There are seven Halstedian fundamentals of surgical wound closure that apply to the management of an acute skin wound.

1. Handle tissues gently and debride only as much as necessary to ensure a clean bed
2. Place incisions to follow tension lines and natural skin folds
3. Ensure complete hemostasis
4. Eliminate tension at the skin edges
5. Evert wound edges
6. Use fine sutures and remove them early
7. Allow time for scars to mature before repeat intervention

HEAD AND NECK INJURIES

20. What is the acceptable management of facial laceration?
Early soft tissue management in cases of maxillofacial and mandibular injuries consists of conservative debridement, conversion of unfavorable wounds to favorable wounds, and meticulous layered closure. Lacerations can be closed pending later surgical fixation of the fractures. If necessary, facial lacerations can be closed up to 24 hours after injury with a good result, owing to the good vascularity of the scalp skin.

21. What is the treatment of orbital blow-out fracture?
The medial wall and floor are the weakest components of the bony orbit and are often injured in blunt orbital trauma. The wall comprises structurally weak lamina papyracea of the ethnoid bone and the sphenoid, maxillary, and lacrimal bones. The maxillary and zygomatic bones form the floor of the orbit and separate it from the maxillary sinus antrum (see figure).

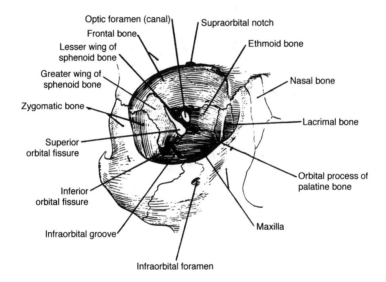

Bony architecture of the orbit with associated foramina. (Reprinted from Ruberg RL, Smith DJ: Plastic Surgery: A Core Curriculum. St. Louis, Mosby, 1994, p 256; with permission.)

Surgical treatment consists of exposure of the orbital contents via a subcilliary or transconjunctival incision. The defect of the floor and/or wall is obturated using a synthetic material, high-density porous polyethylene (Medpor®), or cranial bone graft.

22. Outline the types and management of midface and mandibular fractures.
Le Fort I fractures occur above the level of the teeth and include the entire alveolar process of the maxilla. Le Fort II fractures begin above the level of the apexes of the teeth laterally and extend through the pterygoid plates as in Le Fort I fracture. Medially, it extends to involve a portion of the medial orbit and across the nose. Damage to the ethmoidal area is routine in pyramidal type II fractures. Le Fort III fractures (craniofacial disjunction) are fractures that extend through the zygomaticofrontal sutures and the nasofrontal suture and across the floor of the orbits causing complete separation of the midface from the cranium (see figure, *next page*). Mandibular fractures are classified according to their location (see figure, *next page*). Displaced fractures of the facial skeleton are treated by intermaxillary fixation (IMF) to establish occlusion and by plate and screw fixation to hold the reduction.

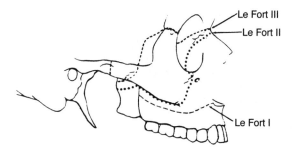

Le Fort fractures. (Reprinted from Ruberg RL, Smith DJ: Plastic Surgery: A Core Curriculum. St. Louis, Mosby, 1994, p 323; with permission.)

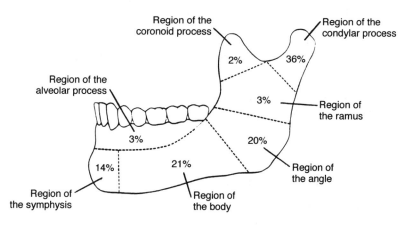

Mandibular fractures. (Reprinted from Ruberg RL, Smith DJ: Plastic Surgery: A Core Curriculum. St. Louis, Mosby, 1994, p 340; with permission.)

23. What is the management of an ear laceration with cartilage involvement?

The anatomy of the external ear comprises elastic cartilage covered by perichondrium and a tightly adherent skin envelope. The topography of the auricle is highlighted by four main cartilaginous convolutions: the helix, antihelix, tragus, and antitragus. The exposed cartilage is sutured with a fine absorbable monofilament suture, such as 5–0 polydiaxonone sutures, to prevent subluxation and maintain the shape of the framework. The skin is approximated using a 6–0 to 7–0 suture. Meticulous hemostasis is necessary as blood accumulation under the perichondrium flap may melt the native structure and go on to organize as a lump cartilage. The cauliflower ear deformity of boxers is an extreme example of this phenomenon.

HAND AND UPPER EXTREMITY INJURIES

24. What are the indications for replantation?

In general, there are no absolute indications for replantation. Each case must be considered on its merits after discussion with the replant team. The patient's age, handedness, sex, occupation, hobbies, wishes, and general health must be addressed in the decision. Clean lacerations are more likely than crushing or avulsed injuries to be successfully reimplanted. Speed is important but is second to a high level of microsurgical skill. Virtually all thumbs should be replanted because of their essential role in hand function. Even a poorly mobile thumb can serve as an excellent post for opposition to the fingers. Most multiple-digit injuries and amputations through the hand or wrist should be treated with reattachment. Replantation of amputated digits distal to the superficialis insertion typically gives excellent results. Amputated parts in children should be reattached because of the excellent results that can be anticipated.

The most important factor in the success rate of replantation is case selection. Patient motivation is important; the patient must have the desire and the capacity to participate in a long period of postoperative rehabilitation.

Relative contraindications include: single digit amputation (especially proximal to the insertion of the flexor digitorum superficialis), avulsion injuries, previous injury or surgery to the part, extreme contamination, lengthy warm ischemia, and advanced age.

25. How should the amputated part be handled prior to replantation?

Completely amputated parts are rinsed thoroughly with cold saline to remove dirt and debris. The part is then wrapped in a sterile gauze that has been soaked in saline and rung out. The wrapped part is placed in a sealed plastic bag. The bag is placed in a solution of ice and water. This avoids freezing the affected part. The part may be x-rayed through the plastic bag.

Partially amputated parts should be left intact! Division of skin bridges may destroy intact channels and ruin the chances for replant success. The nearly divided part should be rinsed and covered with a saline-soaked gauze. A dressing for transport should be placed only after anatomic position has been restored.

26. What do you need to look for with a spiral or oblique metacarpal fracture?

One must look for a rotational deformity of the associated digit. The hand may appear normal when open but on closing, the affected digit will cross into the path of its neighbor, severely compromising hand function. The rotational deformity must be reduced prior to fixation or splinting to avoid a permanent deformity.

27. What is the blood supply to the tendon?

Vincular vessels, which arise from transverse branches of the digital arteries, enter the flexor tendons (FDS and FDP) on their dorsal surfaces (see figure).

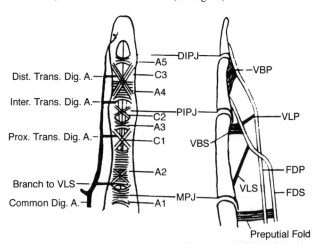

A diagrammatic presentation of the vincular system. DIPJ = distal interphalangeal joint; PIPJ = proximal interphalangeal joint; VBS = vinculum breve superficialis; MPJ = metacarpophalangeal joint; VBP = vinculum breve profundus; VLP = vinculum longum profundus; VLS = vinculum longum superficialis; FDP = flexor digitorum profundus; FDS = flexor digitorum superficialis. (Reprinted from Green DP (ed): Operative Hand Surgery, 3rd ed., Vol 2. New York, Churchill Livingstone, 1993, p 1826; with permission.)

28. What are the pitfalls in the management of tendon lacerations?

The diagnosis of tendon division should be made before the patient goes to the operating room. The flexor and extensor tendons of both the fingers and the wrist are examined. Pitfalls in the diagnosis of tendon injuries:

- If a patient can flex a finger, do not assume that the tendon is intact. Partial tendon division can still move a finger, but usually with pain.
- The index and little fingers have two extensor tendons. The patient can extend these fingers if one tendon is divided.
- If you diagnose tendon injury, look for damage to other structures because you may find an associated nerve and arterial injury.
- Always explain to the patients that after flexor tendon injury they may be off work for a period between 6 weeks and 3 months, depending on their occupation and the nature of the injury.

29. How and where are tendon injuries repaired?

When a tendon is injured, the initial surgery has the greatest influence on the ultimate outcome. Extensor tendons can be repaired in the emergency department provided the surgeon is experienced and there are no other associated hand injuries. Flexor tendons must be repaired in theater.

Preoperatively, antibiotics are given parenterally, tetanus status is assessed, the wound is dressed, and the hand is elevated. The operation should be performed within 6 hours. A bloodless field is essential and is accomplished using a tourniquet. The wound is extended and irrigated with copious saline. The neurovascular bundle is examined and repaired if divided after the tendon is repaired. The tendon ends should be handled carefully. Monofilament sutures are used. A core suture (modified Kessler technique) is followed by epitendonous repair. After wound closure, the hand is immobilized in the position of function and elevated followed by early active mobilization using Klinert splint for 3–4 weeks. A delayed primary repair should be performed within 6 days. The patient should be seen weekly in the clinic to assess finger movements. Patient can return to light duties (office work) after about 6 weeks and to full activities after 3 months.

30. What is the quadrigia effect?

It is the result of an adhesion of one or more previously injured flexor digitorum profundus (FDP) tendons that leads to impaired excursion of the FDPs to other fingers. The cause of quadrigia effect is a common muscle belly shared by all flexor profundus tendons, so an adhesion in one tendon will stop the contraction of the muscle leading to impairment function of the other tendons. Quadrigia is seen after digital amputation, arthrodesis, and tendon repair when adhesions form because of poor technique or lack of proper physical therapy. The treatment of this condition is to divide the adherent tendon proximal to the A1 pulley.

31. Must you remove the nail to evaluate a nail bed injury?

Yes! The treatment of fingernail injuries involves removal of the entire nail with exploration of all portions of the eponychial laceration.

32. How do you manage a distal phalanx fracture associated with a nail bed injury?

The nail bed must be supported by bone throughout its length. If the distal half of the terminal phalanx is fractured it should be anatomically reduced using 18G needle or K-wire. The wire is removed after 3 weeks.

33. What is required to repair a nail bed injury?

The hand should be surgically prepared with an antiseptic solution, and a digital tourniquet is used to allow accurate assessment of eponychium. A blunt-tipped periosteal elevator (Freer) or a fine hemostat is used to avoid traumatizing the uninjured portions of the nail bed. Loupe magnification is required for careful assessment of the nail bed. The nail bed should then be sutured using a 7–0 chromic catgut suture on a fine needle.

Adhesions between the eponychium and the nail bed will result in a grooved or split nail. This is prevented by careful repair of all layers of the nail fold with insertion of the removed nail or a suitable splint to keep the cul-de-sac open during healing. If any nail bed is missing, it is best replaced with a split-thickness nail bed graft taken either from the injured finger or from a toe. If the nail bed is completely destroyed and the distal phalanx remains, length can be conserved by replacing the soft-tissue defect with a reversed de-epithelialized cross-finger flap.

34. What is the treatment of large, full-thickness abdominal wounds from exploratory celiotomy in trauma?

The soft tissue and structural components of the defect must be assessed. The presence of bowel contamination or a fistula will have an influence on the timing and the type of reconstruction.

IV bag closure for edematous bowel or abdominal compartment syndrome is best treated with delayed primary closure of the skin and, when possible, the fascia. If the wound is left open because of contamination or nonoperability of the patient, the wound should be allowed to granulate in a moist antimicrobial environment. Once granulation is established, allograft may be used to test the autograft take. Allograft can be placed at the bedside, avoiding the morbidity of an ICU-to-OR transfer.

In a stable patient, when there is a paucity of fascia, an alloplastic material is often used before free fascia lata grafts. The jury is still out as to the best synthetic material to use among marlex, prolene, Vicryl, Dexon, and Gore-Tex. There seems to be insufficient fibrous ingrowth into the absorbable and Gore-Tex products to result in abdominal wall stability. Marlex and prolene meshes are usually well-incorporated but have been associated with occasional fistula formation. A layered combination of Dexon or Vicryl mesh against the bowel with the overlying nonabsorbable mesh sewn to the remaining fascia has resulted in a reliable closure when covered with local flaps.

Large abdominal defects are difficult to manage, especially when fistulae are present. When distal obstruction is ruled out, small bowel fistulae can be closed primarily provided the anastomosis can be covered with a muscle flap. The rectus muscle or musculocutaneous flap can be fashioned to cover most moderate-sized defects of the abdomen. An external oblique flap is an alternative for some defects. An extended latissimus musculocutaneous flap can be designed to cover some areas of the upper portion of the abdomen. Omental flaps with skin grafts can also be used, providing coverage of extremely large defects. Mid- and lower-abdominal defects may be covered with several flaps including rectus abdominis and rectus femoris. Free tissue transfer for abdominal reconstruction may require vein grafting to establish inflow and outflow.

FOOT AND LOWER EXTREMITY INJURIES

35. What is the classification of lower extremity injuries?

The Gustilo and Byrd classifications of open fractures are the standard classification schemes and have implications for reconstructive treatment (see Table). Type III fractures have extensive soft tissue injury as well as significant periosteal stripping and heavy contamination. It is for this class of fractures that the plastic surgeon is most often consulted for flap coverage. Type IIIC fractures are associated with arterial injury requiring repair. Both the infection rate and the necessity for amputation increase as the classification numbers increase.

Gustilo Classification of Open Tibial Fractures

TYPE	INJURY
I	Open fracture with cutaneous defect < 1 cm
II	Open fracture with extensive soft tissue injury
IIIA	Open fracture with extensive soft tissue lacerations; high energy injury
IIIB	Open fracture with soft tissue loss and periosteal stripping, usually with heavy contamination
IIIC	Open fracture with arterial injury requiring repair

Reprinted from Gustilo RB, Anderson JT: Prevention of infection in the treatment of one thousand and twenty-five open fractures of long bones: Retrospective and prospective analyses. J Bone Joint Surg 58A: 453–458, 1976; with permission.

Byrd Classification of Open Tibial Fractures

TYPE	INJURY
1	Low-energy forces causing a spiral or oblique fracture pattern with skin lacerations less than 2 cm and a relatively clean wound
II	Moderate energy forces causing a comminuted or displaced fracture pattern with skin laceration greater than 2 cm and moderate adjacent skin and muscle contusion but without devitalized muscle
III	High-energy forces causing a significantly displaced fracture pattern with severe comminution, segmental fracture, or bone defect with extensive associated skin loss and devitalized muscle
IV	Fracture pattern as in type III but with extreme energy forces as in high-velocity gunshot or shotgun wounds, a history of crush or degloving, or associated vascular injury requiring repair

Reprinted from Byrd HS, Spicer TE, Cierney G 3rd: Management of open tibial fractures. Plast Reconstr Surg 76:719–730, 1985; with permission.

36. What are the considerations in salvage versus amputation in lower extremity trauma?

Neurovascular examination proceeds with clinical examination including color, temperature, capillary refill, and pulse examination as well as Doppler pulse and pressure checks. If the contralateral lower extremity is uninjured, it represents the best control for comparison. The status of the vasculature can change acutely with fracture manipulation or gradually with the onset of a compartment syndrome. Thus, repeat examinations are necessary. Arteriography is the gold standard for anatomic definition of arterial injury. The neurologic examination must consider the autonomous sensory zones. The medial and lateral plantar nerves are both branches of the posterior tibial nerve and accompany their corresponding vessels in the foot. They provide sensation to the medial and lateral aspects of the plantar surface. The first web space is autonomously innervated by the terminal branch of the deep peroneal nerve, while the remaining sensory nerves have wide areas of overlap: the superficial peroneal nerve, the saphenous nerve, the medial calcaneal nerve, and the sural nerve.

37. Describe the reconstruction options of complex lower extremity open fractures.

Soft tissue coverage of the lower extremity is classically divided into proximal, middle, and distal third territories. The procedure of choice for proximal third lesions is the gastrocnemius muscle rotational flap. The medial and lateral heads of the gastrocnemius muscle are supplied by paired sural arteries and originate from the popliteal artery, thereby giving a type I vascular pattern according to Mathes and Nahai classification. Either the medial or lateral head, or both, may be used for wound coverage with little morbidity.

For middle third lesions, the most useful muscle flap is the soleus. The soleus muscle has a type II vascular pattern with a dominant proximal peroneal artery pedicle and secondary distal branches from the posterior tibial and peroneal arteries. There is no significant donor site morbidity. The soleus muscle flap is reliable and hearty when based proximally but is somewhat more tenuous when based on the distal perforating branches.

Distal third wounds of the lower extremity present the greatest challenge to both orthopaedic and plastic reconstructive surgeons. Free muscle transfers provide the best results when soft tissue coverage of open fracture wounds in the lower leg and ankle is required. Although local muscle and fasciocutaneous flaps have been described for coverage of the foot and ankle, the authors have found them to be of little use because of their unpredictable reliability and the consistently high success rates of free tissue transfers.

Replantation in the lower extremity remains limited. Crush and avulsion mechanisms predominate, and nerve regeneration in the lower extremity (LE) is incomplete. Prosthetic devices provide ambulation with lower risk for blood transfusions, sepsis, and prolonged hospitalization. The goal of lower extremity reconstruction is not a closed wound but a functional lower extremity with ambulation.

38. What local factor in the acute treatment of a long-bone fracture leads to nonunion and osteomyelitis?

Sequestered nonvascular tissue and bone are the principle factors leading to wound infection. Inadequate soft tissue coverage and/or a wound edge brought together under tension may become ischemic because the local trauma leads to edema. Inadequate immobilization, soft interposition, and infection may lead to nonunion of the fracture site.

Surgical debridement is necessary when extensive tissue destruction and vascularity have occurred. Often one might not appreciate on superficial inspection that more extensively damaged tissue lies underneath. Therefore, serial debridements in the OR at 48–72 hour intervals may be necessary until the entire area of injury is appreciated. Along with surgical debridement, broad spectrum antibiotics followed by culture specific antibiotics leads to a significant decrease in infection rates (many prospective randomized studies report infection rates decreased from 15% to less than 5%).

BIBLIOGRAPHY

1. Byrd HS, Spicer TE, Cierney G 3d: Management of open tibial fractures. Plast Reconstr Surg 76:719–730, 1985.
2. Crikelair GF: Surgical approach to facial scarring. JAMA 172:140, 1960.
3. Disa JJ, Carlton JM, Goldberg NH: Efficacy of operative cure in pressure sore patients. Plast Reconstr Surg 89:272–278, 1992.
4. Glass KD: Factors related to the resolution of treated hand infections. J Hand Surg 7A:388–394, 1982.
5. Grabb WC, Smith JW: Basic techniques of plastic surgery. In Smith JW, Aston SJ (eds): Plastic Surgery, 4th ed. Boston, Little, Brown, 1991.
6. Gustilo RB, Anderson JT: Prevention of infection in the treatment of one thousand and twenty-five open fractures of long bones: Retrospective and prospective analyses. J Bone Joint Surg 58A:453–458, 1976.
7. Herrmann JB, Kelly RJ, Higgins GA: Polyglycolic acid sutures. Laboratory and clinical evaluation of a new absorbable suture material. Arch Surg 100:486–490, 1970.
8. Kaye JJ: Vibrio vulnificus infections in the hand: Report of three patients. J Bone Joint Surg 72A:283–285, 1990.
9. Levenson SM, et al: The healing of rat skin wounds. Ann Surg 161:293, 1965.
10. Lindan O, Greenway RM, Piazza IM: Pressure distribution on the surface of the human body. Arch Phys Med Rehabil 46:378, 1965.
11. Madden JW, Peacock EE Jr: Studies on the biology of collagen during wound healing. Ann Surg 174:511–520, 1971.
12. Mathes SJ, Abouljoud M: Wound healing. In Davis JH (ed): Clinical Surgery. St. Louis, Mosby, 1987.
13. McCarthy JG (ed): Plastic Surgery: General Principles. Vol. 1. Philadelphia, W.B. Saunders, 1990.
14. McKenna PJ, Lehr GS, Leist P, Welling RE: Antiseptic effectiveness with fibroblast preservation. Ann Plast Surg 27:265–268, 1991.
15. Peacock EE, Cohen IK: Wound healing. In McCarthy JG (ed): Plastic Surgery. Philadelphia, W.B. Saunders, 1990, pp 161–185.
16. Postlethwait RW: Long-term comparative study of nonabsorbable sutures. Ann Surg 171:892–898, 1970.
17. Ruberg RL, Smith DJ: Plastic Surgery: A Core Curriculum. St. Louis, Mosby, 1994.
18. Stromberg BV: Changing bacteriologic flora of hand infections. J Trauma 25:530–533, 1985.

32. SURGICAL NUTRITION

Gideon P. Naudé, M.B.Ch.B.

1. How long should a physician wait before starting nutrition in a patient who is taking nothing orally?

If it is clear after 3 days that a trauma victim will not be taking anything orally in the immediate future, enteral or parenteral nutrition should be started.

2. What are the usual fluid requirements under basal conditions?

Basal free water requirements are 30 to 35 mL/kg/day.

3. What increases the fluid requirements?

Fluid requirements are increased by fluid loss, as occurs with fever through perspiration and from wounds, burns, fistulas, vomiting, diarrhea, third spacing, and other abnormal losses, including bleeding.

4. What intravenous nutrition is administered through a peripheral vein?

Peripheral parenteral nutrition (PPN) with low dextrose (5%) and a low concentration of amino acids is administered through a peripheral vein. The concentration of dextrose and amino acids must be low, because in higher doses, they are irritating and cause phlebitis. Peripheral nutrition does not usually supply all the patient's needs.

5. What is total parenteral nutrition?

With total parenteral nutrition (TPN), the concentrations of dextrose and amino acids are sufficiently high to supply all the patient's needs. The problem of phlebitis does not occur because the flow in a central vein is very high and dilution occurs almost instantly.

6. What is the indication for TPN?

TPN is administered when no functional gastrointestinal tract is available.

7. Are complications associated with central vein catheter placement?

Central vein catheter placement usually is a relatively safe procedure, but the following complications may occur:

Early complications:
- Pneumothorax and hemothorax can occur if the needle enters the pleural cavity (particularly subclavian catheters). A chest drain may be necessary.
- Arterial puncture is indicated by bright red bleeding. Apply pressure for a few minutes, and check distal pulses.
- The catheter may track up the jugular vein. Reposition and check the new position with a radiograph.
- Cardiac arrhythmia may occur if the catheter is intracardiac. Pull the catheter back.
- Brachial plexus injury
- Thoracic duct injury
- Cardiac perforation and tamponade
- Mediastinal hematoma
- Embolism (e.g., catheter, air)

Late complications:
- Thrombosis with embolization
- Infection and septic emboli

8. What are the usual daily calorie requirements?
The usual daily calorie requirements are 30 to 35 cal/kg.

9. How do you calculate daily calorie requirements?
Use the Harris-Benedict equation to calculate the daily calorie requirements:
Male = 66.5 + (13.7 × wt [kg]) + (5 × ht [cm]) − (6.7 × age [yr]) × activity factor × injury factor
Female = 665.1 + (9.6 × wt [kg]) + (1.8 × ht [cm]) − (4.7 × age [yr]) × activity factor × injury factor
The daily calorie requirements also can be estimated:
To maintain weight: 30 to 35 cal/kg
To lose weight: 25 to 30 cal/kg
To gain weight: 35 to 40 cal/kg

10. What increases the calorie requirements?
The factors influencing the calorie requirements are activity and injury.

Activity	Activity Factor	Injury	Injury Factor
Basal	1.2	Trauma	1.2–1.8
Normal	1.3	Surgery	1.1–1.2
Fever	1.3	Sepsis	1.4–1.8

11. How is the increased calorie requirement calculated?
The activity factor and injury factor are multiplied in the Harris-Benedict equation (see Question 9).

12. What is the daily protein requirement?
The daily protein requirement is 1 to 1.5 g/kg of lean body weight.

13. How is the daily protein requirement administered?
It is given in the form of amino acids. The usual amount is 1 to 1.5 g/kg, but it may be as high as 3 g/kg. Branched-chain amino acids (i.e., leucine, isoleucine, and valine) are thought to decrease the breakdown of muscle during catabolism.

14. What are the average daily requirements of electrolytes for adults, and how are they given?
The normal daily requirements of electrolytes for an average adult may be given intravenously:
- Sodium: 60 to 150 mEq
- Potassium: 60 to 100 mEq
- Calcium, magnesium, and phosphate administration depends on the need as determined by the blood concentration of the substance.

15. How does an essential fatty acid deficiency manifest during intravenous nutrition, and how is it prevented?
It manifests mostly in the skin and its appendages as dry and scaly skin and as hair loss. Giving lipid solutions prevents this deficiency.

16. How are lipids administered?
Lipids are administered in the form of long-chain fatty acids. These consist of linolenic acid (60%) and stearic, oleic, palmitic, and linoleic acids. They are prepared in the form of a 10% or 20% solution. Before starting a lipid infusion, the patient's serum lipid levels are determined, and if they are elevated, lipid administration is contraindicated because it causes pancreatitis. Lipid

administration is started at 0.5 g/kg/day and increased by 0.5 g/kg/day every few days to a maximum of 2.5 g/kg/day.

17. Which vitamins are added to TPN, and how much of each is administered to an adult?

Vitamin	Amount
Fat soluble	
A	2500 IU/day
D	250 IU/day
E	10–15 IU/day
K	10 mg/wk–10 mg/day
Water soluble	
B_1 (thiamine)	5 mg/day
B_2 (riboflavin)	5 mg/day
B_3 (niacin)	50 mg/day
B_6 (pyridoxine)	5 mg/day
B_{12} (cyanocobalamin)	12 μg/day
Biotin	60 μg/day
Folic acid	600 μg/day
Pantothenic acid	15 mg/day
C	50–300 mg/day

18. What are the necessary trace elements?
Chromium, cobalt, copper, iodine, iron, manganese, selenium, and zinc are required trace elements.

19. How are trace elements administered?
Chromium, copper, iodine, iron, selenium, and zinc are administered with the TPN. Cobalt is given in the form of vitamin B_{12}, and manganese deficiency does not occur while on parenteral nutrition.

20. How is TPN calculated?
Because exact calculation of TPN is difficult, a slight excess of all nutrients is given. Water is given in a volume of 30 to 35 mL/kg, and more is given if increased losses occur. Caloric intake should be 30 to 35 cal/kg, more if stressed, given in the form of carbohydrates (dextran) or fats (intralipid). Proteins are given as amino acids in a dose of 1.5 g/kg, but the amount needed may be as high as 3 g/kg. Electrolytes, vitamins, and trace elements are given as described earlier.

21. What are the indications for enteral feeding?
The patient has a functional alimentary tract but is unable to take meals orally because of the following conditions:
Major head and neck injuries and reconstruction procedures
Esophageal injuries or obstructions
Chronic starvation and debilitation because appetite is lacking

22. How can enteral feeding be administered?
Enteral feeding is administered by long tubes, such as the nasogastric or nasoduodenal tubes, that can be placed while the patient is in the ward. The tubes may also be placed operatively in the form of gastrostomies and jejunostomies.

23. Are there complications to the placement of an enteral feeding tube?
• Nonoperatively placed (nasogastric and nasoduodenal) tubes may be misplaced in the trachea or curl up in the esophagus, causing aspiration when feeding is started. In unsuspected cases of ileus, gastric dilatation and subsequent vomiting may occur.

- Perforation of the esophagus may occur.
- As with any surgical procedure, complications can occur with the placement of gastrostomy and jejunostomy tubes. The most common complications of operatively placed (gastrostomy and jejunostomy) tubes are bleeding, infection, and dislodgment of the tube with intraperitoneal soiling of bowel contents and nutritional formula, which leads to peritonitis.

24. When are nasogastric tubes used, and when are nasojejunal tubes used?

Nasogastric feeding can be used if there is a low risk of aspiration, if the patient is conscious and alert, and if there is no history of reflux esophagitis. Nasojejunal feeding is used if there is a high risk of aspiration.

25. What are the causes of diarrhea in patients receiving enteral nutrition?

- Diarrhea is common with any form of enteral feeding. Mechanical causes are solutions that are too cold, hypertonic solutions, boluses that are too large, and low- or no-salt solutions.
- Infective causes include bacterial contamination of the bag or, if antibiotics have been used, staphylococcal or fungal overgrowth or *Clostridium difficile* infection.
- Medications, fat intolerance, and lactose intolerance also produce diarrhea.

26. What are the basic types of enteral nutrition?

Polymeric, elemental, and modular types of enteral nutrition are available.

27. How would you differentiate the types of enteral nutrition?

- *Polymeric diets* contain large molecular forms of protein, carbohydrates, and fat. Proteins are in the form of whole proteins, sugar is in the form of sucrose and corn sugar, and fat is in the form of oils. This is the most physiologic form of enteral nutrition for patients with normally functioning alimentary tracts who are unable to eat.
- *Elemental diets* (i.e., defined formulas) are predigested. The sugars are in the form of monosaccharides and disaccharides, protein is in the form of amino acids, and fat is in the form of medium- and long-chain triglycerides. These diets are for patients without the ability to digest their food normally, such as those with short bowel syndrome, intestinal fistulas, or pancreatic insufficiency in which the digestive enzymes are lacking. They are less physiologic than polymeric diets, do not maintain the intestinal mucosa as well, and cost more.
- *Modular diets* are broken down to their component parts—separate containers of protein, fat, carbohydrate, essential trace elements, and electrolytes. These components can be combined to suit specific needs, such as for patients with diabetes, liver, or renal failure and for patients with various forms of nutritional intolerance.

28. What is an indication that enteral feeding would not be tolerated?

Obstruction, high-output ileus, fistulas, diarrhea, or any condition producing a gastrointestinal loss of more than 600 mL/day (i.e., nasogastric, fistula, or rectal loss) may contraindicate enteral feeding.

29. Are enteral nutrition and TPN superior to oral feeding?

No. Oral feeding is superior to any artificial method because the stimulus of eating causes the secretion of enzymes and hormones vital for digestion, absorption, and use of nutrients. Enteral feeding is less effective than oral feeding, and TPN is less effective than either.

30. How would you assess the results of surgical nutrition?

Catabolism is converted to anabolism as evidenced by the nitrogen balance, which can be calculated as follows:

$$\text{Nitrogen balance (g/day)} = \frac{\text{Protein intake (g/day)}}{6.25} - (\text{Urinary urea nitrogen [g/day]} + 4)$$

A positive result greater than $+2$ g/day indicates anabolism. Albumin is a good indicator of nutrition, and albumin increasing to normal levels (>3.5 g/dL) is a sign of adequate nutritional support. Weight gain is not reliable because edema may cause weight gain.

31. When may surgical nutrition be stopped?
    Surgical nutrition may be stopped when the patient is able to ingest adequate amounts orally or when a patient on TPN is changed to enteral feeding of sufficient volume to adequately satisfy all of the nutritional needs. When TPN is stopped, it should be reduced gradually over many hours to prevent reactive hypoglycemia.

BIBLIOGRAPHY

1. Apelgren KN, Dean RE: Enteral Feeding in Long-Term Care. Chicago, Precept Press, 1990.
2. Barker LR, Burton JR, Zieve PD: Ambulatory Medicine, 4th ed. Baltimore, Williams & Wilkins, 1994.
3. Bongard FS, Stamos MJ, Passaro E: Surgery: A Clinical Approach. New York, Churchill Livingstone, 1997.
4. Civeta JM, Tatlor RW, Kirby RR: Critical Care, 2nd ed. Philadelphia, Lippincott-Raven, 1992.
5. Skipper A (ed): Dietitian's Handbook of Enteral and Parenteral Nutrition, 2nd ed. Gaithersburg, MD, Aspen, 1998.

XI. Special Types of Trauma

33. BURNS

Stefan R. Schirber, M.D., and Kenneth Waxman, M.D.

1. What is the incidence of burn injury in the United States?

Burn injuries have declined steadily over the past decades. Approximately 1.25 million people are treated annually for burns. Seventy-five percent of these patients have burns that cover less than 10% of total body surface area (TBSA).

2. What are the causes of burn injury?

Burns result from contact with thermal substances (i.e., heat) and from chemicals. Liquids, solids, flame, radiation, and electricity can all produce burns.

3. What is the first priority of burn resuscitation?

As with any trauma, life-threatening injuries take first priority. ABCs (airway, breathing, and circulation) should be evaluated and stabilized. The extent of the burn can then be estimated (% TBSA) and appropriate fluids begun. The secondary survey should then take place so that attention to associated injuries can be performed. Warm dressings and tetanus status are also provided at this stage.

4. What is the tissue response to a burn injury?

After a burn, fluid accumulates rapidly in the wound and, to a lesser extent, in the unburned tissues. A burn of 15–20% TBSA or greater will cause hypovolemic shock if not adequately resuscitated. Edema response is most rapid in the first 6–8 hours postburn, but continues for at least 18–24 hours. Locally released inflammatory mediators from platelets, macrophages, and leukocytes contribute to hyperpermeability of the microcirculation. Regional blood flow increases with a concomitant rise in capillary pressure. Denatured protein (coagulated by heat) may further perpetuate wound edema via osmotic and hydrostatic gradients.

5. What is eschar?

Eschar is nonviable, inelastic skin destroyed by intensive thermal damage. Early excision of eschar is important in preventing neurovascular constriction of extremities or ventilatory compromise when the chest is involved. Additionally, eschar may harbor pathogenic bacteria.

6. How are burns classified?

Burns are classified according to depth as follows:

Burn Classification

	SIGNS AND SYMPTOMS	RESULT
First degree	Erythema, pain	Healing within 1–2 weeks
Second degree	Erythema, pain, bullae, and moisture from fluid extravasation	Spontaneous healing from residual epithelial cells
Third degree	Dark, charred eschar; white dry patches; insensitive to pain	Requires topical antibiotics; susceptible to infection; healing via contracture or grafting
Fourth degree	Involvement with muscle or bone	Major reconstruction or amputation required

7. How do you determine the percentage of body surface area involved?

The common clinical means to estimate TBSA involved in a burn is by the "rule of nines." In the rule of nines, the TBSA is divided into areas of 9% each. Head and upper extremities are 9% each, each lower extremity and anterior and posterior torso is 18%. The palm of the hand is approximately 1% TBSA. Because of the relatively greater surface area occupied by the head during infancy and early childhood, a Lund-Browder chart allows a more accurate estimate for this subgroup.

8. What are the signs and symptoms of an inhalation injury?

History and high index of suspicion should alert one to the possibility of an inhalation injury. Laryngoscopy should be performed in any patient with possible inhalation injury. Evidence of supraglottic edema or erythema heralds such an injury, and early, prophylactic endotracheal intubation should be performed to prevent loss of airway. Later, upper airway obstruction may be manifested by altered phonation, stridor, intercostal retractions, and cyanosis.

9. What produces an inhalation injury?

Inhalation injury may be attributed to three components: thermal injury, carbon monoxide (and HCN) poisoning and chemical injury. The thermal injury results from direct heat exposure and is usually limited to the supraglottic area. Carbon monoxide, a byproduct of organic combustion, is commonly inhaled. The affinity of CO for hemoglobin is 300 times greater than that of O_2. CO also binds the cytochrome system, thereby decreasing oxygen delivery. Subsequent hypoxia may lead to encephalopathy and renal failure. Treatment involves 100% O_2, which decreases the half-life of carboxyhemoglobin from 4.5 hours to 50 minutes. Chemical injury stems from corrosive gases and chemical irritants, which are inhaled and are subsequently drawn deep into the lungs. Damage to type 2 pneumocytes will then lead to loss of surfactant production and alveolar volume.

10. How does one cover a burn?

Superficial, partial-thickness burns may be treated with daily dressings, local wound care, and topical antibiotics until epithelialization occurs. Temporary coverage with allograft or xenograft may also be performed and may decrease pain and the need for daily dressing changes. These grafts are particularly well-suited to young children and uncooperative patients. Deep, partial-thickness burns have also been shown to have better functional outcome (i.e., improved joint mobility and decreased hypertrophic scarring) when early, aggressive debridement and grafting is performed. Twenty years ago, Janzekovic demonstrated that early removal of burned tissue by tangential excision reduced pain, number of operations, mortality, blood loss, and the length of hospital stay. Full-thickness burns should be treated by removal of devitalized tissue (debridement) and grafting with autologous skin grafts, if possible.

11. How should fluid resuscitation be performed?

Historically, burn shock (hypovolemia) due to inadequate fluid resuscitation was the main cause of mortality with major burns. Aggressive fluid resuscitation techniques were started in the 1960s and '70s primarily with crystalloids such as lactated Ringer's solution (LR) or normal saline (NS). These techniques have shifted the mortality away from burn shock to burn sepsis. Many formulas exist for fluid resuscitation in burn patients and are based on burn size (TBSA). The most common is the Parkland formula, which calculates the 24-hour fluid requirements as 4 ml/kg/% TBSA using LR solution. One half of this total is given during the first 8 hours, and the remaining half is given over the subsequent 16 hours postburn. However, fluid rates in practice must be continuously titrated to the patient's physiologic responses.

12. What is the role of antibiotics in burn cases?

Prophylactic intravenous antibiotics are not justified in burn cases and serve only to select out resistant bacteria. Topical antibiotics should be used in second and third degree burns. Of the available topical agents, three have proven efficacy. Mafenide acetate has excellent penetration of eschar, but acts as a carbonic anhydrase inhibitor and is associated with metabolic acidosis. Silver nitrate is also acceptable, yet leaches electrolytes and stains local tissues. The most common agent, silver sulfadiazine (Silvadene), has excellent coverage with low toxicity. Silvadene can cause a transient leukopenia as well.

13. What should be the initial challenge in the traumatic, hypovolemic burn patient?

Infusion of 2–3 L of warmed LR and reassessment of vital signs should be performed. If the patient remains hypotensive, type specific or O negative blood should be ordered. Additionally, clotting factors and platelets should be available in anticipation of a potential consumptive coagulopathy (DIC). If external bleeding is not present and hypotension persists, an internal bleeding source has to be ruled out.

14. What is the best IV access in a multitrauma burn patient?

At least two large-bore (16-gauge or larger) peripheral IVs are required. If no veins are available percutaneously, a venous cutdown should be performed as far distally on the extremity as possible to allow for serial IV changes via more proximal cutdowns on that extremity. Small children may require intraosseous IV access by a large-bore needle distal to the tibial tuberosity into the marrow.

15. Are traditional ventilators the best treatment option in the severely burned patient with inhalation injury?

High-frequency percussive ventilation (HFPV) is currently the only proven treatment method for lowering morbidity and mortality with inhalation injury. HFPV prevents pneumonia, decreases intrapulmonary shunt, lowers peak inspiratory pressure, and, to some degree, decreases PEEP and mean airway pressure.

16. Should patients with inhalation injury be given prophylactic antibiotics or steroids?

Neither IV antibiotics nor steroids have been shown to be beneficial prophylactically. In the case of a known pathogen, specific IV antibiotic therapy is clearly indicated. Otherwise, topical antibiotics should be applied to burned areas.

17. Is urine output (UOP) a reliable indicator of adequate fluid resuscitation?

In smaller burns (< 30% TBSA), a UOP of 1 ml/kg/hr may be adequate for assessing perfusion and indeed is the basis, along with vital signs, for the fluid resuscitation formulas. For larger burns, UOP is an unreliable indicator and invasive monitoring is required.

18. When is a Swan-Ganz catheter indicated?

All severe and most moderate burns require placement of a Swan-Ganz or pulmonary artery (PA) catheter for optimal volume resuscitation. The PA catheter allows improved guidance in delivering fluid or blood to increase the cardiac index and oxygen delivery (DO_2) to achieve a venous saturation greater than 65%. Once hypovolemia is corrected, inotropic agents may be introduced to increase cardiac output if necessary. Measurement of PA parameters allows careful adjustment of cardiac performance.

19. Does cardiac output (CO) decrease in the traumatic burn patient?

Cardiac output can decrease as much as 50% by 1 minute postburn and return to 33% of baseline at 1 hour postburn in a patient with a 50% TBSA burn. Decreased cardiac contractility has been demonstrated as left ventricle dysfunction via ultrasound studies specifically in postburn rather than nonburn trauma patients.

20. What happens to normal metabolism in the burned patient?

Burn patients exhibit a prolonged hypermetabolic state lasting several weeks. Massive protein catabolism and lipolysis occur during this time. Increased catecholamines, loss of water and heat, and sepsis all contribute to this accelerated metabolism.

21. What is the role of nutrition in the burned patient?

Enteral nutrition is the preferred route and is second only to adequate fluid resuscitation in reducing septic complications and improving overall survival. Nasogastric tube (NGT) placement with subsequent feeding should take place immediately. A diet of 80–100:1 calorie-to-nitrogen ratio with omega-3 and omega-6 fatty acids, glutamine, and fiber should be implemented. Decreased translocation of gut bacteria and fewer septic complications have been shown with this regimen.

22. Do feeding jejunostomy tubes play a role?

Patients with multitrauma undergoing abdominal exploration should have jejunostomy tubes (J-tubes) placed even with ileus and anastomoses. Gastric residuals are checked every 4 hours and tube feeds held if greater than 150 cc. Persistent residuals may be treated with metoclopramide, cisapride, or IV erythromycin, in that order, with the caveat that increased residuals may signal a septic event.

23. How does one achieve adequate pain control with burned patients?

Pain control is extremely important in burn cases and should include frequent reassessment and patient-controlled analgesia, when possible. Visual analog scales (e.g., assigning values to poker chips for children and using numbers 1–10 for adults) may be implemented. Infants and verbally impaired patients require an observer pain scale. Additionally, patients with significant trauma or burns who are intubated may require opiates, amnestics, or paralysis.

24. How can one avoid catheter sepsis?

It is important to change all lines placed on admission within 24 hours. One should use clinical judgment in guiding line changes and culture catheter tips for temperatures greater than 102°F or other signs of sepsis.

25. When should rehabilitation begin?

Rehabilitation should begin on the day of injury and proceed with a multidisciplinary approach. Physical therapy should begin early on with particular attention to the areas of the head, neck, and hands. This should help prevent the most costly aspects of burn injuries: loss of work productivity and chronic rehabilitation.

26. Should cultured epidermal autografts be used?

In patients with massive burns, cultured cells are an option. However, cultured cells are expensive and result in high failure rates, scarring, and poor coverage. Their use should be reserved for selected cases of massive burn injury.

27. How can one decrease scarring?

Scarring is variable depending on many different skin types, but keeping the wounds moist and applying pressure garments have been shown to help.

BIBLIOGRAPHY

1. Achauer BM: Treating the burn wound. In Achauer BM (ed): Management of the Burned Patient. Norwalk, CT, Appleton & Lange, 1987, pp 93–109.
2. Dougherty W, Waxman K: The complexities of managing severe burns with associated trauma. Surg Clin North Am 76:923–958, 1996.
3. Janzekovic Z: A new concept in the early excision and immediate grafting of burns. J Trauma 15:42–62, 1975.
4. Monafo WW: Initial management of burns. N Engl J Med 335:1581–1586, 1996.
5. Nguyen TT: Current treatment of severely burned patients. Ann Surg 223:14–25, 1996.

34. CHEMICAL BURNS

Thuan T. Nguyen, M.D., and Justin D. Merszei, M.D.

1. What are the common sources of chemical exposures leading to chemical burns?

A chemical injury may be encountered by all walks of life. More than 25,000 products capable of causing serious chemical injuries are currently marketed for use in the home and for agriculture and industry. Many of these chemicals are used daily to clean kitchens, bathrooms, and to bleach hair and laundry. Dangerous exposures may follow occupational use of industrial chemicals because of their increased concentration. In addition, these burns are commonly associated with injury to a large total body surface area (TBSA).

2. How does the pathophysiology of a chemical burn differ from a thermal burn?

Application of heat or chemicals, especially pH disturbances, can cause biological structures to break down. In thermal injuries, there is a rapid coagulation of proteins due to irreversible cross-linking reactions during thermal contact; with chemical burns the protein destruction continues long after the initial insult. Therefore, the primary difference between chemical burns and thermal burns is that chemical burns do not necessarily destroy tissue by hyperthermic activity, rather chemical agents cause injury by altering tissue proteins, disrupting cellular metabolism, and a variety of other chemical reactions.

3. How are the common agents involved in chemical burns classified?

Chemical agents that cause burns are classified based on the reactions that the chemical is prone to initiate. In general, there are four broad chemical classes. **Acids** lower pH by donating protons. Free hydrogen ions can protonate any amine or carboxylic site thereby destroying protein structure. In addition, concentrated acids can injure tissue through heat generation and desiccation. **Bases** are hydrogen ion acceptors. Bases will strip protons from amine and carboxylic groups destroying protein structure. Furthermore, bases can form salts and soaps, causing additional tissue damage. **Organic compounds** such as phenol and petroleum-based compounds cause protein destruction by chemical reactions, heat production, and possibly by acting as a solvent. **Inorganic agents** such as sodium, phosphorus, and chlorine damage tissue by direct binding, salt formation, and heat production. As a general rule, concentrated solutions are more viscous, more reactive, more hygroscopic, and liberate more heat during lavage or neutralization. Since all four classes of chemicals cause damage by more than one chemical reaction, it is more useful to group each chemical agent by its predominant mechanism of tissue destruction. The six primary mechanisms of tissue destruction are:

1. **Reduction:** caused by the reduction of the amide linkages following exposure to reducing agents. These agents are rare, highly reactive chemicals, such as metal hydrides.

2. **Oxidation:** damages tissue by adding an oxygen, sulfur, or halogen to proteins, thereby altering or destroying physiological function. Examples are sodium hypochlorite, potassium permanganate, chromic acid, and peroxides.

3. **Corrosive agents:** compounds such as phenols and metallic hydroxides act to corrode skin and denature proteins, by a variety of mechanisms not completely understood.

4. **Protoplasmic poisons:** some compounds such as formic and acetic acid destroy protein function by forming esters. Other compounds in this class, such as oxalic and hydrofluoric acid, bind inorganic ions thereby interfering with normal cellular function.

5. **Desiccants:** concentrated sulfuric acid and other hygroscopic agents cause tissue damage by extracting water. In addition, desiccants can generate heat by an exothermic reaction causing additional tissue damage.

6. **Vesicants:** include chemical warfare agents such as mustards, arsenicals, and halogenated oximes that are typically characterized by their ability to cause blisters. Vesicants damage tissue

by a variety of mechanisms including the alkylation of DNA and perhaps the release of proteases from lysosomes.

4. What is the appropriate emergency management of a patient suspected of having a chemical burn?

Whether at the geographic site of injury or in the emergency department, it is important to know the exact causative agent as soon as possible because the degree of local tissue damage and the level of systemic toxicity are determined by the duration of skin contact. In addition, the anatomic location of the burn, the amount of surface area exposed, its mechanism of injury, and the chemical concentration are all factors that influence the extent of local and systemic injury. Since the duration of chemical exposure can be manipulated, it is extremely important to promptly remove the chemical to prevent further tissue damage. This includes removal of all clothing and brushing dry chemicals off the skin, followed by copious lavage at the scene of injury or in the emergency department. Lavaging is believed to dilute the chemical agent, attenuate the chemical reaction, suppress any elevated tissue metabolism, have an anti-inflammatory action, suppress hygroscopic action, and return pH to normal levels. In addition, constant water flow will dissipate any heat of dilution that is produced. Delaying treatment for such injuries until resuscitation has been successfully completed may be harmful, because the chemical may have a prolonged action and produce serious metabolic effects. In one study, the incidence of full-thickness burns was five times greater among patients who did not receive irrigation within 10 minutes of chemical contact (see algorithm).

5. In what situations is water lavage not indicated initially and what special methods should be used to minimize the absorption of these chemical agents?

As stated in the previous question, early water lavage effectively reduces the severity of injury from chemical burns. However, chemicals such as muriatic acid, hydrosulfuric acid, hydrochloric acid, and sodium metal create significant exothermy in combination with water, and, therefore, should not be lavaged. Since muriatic acid, concentrated sulfuric acid, and hydrochloric acid produce heat when water is added, these burns should be neutralized with soap or lime water before lavage. Sodium metal forms sodium hydroxide and heat in the presence of water; it has a propensity to explode. Accordingly, sodium metal burns should be covered with oil and, when indicated, should be excised. Other chemicals, such as phenol, are insoluble in water and should be diluted with an oil-based solubilizing agent such as polyethylene glycol. In addition, dry lime reacts with water to form an injurious alkali and, therefore, should be brushed off the skin before lavage.

6. Describe the process of lavaging or dilution.

The immediate treatment after a chemical injury consists of lavaging the burned area with copious volumes of tap water. "Tubbing" or immersion therapy in a burn tank is not recommended because it increases the risk of nosocomial infection, electrolyte imbalances, and hypothermia. Furthermore, tank immersion risks introducing chemicals diluted by the tank water to other areas of the body.

A shower lavage by a hand-held unit over a hydrotherapy tank is recommended. Some authors recommend irrigating up to 6–8 hours for alkali burns and beyond for patients with continued pain. Since acid burns are generally less invasive, the duration of irrigation can be shorter than that required for a similar alkali burn. Some clinicians believe that a gross endpoint to lavaging is when the patient no longer experiences pain. However, it must be remembered that some chemical burns are not associated with pain yet still require copious irrigation. These patients must be managed based on the severity of the burn and the concentration of the involved chemical.

7. Describe the typical appearance of a chemical burn.

Chemical injuries may appear deceptively harmless and superficial immediately after exposure. The unusual tanning and local anesthetic properties of some chemicals make it notoriously

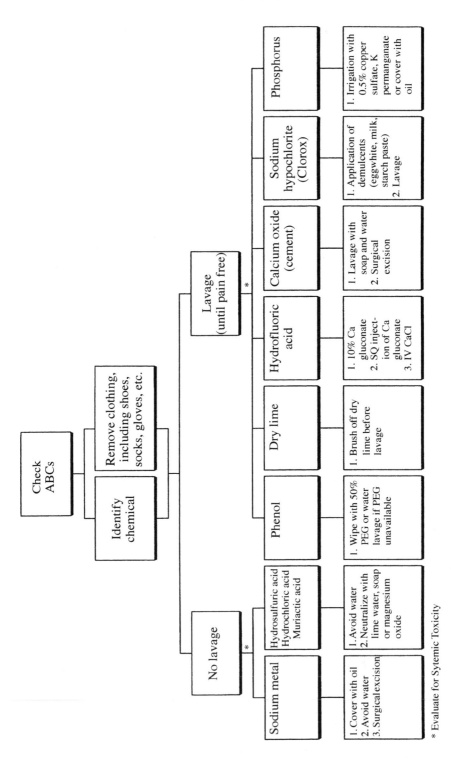

Algorithm for the emergency treatment of chemical burns.

difficult to estimate the depth and extent of these burns. Moreover, different chemical burns present with unique characteristics making it harder for a clinician to manage cases based on experience. After the first 48–72 hours following injury, changes in the appearance of the surface wound frequently reflect the true depth of necrosis. Frequently, the extent and depth of the burn are underestimated resulting in insufficient fluid resuscitation.

8. What common systemic toxicities are related to chemical burns?

Systemic toxicities are associated with ingestion or cutaneous contact through the wound. Although the more common chemicals involved in burns are associated with specific manifestations, systemic symptoms may overlap and present in an odd manner. Chemical burns often do not cause pain initially. Since the injury is subtle, the patient is not aware of the burn until an extended duration of exposure has passed. This can lead to a delay in diagnosis resulting in a more severe injury, locally and systemically.

Chemical burns are commonly associated with specific toxicities. Hydrofluoric acid causes hypocalcemia inducing cardiac arrhythmias, especially ventricular fibrillation. Absorption of petroleum distillates may cause pulmonary hemorrhages, cardiac arrhythmias, and renal and hepatic damage. Absorption of formic acid can cause intravascular hemolysis, renal failure, and necrotizing pancreatitis. White phosphorus can cause ventricular arrhythmias and hepatic and renal damage. In addition, chemical burns can cause inhalation injury either because of smoke or an aerosolized chemical. These injuries are managed like smoke inhalation injuries, with airway protection and supplemental oxygen. Prophylactic steroid and antibiotic treatment is not indicated for chemical inhalation injuries.

9. What are alkali burns, and what is their typical clinical course?

Multiple chemical agents are involved in caustic alkali burns. Alkalis are the most common chemicals around the home. They are the active products used in cleaning agents, garden lime, fertilizers, cement, and unblocking drains. Some examples of these agents are lime, potassium hydroxide, and sodium hydroxide. As a rule, alkalis produce less immediate damage than acids, but ultimately cause more tissue destruction owing to three predominant mechanisms of injury: saponification of fat, extraction of water from cells, and dissolving tissue proteins to form alkaline proteinates, which are involved in further chemical reactions. As already mentioned, alkali burns initially appear superficial and benign, but if left untreated they can progress to a full-thickness injury. Since alkalis liquefy tissue, deeper penetration of the agent occurs that frequently requires excision of necrotic tissue and resurfacing. Note that neutralizing agents should not be used to treat alkali burns. The heat of neutralization may only accentuate the severity of injury. Treatment consists of copious water lavage for 6–8 hours, or longer if pain persists.

10. How do acid burns differ from alkali burns?

Acids lower pH by donating protons. These protons are reactive and will destroy protein structure in the wound. Eventually, hydrogen ions will catalyze protein hydrolysis into constituent amino acids. Classifying a chemical burn as an acid burn is a very broad classification. Keep in mind, there are other mechanisms involved in tissue damage. For example, sulfuric acid injures tissue by heat generation and desiccation. Phosphoric acid can cause a mixed chemical injury by chelating calcium. In general, acids form a hard eschar that may help protect the underlying tissue from further chemical burn. As with alkali burns, neutralizing agents are contraindicated owing to the possibility of generating an exothermic reaction augmenting tissue injury.

11. Describe wet cement burn.

Calcium oxide (cement) is an alkali that, when mixed with water, sand, and gravel, becomes concrete. Wet cement is caustic, with a pH as high as 12.9, and can cause a full-thickness alkali burn. Such injuries usually occur in amateur cement workers who handle, kneel, or walk barefoot in wet cement. In addition to alkali injury, cement can also penetrate clothing and react exothermically with sweat. The dry cement powder is very hygroscopic and can cause a desiccation re-action injuring the skin. Typically, the symptoms of pain and burning to not appear until several hours after exposure. Prolonged irrigation of the area is essential. Often surgical excision of these burns is required owing to the depth of injury.

12. Describe the typical presentation, mechanism, and treatment of a Clorox burn?
Sodium hypochlorite (household liquid chlorine bleach such as Clorox) is used as a disinfectant, deodorant, and bleach. Although there is no clinical data, typical household solutions of 4–6% are probably only lethal to adults in extremely large doses. On the contrary, as little as 30 ml of 15% available chlorine concentration may cause a severe injury. Tissue damage occurs by corrosion and protein coagulation of skin and mucus membranes. Sodium hypochlorite is a potent oxidizing agent in an alkaline solution; the mechanism of injury is thought to be through its own oxidation. Clinically, burn severity is determined by concentration rather than the duration of tissue contact. Early symptoms are pain, inflammation, and irritation at the site of injury. Therapy comprises immediate ingestion or application of demulcents such as milk, eggwhite, starch paste, milk of magnesia, and aluminum hydroxide followed by lavage. Sodium bicarbonate is contraindicated because it causes the release of carbon dioxide.

13. Describe the typical clinical presentation and the initial treatment of a patient with phenol burn.
These chemical burns generally present as a benign partial-thickness lesions. At times, phenol imparts a dull gray color to the skin that may progress to black gangrene. Phenol is absorbed through intact skin and across the lungs as a vapor. Systemically, phenol is a central nervous system (CNS) stimulant that can cause hyperreflexia and convulsions. CNS depression follows, and respiratory arrest may occur. In addition, phenol demyelinates and destroys peripheral nerves causing anesthesia at the site of contact. Phenol also causes cardiac depression, liver necrosis, and renal failure. Smoky colored urine is often associated with phenol burns owing to systemic toxicity. Since phenol is not soluble in water, topical application of polyethylene glycol (PEG) or vegetable oil is beneficial in these injuries followed by lavage. Even though undiluted PEG is the best solvent, copious water irrigation should be initiated when PEG is not immediately available. Immediate recognition of the severity of phenol burns and correct initial treatment may prevent significant morbidity and mortality in these burn patients.

14. In what settings are phosphorus burns seen? What is the mechanism of injury and how should these injuries be treated?
Organic phosphorus is an incendiary agent used in a variety of weapons including hand grenades, motor bombs, and artillery shells. Phosphorus is also found in fireworks and fertilizers, which is the likely source for burns in a civilian population. Red phosphorus is insoluble, nonabsorbable, and nonvolatile and therefore nontoxic. Yellow phosphorus, which is commonly called white phosphorus, is insoluble in water but readily soluble in most oils. On exposure to air, phosphorus fumes may spontaneously burst into flames. Contact with skin is associated with a painful second or third degree burn due to both the chemical and thermal components of the agent. In addition, the combustion products of phosphorus are a variety of oxides and polyphosphates that can bind calcium, causing systemic toxicity. The chemical mechanism will progress until all the phosphorus is oxidized or starved of oxygen when immersed in water.

The phosphorus burn injury is typically yellow, necrotic, and painful, and smells of garlic. As with other chemical burns, the patient's clothing must be removed immediately. Care must be taken with the clothing of patients involved in phosphorus burns because the clothing may ignite. If lavage is not possible during transportation, the burn wound should be covered with saline, or water-soaked dressing until the patient reaches the hospital. The wound should then be irrigated with copious amounts of saline or water while removing large particles of phosphorus. Specific therapy of phosphorus burns is irrigation with 0.5% copper sulfate solution or potassium permanganate (1:5000) or by covering the wound with liquid petrolatum. This antidote forms a black film of cupric oxide on the surface of the wound, impeding oxidation and allowing the easy removal of the white phosphorus. Solutions stronger than 1% copper sulfate have caused intravascular hemolysis and renal failure and are, therefore, contraindicated.

Organic phosphorous compounds such as parathion are toxic cholinesterase inhibitors and are associated with severe systemic toxicity. In addition, hypocalcemia and hyperphosphatemia further augment electrolyte disturbances and have been reported to cause fatal cardiac arrhythmias. Acute fatty degeneration of the liver due to phosphorous toxicity can cause jaundice, decreased protein synthesis, hypoglycemia, and hemorrhage because of the depletion of clotting factors.

15. In what occupational setting are hydrofluoric acid burns seen? Describe its mechanism of injury.

Hydrofluoric acid is a very corrosive, inorganic acid of elemental fluorine that is used in the manufacturing of many products including plastics, pottery glazing, and rust removers. Burns can occur through small perforations in a work glove, accidental splashing, or the failure of workers to recognize the threat of the benign-looking solution of acid.

There are two mechanisms of injury. The immediate injury is due to the high tissue hydrogen ion concentration that occurs in all acid burns and produces a typical caustic skin injury that alters the skin's normal protective barrier. The second mechanism is subtle yet more serious: soluble free fluoride ions penetrate the damaged skin and cause a liquefactive necrosis of the soft tissues, decalcification of bone, and local dehydration. The process of destruction can go on for many hours or even days resulting in extensive damage and systemic toxicity if treatment is delayed.

16. What is the appropriate treatment for a hydrofluoric acid burn? When is one treatment more appropriate than the other?

Less severe hydrofluoric acid (HF) burns (less than 5% TBSA contact with concentrations less than 20% HF) are usually associated with no symptoms for 24 hours. After lavage with copious water, these burns are treated with a paste of 35 ml of injectable calcium gluconate (10%) in 150 gm of K-Y jelly, applied over the affected area and changed every hour as needed.

When pain persists or more severe injuries are suspected (greater than 1% TBSA contact with greater than 20% concentration of HF), the burned tissue may require subcutaneous injection of calcium gluconate into painful areas. This pain and erythema typically occurs immediately or within the first 8 hours of exposure. Calcium gluconate injection is an effective method of binding fluoride anions. The injections should be carried out using a 27- or 30-gauge needle. The subcutaneous tissues under the involved skin should be injected from sites on the periphery of the lesion. A dose of 0.5 ml/cm^2 of 10% calcium gluconate is used. Although calcium chloride has more milliequivalents per milliliter of calcium, subcutaneous infiltration is contraindicated owing to its tissue irritating properties. This method has been shown to result in dramatic relief of pain and immediate improvement of lesion appearance.

Severe HF contact burn or inhalation greater than 60% HF fumes are usually associated with systemic toxicities. The systemic manifestation of hydrofluoric acid exposure comes primarily from serum hypocalcemia and hypomagnesemia. However, the hypocalcemia seen in HF does not produce the typical signs of hypocalcemia. The serum calcium level and the electrocardiogram are the most reliable indicators of hypocalcemia. In addition, the hypocalcemia induces cardiac arrhythmia, such as refractory ventricular fibrillation, that is particularly resistant to treatment. Systemic toxicities due to HF exposures should be treated with intravenous calcium (1 g CaCl every 15–30 minutes) until normal serum calcium levels are achieved.

17. How is a chemical burn to the eye managed?

The eye is frequently involved in chemical burns. Some centers report that almost half of their patients with chemical burns have ocular involvement. A chemical burn to the eye is an emergency, and an ophthalmologist must be contacted immediately. Copious irrigation with water must be started immediately and continue throughout transportation to the hospital. This can be easily accomplished by immersing a patient's face in a bowl of water and having him open and close his eyes continuously. Once the patient arrives at the hospital, one staff member should be designated to irrigate the eye with a continuous stream of 1–2 liters of normal saline. This can be accomplished with the use of intravenous tubing and an 18-gauge angiocatheter.

BIBLIOGRAPHY

1. Anderson WJ, Anderson JR: Hydrofluoric acid burns of the hand: Mechanism of injury and treatment. J Hand Surg 13A:52–57, 1988.
2. Bromberg BF, Song IC, Walden RH: Hydrotherapy of chemical burns. Plast Reconstr Surg 35:85–95, 1965.
3. Cartotto RC, Peters WJ, Neligan PC, et al: Chemical burns. Can J Surg 39:205–211, 1996.
4. Curreri PW, Asch MJ, Pruitt BA Jr: The treatment of chemical burns: Specialized diagnostic therapeutic and prognostic considerations. J Trauma 10:634–642, 1970.
5. Fitzpatrick KT, Moylan JA: Emergency care of chemical burns. Postgrad Med 78:189–194, 1985.
6. Milner SM, Lindsey RTA, Nguyen TT, et al: Chemical burns. In Herndon DN (ed): Total Burn Care. Philadelphia, W.B. Saunders, 1996, pp 415–424.
7. Jelenko C III: Chemicals that burn. J Trauma 14:65–72, 1974.
8. Kirkpatrick JJR, Enion DS, Burd DAR: Hydrofluoric acid burns: A review. Burns 21:483–493, 1995.
9. Leonard L, Scheulen J, Munster A: Chemical burns: Effect of prompt first aid. J Trauma 22:420–423, 1982.
10. Mozingo DW, Smith AD, McManus WF, et al: Chemical burns. J Trauma 28:642–647, 1988.
11. Rodeheaver GT, Hiebert JM, Edlich RF: Initial treatment of chemical skin and eye burns. Compr Ther 8: 37–43, 1982.
12. Sawhney CP, Kaushish R: Acid and alkali burns: Considerations in their management. Burns 15: 132–135, 1989.
13. Saydjari R, Abston S, Desai MH, Herndon DN: Chemical burns. J Burn Care Rehabil 7:404–408, 1986.
14. Vance MV, Curry SC, Kunkel DB, et al: Digital hydrofluoric acid burns: Treatment with intraarterial calcium infusion. Ann Emerg Med 15:890–896, 1986.
15. Wale R: Chemical burns: First aid and prevention. Aust Fam Physician 15:425–426, 1986.

35. ELECTRICAL BURNS

Bruce E. Zawacki, M.D., and Warren L. Garner, M.D.

1. What sources of electrical power commonly produce electrical burns, and roughly what voltage is each capable of delivering?

A direct strike by a several million–volt lightning bolt can split a tree or kill a human in a fraction of a second. Surviving victims are usually those near the strike; their burns, if present at all, rarely involve deep tissues and are not discussed here. Power transmission lines can carry 230,000 volts and often deliver 7000 to 8000 volts to residential and industrial locations. Home voltages in the United States are typically 120 volts, although 240 volts are available between two separate hot wires that are present in many homes. Industrial batteries can deliver more than 100 volts, and automobile batteries typically deliver 12 volts but are capable of delivering large currents.

2. How are "low-voltage" and "high-voltage" electrical burns defined conventionally, and in what ways do they differ clinically?

By convention, low-voltage injuries are defined as those caused by less than 1000 volts, and high-voltage injuries are those caused by more than 1000 volts. Death at the site of electrocution can occur after exposure to high or low voltages, but physical burns are more likely to be present after high-voltage injury (96%) than low-voltage injury (57%). Characteristics of patients with high- or low-voltage electrical burns surviving and admitted to the hospital are summarized in the following Table.

Characteristics of Electrical Burns Requiring Hospital Admission

CHARACTERISTIC	LOW-VOLTAGE BURNS (<1000 V)	HIGH-VOLTAGE BURNS (≥1000 V)
Relative frequency	70%	30%
Cardiac dysrhythmias	Up to 30%	~30%
"Progressive tissue necrosis"	Reported rarely, if ever	Frequently reported
Fluid resuscitation needs	As in thermal burns	Typically much more than thermal burns of similar surface area
Surgery required	50%	Virtually all
Fasciotomy required	Reported rarely, if ever	Very common
Amputation required	1–2%, relatively minor	~50%, often major
Wound coverage at surgery	Skin graft (occasional flap coverage)	Skin graft (often flap coverage)
Average operations per patient	0.5	2–3
In-hospital mortality	Rare	0–15%
In-hospital morbidity	Very low	Very high
Long-term neurologic sequelae	9%	70%
Ability to return to previous work	Virtually 100%	Approximately 5%

3. Describe the appropriate management of typical low-voltage electrical burns.

A careful history is necessary to discover whether the injury might be caused by high voltage from a capacitor (e.g., as in repair of a television or microwave oven). The history should include information about unconsciousness, cardiac or pulmonary arrest, abnormal pulse rate or rhythm and dysrhythmias identified on the electrocardiogram (ECG) in the prehospital or emergency room setting, and chest pain. A 12-lead ECG should be obtained.

Three types of low-voltage burns have been described in the literature. They may be difficult to distinguish in the emergency department immediately after injury, and more than one type may be seen in the same patient:

1. *Contact with materials heated by touching a low-voltage source* such as an automobile battery or electroplating equipment. Usually superficial, this burn is treated as a thermal burn.

2. *Low-voltage arcing* (i.e., a bright flash due to photons released by electrons pulled from their orbital shells by an electrical field) may produce temperature of up to 4000°C for brief periods. Occurring some distance from the patient, the heat of the flash may produce a superficial, partial-thickness burn. Occurring closer to the patient, clothing can be ignited , although this is more common with high-voltage injuries. These injuries also are treated as thermal burns.

3. *Low-voltage burns producing deep local injury* typically show little or no evidence of distinguishable source- and grounding-contact points and are characterized by the absence of injury at a distance from areas of contact. They are common and typically caused by biting on electrical cords or sucking on electrical outlets or sockets by young children. Injury to oral commissures, tongue, and gums is common and can occasionally lead to airway compromise early due to intraoral edema or late due to microstomia because of wound contracture. These injuries are treated like thermal burns but without early excision. Most heal with conservative treatment. Topical antibacterial cream and splinting are typically applied to prevent or reduce the magnitude of reconstructive surgery necessary to correct microstomia after the scar matures. The patient's family should be instructed that delayed bleeding from the labial artery occurs, albeit rarely, when eschar separates. This can be controlled by local pressure and return to the burn center.

4. In addition to burns, exposure to high-voltage electricity is often accompanied by other injuries important to diagnose and manage. Describe these.

Virtually any organ of the body that is in proximity to the source or ground of electrical current (e.g., brain, gallbladder, bowel) may be injured by high-voltage currents passing through it. Other less obvious types of injury can also occur and must be looked for and dealt with by a detailed "trauma workup."

Head and neck injury. Blunt injury to the cranium, intracranial contents, or cervical spine may occur as the patient falls or intense muscular contractions throw the patient clear of the electrical source. Cataracts can occur immediately or after a delay. Hypoxia due to cardiac or respiratory arrest may also produce brain damage.

Cardiovascular injury. Asystole, ventricular fibrillation, premature ventricular contractions (PVCs), atrial fibrillation, S-T and Q wave abnormalities, bundle-branch block, and myocardial infarction may be present on admission. Cardiac abnormalities may also develop after admission. Delayed arterial occlusion due to electrical injury or increased compartmental pressure can develop early or after considerable delay.

Respiratory damage. Respiratory arrest can result from tetanic muscular spasms, spinal cord injury, aspiration, airway obstruction, pneumothorax, or other sequelae of a fall or other mechanical injury.

Abdominal and genitourinary injury. Blunt trauma, as with other types of injuries, has been recorded, and renal failure due to release of myoglobin or hemoglobin into the blood stream may occur.

Musculoskeletal and neurologic injury. Fractures of the long bones and spine and dislocation of the shoulders and other joints have been recorded, and more than one level of spinal fracture can occur at the same time. A computed tomography (CT) scan or magnetic resonance imaging (MRI) is appropriate to rule out intracranial injury in the presence of clouded mental status, seizures, or unconsciousness. Even in the absence of spinal fractures, immediate or delayed spinal cord damage can occur, and peripheral nerve damage is quite common early and late after the injury.

Fetal injury. Fetal injury and death have been described in pregnant women who suffer apparently minor electrical shocks without loss of consciousness or cutaneous wounds.

5. Describe typical high-voltage electrical burns and the general management approaches appropriate to them.

The first three types of high-voltage electrical burns are analogous to low-voltage injuries (see Question 2). A fourth, "true" or "deep-conductive" injury is distinctly different from thermal injuries and low-voltage electrical injuries. More than one type may be seen in the same patient.

1. *Contact with materials heated by high-voltage electricity* (e.g., vaporized or liquefied metal, plastic or wire insulation). These injuries may be treated as a thermal burn.

2. *High-voltage arcing* may produce larger, superficial partial-thickness flash burns and may ignite clothing more often than similar injuries caused by low voltage. These can also be treated as thermal burns.

3. *High-voltage burns producing deep local injury* without separately distinguishable source- and grounding-contact points or electrical injury distant therefrom. Analogous to perioral low-voltage burns but more severe, these injuries can produce burns at least to bone, often occurring with visible and audible arcing. Persons climbing atop railway cars and approaching overhead high-tension cables can sustain this type of injury to the head. These burns are typically treated as very deep local thermal burns.

4. *High-voltage, deep-conductive electrical injuries* (so-called true electrical injuries) constitute approximately 50% of high-voltage electrical burns. They are characterized by distinguishable source- and grounding-contact points and electrical injury to intervening tissues or organs. They require management techniques that are different from typical thermal burns and often unique in trauma care.

6. What is the appropriate emergency management of a typical high-voltage, deep-conductive ("true") electrical injury at the geographic site where the injury occurred?

Great care must be taken to extricate the victim from the scene without rescuers or bystanders sustaining electrical injury. Extinguish and remove any burning clothing. Begin the ABCs of emergency care. Respiratory insufficiency or arrest (which may be prolonged) or severe cardiac dysrhythmias are common and require cardiopulmonary resuscitation, which is often successful if promptly applied. Immobilization of possible spinal fractures is necessary until spinal stabilization can be ensured. If the patient is hypotensive, start a large-bore intravenous line, and give 10 to 20 mL/kg of Ringer's lactate. A brief history, secondary assessment, splinting of fractures, hypothermia precautions, and prompt delivery to the emergency room are all appropriate.

7. What is the appropriate management in the emergency department of a high-voltage, deep-conductive injury?

Often, a combination of the well-established trauma-, burn-, and cardiac-emergency protocols described elsewhere are necessary, followed by obtaining history from bystanders, insertion of a Foley catheter, and continuation of fluid resuscitation. Secondary assessment should focus especially on the types of injury described in Question 4. Appropriate radiographs to rule out spinal, cranial, or other fractures are necessary. An ECG, ECG monitoring, cardiac isoenzyme level studies, complete blood cell count (CBC), urinalysis for myoglobin or hemoglobin, and any tests appropriate for particular injuries identified should be performed. Other tests should include serum electrolytes, blood urea nitrogen (BUN), creatinine, liver chemistries, urinalysis, tests for consumptive coagulopathy and liver function, and blood gas determinations. Drawing blood for type and crossmatch should be considered, and a nasogastric tube should be inserted.

8. Describe appropriate intravenous fluid therapy for resuscitation of shock associated with high-voltage, deep-conductive electrical burns.

Fluid resuscitation formulas appropriate to thermal burns often underestimate the fluid requirements of high-voltage, deep-conductive electrical burns. Ringer's lactate, as much as 9 mL/kg/% body surface area (BSA) burned or more, may be necessary in the first 24 hours to maintain urine output of 0.5 to 1 mL/kg/hr or 1 to 1.5 mL/kg/hr when urine contains evidence of myoglobin or hemoglobin. When these hemochromogens are present in the urine, a relatively rapid intravenous infusion of mannitol is appropriate to initiate this level of diuresis. Intravenous bicarbonate to maintain a urine pH of greater than 7 helps minimize pigment precipitation in the urine. If possible to achieve quickly, cardiovascular stability and good urine output should be accomplished before escharotomies or fasciotomies are performed, because such procedures are often associated with a marked transient increase in serum levels of hemochromogens. Undue delay, however, is inappropriate.

9. Which patients with electrical injury should be monitored for delayed appearance of cardiac injury, and how should they be monitored?

There appears to be a general agreement that ECG monitoring is appropriate if any of the following risk factors are present:

- Significant risk factors for or history of cardiac disease
- Cardiac arrest
- Documented loss of consciousness
- Dysrhythmia observed in the prehospital or emergency department setting
- Hypoxia
- Chest pain
- Concomitant injuries severe enough to warrant admission to the ICU
- Suspicion of conductive injury (i.e., presence of separate source and ground burns)

Several largely retrospective studies have suggested that neither an ECG nor ECG monitoring may be necessary in the absence of any of the factors indicated in the previous list, although there are anecdotal reports of delayed onset of serious dysrhythmias after low-voltage and high-voltage injuries. A conservative approach would involve an initial ECG and ECG monitoring for 8 to 12 hours in all electrical injuries of high or low voltage and more prolonged monitoring of patients with any of the listed risk factors. Interestingly, myocardial infarction by ECG criteria is rare after electrical injury, even though elevations of serum creatine kinase and the creatine kinase-MB fraction are quite common.

10. How should patients with high-voltage, deep-conductive electrical injuries be monitored for evidence of increased compartmental pressure in burned extremities? How should a compartment syndrome be managed after diagnosis?

As described under Question 5, not all high-voltage electrical injuries are "true" or deep-conductive injuries, and not all are at risk for elevated intracompartmental pressure. Indications for escharotomies or fasciotomies are as follows:

- Charred or mummified distal limb
- Diminished or absent distal pulses or arterial Doppler flow signal
- Loss of sensation or motor function in the distal limb
- Gross limb swelling
- Pain or abnormally firm or hard muscle tone
- Compartment pressures of more than 30 mmHg or differing from mean arterial pressure by less than 40 mmHg

Repeated measurements of pressures in compartments of the arm, leg, and the volar and dorsal intrinsic muscular compartments of the hand are typically accomplished with a Stryker-type apparatus. Repeated measurements over 48 hours may be necessary to avoid missing delayed damage due to increased compartmental pressure, which may recur even after escharotomies or fasciotomies have been performed. Standard tests or orthopaedic and vascular consultations should be obtained before carrying out fasciotomies to ensure that the fasciotomies are adequate and that adequate releases of ulnar and median nerves at the wrists and elbows are performed. Standard escharotomy incisions are regularly inadequate for this purpose. To ensure completeness and control of pain and bleeding, general anesthesia is usually required, and thorough exploration of the deepest compartments of the arm and leg is necessary to avoid unnecessary necrosis due to unrelieved high pressure.

11. What is meant by progressive tissue necrosis in high-voltage, deep-conductive electrical injuries?

Cutaneous and deep-tissue damage are related to current density. Traversing currents converge at source- and grounding-contact points and near joints where the cross-sectional area of highly conductive muscles is very small. Tissue necrosis at these points is typically severe and immediately obvious at operation soon after injury. This necrotic tissue and any other visibly necrotic tissue present are débrided, usually at the initial operation. When the site of injury is reassessed a few days later at reoperation, however, muscle tissue that appeared normal at the first operation often appears obviously necrotic, apparently because of delayed, *de novo,* or progressive necrosis.

12. Discuss the possible mechanisms involved in producing progressive tissue necrosis and the suggested approaches to management of each.

Inadequate fluid resuscitation. This requires education and increased conscientiousness in the use of available techniques.

Delayed or inadequate decompression of elevated intracompartmental pressure. Repetitive measurements of intracompartmental pressure, early escharotomies and fasciotomies, and postfasciotomy and escharotomy repeat measurements of compartmental pressures have been recommended to prevent recurrent intracompartmental hypertension.

Wound drying. After early fasciotomy and débridement (typically in the first hours after injury), wound drying can be prevented by application of split-thickness skin allograft or xenograft or with the application of moist dressings.

Wound infection. This may be diminished by scrupulous débridement and application of topical antibacterial agents (especially mafenide acetate) to penetrate dead tissue.

Products of arachidonic acid cascading. Topical and systemic agents designed to interfere with the arachidonic acid cascade have been reported to improve tissue survival experimentally.

Electroporation. Surfactant materials administered intravenously to correct electroporation (i.e., holes in cell membranes caused by electrical currents too weak to cause thermal injury) have been reported to improve tissue survival experimentally, but no systematic clinical studies are yet available.

Reperfusion injury. This has been extensively studied experimentally in other disease processes, but not clinically in electrical injury.

Delayed occlusion of small blood vessels. This is difficult to demonstrate by conventional angiography, although there are several reports that quite large vessels diagnosed as being in danger of occlusion and limbs or parts of limbs have been rescued by early or prophylactic saphenous vein–arterial interposition grafts.

13. Describe and evaluate available methods for distinguishing necrotic from living tissue in electrical burns preoperatively and intraoperatively.

Preoperative pain, tenderness, paresthesias, and swelling with or without evidence of ischemia suggest the presence of necrotic tissue. Studies of xenon 133 washout, MRI, measurement of electrical resistivity, and nuclear magnetic resonance (NMR) spectroscopy have limited clinical value. Technetium-99 stannous pyrophosphate scintography is helpful in identifying dead bone and dead or irreversibly injured muscle. Its high sensitivity and limited resolution limit its value in intraoperative assessment of viability, but it can be helpful in planning amputations, obtaining informed consents, and planning operations. Intraoperative clinical assessment of viability remains the most reliable source of information available in deciding which portion of muscle is to be débrided.

Intraoperatively, gross feel of muscle (i.e., very hard or very mushy), color (i.e., black, brown, or pale, cooked–fish-flesh discoloration), absence of bleeding on incision, and absence of contraction when pinched or stimulated electrically remain the final indications for excision or débridement of questionably viable muscle. Frozen-section or permanent-section histology is available in some centers to confirm nonviability but is seldom used.

14. Discuss delayed, immediate, and early approaches to wound closure after excision of necrotic tissue found at exploration of high-voltage, deep-conductive electrical burns.

Delayed closure of such wounds has been traditional for many years. Whereas operative fasciotomies and release of pressures in muscle compartments and essential points of compression of nerves is appropriate whenever clinically indicated, débridement of obviously dead tissue may be performed at the initial fasciotomy operation or can be delayed for a few days. Topical antibacterial agents in cream or solution form are typically applied, and repeated surgical explorations and débridements are continued in the operating room at 24- to 48-hour intervals until it is obvious that all nonviable tissue has been removed or until amputation is performed. A week or more after injury, when the wound appears free of necrotic tissue likely to produce infection, the wound is closed by skin graft, flap coverage, or more proximal amputation. This technique is designed to conserve all possible viable tissue, increase the certainty of graft survival, and avoid infection. It tends to be associated with longer hospitalization and is thought to increase rehabilitative problems.

In some cases, patients have been brought to the operating room a few hours after injury for *immediate* decompression and débridement, and after removal of all necrotic tissue evident, flap closure of the wound has been accomplished at the same operation. Theoretical advantages of this approach are reduction of infection by early removal of necrotic tissue and closure and more rapid mobilization of joints and less exposure of vital structures, potentially shortening hospitalization. A possible disadvantage of this is overlooking retained dead tissue or tissue that goes on to become necrotic because of progressive tissue necrosis. Theoretically, injured tissue that might otherwise become necrotic can be rescued by application of well-vascularized tissue, although reported examples of this immediate approach are rare and must be considered anecdotal.

The *early* approach to this problem typically involves compartmental decompression or débridement-amputation either immediately or in the first 48 to 72 hours, followed as necessary by application of split-thickness allograft or xenograft with or without topical antibacterial preparations. This is followed by repeated operations as required and definitive closure as necessary by skin graft or flap between the third and the fifth day after injury. Some recommend giving topical antithromboxane preparations or other materials designed to diminish progressive necrosis up to the time of definitive closure. This approach seeks to split the difference between immediate and delayed approaches but gives adequate time for delayed, progressive necrosis to occur and be diagnosed before definitive closure occurs.

15. Which of the three approaches described in Question 14 has been demonstrated to be superior in adequate clinical trials?

None. Although each approach has its impassioned advocates, valuable objective measures such as the rate of return to work are only sparsely reported. Controversy over which of these or other approaches are optimal persists.

16. Describe the delayed neurologic and ophthalmologic sequelae peculiar to electrical burns.

Seizures, corticoencephalopathy, hemiplegia, aphasia, and brain stem dysfunction may be delayed as long as 6 to 9 months after injury. Spinal cord damage up to and including transverse myelitis has appeared after days to months. Peripheral motor and sensory nerve abnormalities are common in high-voltage and low-voltage injuries, and onset can be delayed up to 3 years after injury.

Cataracts are much more common in high-voltage injuries but also have been observed in low-voltage injuries. They appear to occur more frequently in more severe injuries and when a contact point occurs above the clavicle. Incidence is probably between 5% and 20% in high-risk patients. Most affected patients develop initial vision loss within 12 months of the injury, with gradually increasing vision loss thereafter. Delays as long as 12 years have been reported for the onset of cataracts. Thorough examination and careful follow-up are therefore indicated. Response to surgical repair is usually very satisfactory.

BIBLIOGRAPHY

1. Block TA, Aarsvold JN, Matthews KL, et al: Nonthermally mediated muscle injury and necrosis in electrical trauma (the 1995 Lindberg Award). J Burn Care Rehab 16:581–588, 1995.
2. Chick LR, Lister GD, Sowder L: Early free-flap coverage of electrical and thermal burns. Plast Reconstr Surg 89:1013–1019, 1992.
3. Cooper MA: Emergent care of lightning and electrical injuries. Semin Neurol 15:268–278, 1995.
4. Hammond J, Ward CG: The use of technetium-99 pyrophosphate scanning in management of high-voltage electrical injuries. Am Surg 60:886–887, 1994.
5. Hanumadass ML, Voora SB, Kagan RJ, Matsuda T: Acute electrical burns: A 10-year clinical experience. Burns 12:427–431, 1986.
6. Hussmann J, Kucan JO, Russell RC, et al: Electrical injuries—Morbidity, outcome, and treatment rationale. Burns 21:530–535, 1995.
7. Kyriacou DN, Zigman A, Sapien R, Stanitsas A: Eleven-year-old male with high-voltage electrical injury and premature ventricular contractions. J Emerg Med 14:591–597, 1996.
8. Lee RC, Capelli-Schellpfeffer M, Kelly KM (eds): Electrical Injury: A Multidisciplinary Approach to Therapy, Prevention, and Rehabilitation. New York, The New York Academy of Sciences, 1994.
9. Lee RC, Cravalho EG, Burke JF (eds): Electrical Trauma: The Pathophysiology, Manifestations and Clinical Management. Cambridge, University Press, 1992.
10. Purdue GF, Hunt JL: Electrocardiographic monitoring after electrical injury: Necessity or luxury. J Trauma 26:166–167, 1986.
11. Quinby WC, Burke JF, Trelstad RL, Caulfield J: The use of microscopy as a guide to primary excision of high-tension electrical burns. J Trauma 18:423–430, 1978.
12. Robson MC, Murphy RC, Heggers JP: A new explanation for the progressive tissue loss in electrical injuries. Plast Reconstr Surg 73:431–437, 1984.
13. Saffle JR, Crandall A, Warden GD: Cataracts: A long-term complication of electrical injury. J Trauma 26:17–21, 1985.
14. Yang J-Y, Noordhoff S: Early adipofascial flap coverage of deep electrical burn wounds of upper extremities. Plast Reconstr Surg 91:819–827, 1993.

36. SOFT TISSUE INJURIES AND CRUSH SYNDROME

George C. Velmahos, M.D., Ph.D., and Jesús I. Ramírez, M.D.

1. What is crush syndrome?

Crush syndrome refers to the systemic manifestations associated with crush injuries. These injuries are caused by prolonged continuous pressure on the body, with the extremities being most often affected.

2. When was crush syndrome first described?

Description of the crush syndrome is commonly attributed to Bywaters and Beall, who reported it after the London air raids of 1940. They described four cases where civilians had been buried for several hours under the debris of collapsed buildings. Initially the victims seemed to be "in good condition, except for swelling of the limb and some local anesthesia." Then they rapidly deteriorated over a few days with shock, urine pigmentation, oliguric renal failure, and sudden death.

In the German literature, the syndrome had previously been described after the 1909 Messina (Sicily) earthquake.

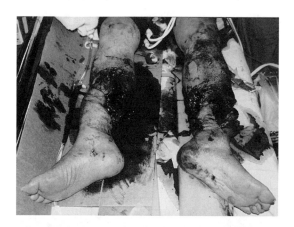

Crushed extremities with bilateral open tibial fractures, Gustilo type IIIC.

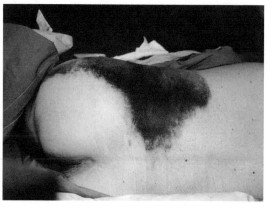

Major soft tissue injury of the flank and gluteal area, producing gluteal compartment syndrome.

3. **When can crush syndrome reach epidemic proportions?**

During mass disasters. Such was the case after the earthquakes of Tangshan (China, 1976), Spitak (Armenia, 1988), Hanshin-Awaji (Japan, 1995), and Marmara (Turkey, 1999).

4. **Mass disasters aside, when may crush injury present?**

Crush injuries present in victims of severe beatings, motor vehicle accidents (especially with delayed extrication), pedestrian accidents (especially with pinning), or industrial and agricultural accidents.

5. **Why is a high index of suspicion necessary after soft tissue injuries?**

The severity of injury is impossible to determine on initial examination and may only become apparent after a significant lapse of time. Underestimating the extent of underlying muscle injury may lead to inadequate treatment and multiple organ system failure.

6. **What are the early symptoms and signs of crush injuries?**

Shortly after crush injury, symptoms and signs may be nearly absent. Patients may have no pain, no swelling, and strong distal pulse. The only sign may be a neurologic deficit in the form of patchy sensory loss or flaccid paralysis. It is not for several hours that edema develops and dominates the clinical picture.

7. **What are the three common local complications of extensive soft tissue injuries?**
- Edema, which may be accompanied by cellulitis
- Hematoma, which may be accompanied by abscess formation
- Compartment syndrome

8. **What is compartment syndrome?**

Compartment syndrome describes the effects of increased pressure within an enclosed tissue space, such as muscle compartments bound by fascia. The initial injury produces cell lysis and microvascular disruption, resulting in edema. When the interstitial pressure from edema exceeds capillary perfusion pressure, ischemia develops and leads to further cell death and edema. Ultimately, tissue viability is compromised.

9. **What is the treatment of choice for compartment syndrome?**

Decompression by fasciotomy, which breaks the cycle described above.

10. **How is the intracompartmental pressure of the extremities commonly measured?**

The most commonly used method of involves insertion of a needle connected to a handheld solid-state transducer, such as the Intracompartmental Monitoring System (Stryker® Instruments, Kalamazoo, MI) or PressureSense™ (Millenium Medical Technologies, Santa Fe, NM).

11. **What pressure values are considered normal and what values are considered abnormal?**

Normal intracompartmental pressure is 10 mmHg in resting muscle. The threshold level for performing fasciotomy is debated. Pressures below 20 mmHg are rarely associated with ischemia and pressures greater then 40 mmHg are generally considered at high risk for ischemia. Pressures in between are considered to be in a "gray zone," where compartment syndrome may develop, particularly in the presence of other ischemic factors (such as hypotension or hypoxemia).

12. **Does the presence of crush injury alter the treatment of increased compartmental pressures?**

Patients with crushed extremities and equivocal pressure measurements (in the gray zone) may be better served by close monitoring than by fasciotomy. Once the skin barrier is broken, devitalized muscle is prone to infection, which may spread rapidly. Thus, some authors have reported increased amputation rates and mortality with liberal use of fasciotomy in this setting. On the other hand, delaying a necessary fasciotomy allows ischemic damage to progress.

13. Can compartment syndrome be quantitatively assessed without breaking the skin? How?
    Yes, by using near-infrared spectroscopy (NIRS). This technology is not widely available and is considered investigational.

14. How does near-infrared spectroscopy work?
    NIRS combines features of pulse oximetry and ultrasound. It assesses tissue oxygenation by measuring the difference in color between oxyhemoglobin and hemoglobin, similar to the way pulse oximetry assesses arterial blood oxygenation. The assessment is made beneath the level of the skin by a device that emits photons and measures their transmission through tissue at a certain depth, similar to the way ulrasound creates images by emitting sound waves and measuring their transmission through subcutaneous structures.

15. What four advantages are claimed for NIRS, compared with direct pressure measurement?
    NIRS is not widely available and still considered investigational. Proponents argue the following advantages:
- It is noninvasive.
- It provides continuous monitoring, as opposed to "spot checks" by handheld transducers.
- It provides a more physiologic measure of ischemia.
- It can detect ischemia in the presence of hypotension or hypoxemia because it directly measures tissue oxygenation. In this setting, compartment pressure measurements have been demonstrated to be less sensitive for neuromuscular compromise.

16. What are the five common systemic complications of extensive soft tissue injuries?
- Hypovolemia
- Electrolyte changes
- Disseminated intravascular coagulation
- Renal failure
- Arrythmias

17. Describe the pathophysiology for each of the previous complications.
- Hypovolemia results from fluid extravasation into injured tissue. Sufficient fluid to produce hypovolemic shock may extravasate into a single lower extremity.
- Electrolyte changes are mainly seen as hyperkalemia, hyperphosphatemia, and hypocalcemia. Potassium and phosphorus are released from the intracellular compartment as a direct result of cell death, while calcium is trapped in muscle cells that lack energy to normally extrude it from the cytosol.
- Disseminated intravascular coagulation may result from substances released by injured tissue which activate the coagulation cascade.
- Renal failure develops as a result of vasoconstriction, direct nephrotoxicity, and tubular cast formation. Vasoconstricton is in response to hypovolemia. Nephrotoxicity is caused by iron-containing myoglobin breakdown products, which are released in an acidic environment and cause tubular cell lipid peroxidation. Casts form in the renal tubules from precipitates of both myoglobin and uric acid.
- Arrythmias may result from electrolyte abnormalities, particularly the combination of hyperkalemia and hypocalcemia.

18. What tests should routinely be included in the evaluation of the soft tissue injury victim?
- Hematocrit
- Electrolytes (K, Na, Ca, Mg, and P_i)

- Coagulation panel (PT, aPTT, and platelets)
- Blood urea nitrogen & creatinine
- Urinalysis (for myoglobin/pigment)
- Creatine phosphokinase
- Arterial blood gas
- Radiographs of injury site

19. What is the incidence of renal failure for patients with soft tissue injuries?

Renal failure is reported to develop in 5–15% of patients with soft tissue injuries. The incidence is thought to increase with the extent of muscle injury.

20. What are four risk factors for renal failure after soft tissue injury?

- The presence of myoglobinuria
- Venous bicarbonate less than 17 mmol/L
- Delay in treatment greater than 12 hours after injury
- Creatinine phosphokinase (CPK) level greater than 10,000 IU/mL

21. What treatment may be instituted to prevent renal failure?

- Aggressive fluid resuscitation is the mainstay of treatment. A balanced crystalloid solution should be administered at a rate sufficient to maintain urine output of at least 100 mL/hr.
- Mannitol should be given as a bolus of 1 gm/kg, than as a continuous infusion of 0.1 g/kg/hr.
- Bicarbonate should be given as a 100 mEq bolus and then as an infusion of 0.5 mL/kg/hr.
- If anuria develops, dialysis is required and may help prevent chronic renal failure as the final outcome.

22. What is the effect of mannitol?

Mannitol potentially counteracts the three toxic effects of crush injury on the kidney: vasoconstriction, direct nephrotoxicity, and tubular cast formation. It decreases blood viscosity, thereby increasing renal blood flow. It acts as a free-radical scavenger, protecting renal tubule cells from oxidative injury. Finally, it acts as a diuretic, thereby diluting and flushing out renal tubule precipitates.

23. What is the effect of bicarbonate?

Bicarbonate alkalinizes the urine, inhibiting formation and precipitation of toxic myoglobin breakdown products.

24. There may be a role for hyperbaric oxygen therapy in crush injuries. What three physiologic effects of hyperoxygenation may be beneficial in crush injuries?

- It produces hyperoxic vasoconstriction, thereby reducing vasogenic edema and intracompartmental pressure.
- It increases the amount of oxygen dissolved in plasma, improving oxygen delivery by creating a steep diffusion gradient from plasma to tissue. This has three potentially beneficial effects:
    Preserved tissue viability in ischemic areas
    Enhanced wound healing by fibroblasts
    Enhanced bactericidal activity of polymorphonuclear leukocytes
- It decreases reperfusion injury by limiting ischemia time—the extent of reperfusion injury is directly proportional to the duration of ischemia. With timely use of hyperbaric oxygen after ischemic injury, decreased lipid peroxidation and neutrophil sequestration have been reported.

25. Is there any clinical evidence to support the theoretical benefits of hyperbaric oxygen therapy in crush injuries?

Most research on hyperbaric oxygen therapy for crush injuries has been conducted in the laboratory, either in animals or *in vitro*. Recently, the first controlled human trial, involving 36 patients, reported complete healing in 94% of patients with soft-tissue injuries treated by hyperbaric oxygen as opposed to 59% of control patients ($p < 0.01$). Also, improved renal function was recently reported in four crush injury patients treated with hyperbaric oxygen therapy after a hotel collapse in Thailand.

26. What is the prognosis after soft tissue injury? Specifically, what is the incidence of renal failure and what is the mortality?

Approximately 10% of patients will require dialysis. With appropriate treatment, the majority will recover renal function. Death occurs in 1–2% of patients and is caused predominantly by hyperkalemia, sepsis, or delay in institution of dialysis. The prognosis varies with the extent of the injury and the number of risk factors present.

BIBLIOGRAPHY

1. Arbabi S, Brundage SI, Gentilello LM: Near-infrared spectroscopy: a potential method for continuous, transcutaneous monitoring of compartmental syndrome in critically injured patients. J Trauma 47:829–33, 1999.
2. Better OS, Stein JH: Early management of shock and prophylaxis of acute renal failure in traumatic rhabdomyolysis. N Engl J Med 322:825–829, 1990.
3. Bouachour G, Cronier P, Gouello JO, et al: Hyperbaric oxygen therapy in the management of crush injury: a randomized double-blind placebo-controlled clinical trial. J trauma 41:333–9, 1996.
4. Bywaters EGL, Beall D: Crush injuries with impairment of renal function. Br Med J 1:427–32, 1941.
5. Gentilello LM, Sanzone A, Wang L, et al: Near-infrared spectroscopy versus compartment pressure for the diagnosis of lower extremity compartmental syndrome using electromyography-determined measurements of neuromuscular function. J Trauma 51:1–9, 2001.
6. Knottenbelt JD: Traumatic rhabdomyolysis from severe beating: Experience of volume diuresis in 200 patients. J Trauma 37:214–219, 1994.
7. Michaelson M: Crush injuries and crush syndrome. World J Surg 16:899–903, 1992.
8. Muckart DJJ, Moodley M, Naidu AG, et al: Prediction of acute renal failure following soft tissue injury using the venous bicarbonate concentration. J Trauma 33:813–817, 1992.
9. Odeh M: The role of reperfusion induced injury in the pathogenesis of the crush syndrome. N Engl J Med 324:1417–1421, 1991.
10. Ward MM: Factors predictive of acute renal failure in rhabdomyolysis. Arch Intern Med 148:1553–1557, 1988.

37. HYPOTHERMIA

Ian C. Carmody, M.D., and Thomas V. Berne, M.D.

1. What are some of the causes of hypothermia?

Causes include hypovolemic shock, exposure to cold environments, submersion in water, surface evaporation, anesthesia, and hypothyroidism. Countries with colder climates have a higher incidence of hypothermia admissions. Prolonged exposure to outdoor aquatic environments, even in warm climates, can lead to hypothermia. Surface evaporation related to air currents or the topical use of isopropyl alcohol occasionally is causative. General and local anesthesia cause hypothermia by reducing the shivering mechanism.

2. What mechanisms of injury are risk factors for hypothermia?

Significant blood loss, burns, spinal cord injury, submersion, and avalanche are risk factors.

3. Which populations are at higher risk for developing hypothermia?

The elderly, pediatric, and substance-abuse populations are at higher risk for hypothermia.

4. What symptoms and physiologic changes occur with mild hypothermia (down to 33°C [91.4°F] core body temperature)?

At a core body temperature of 35°C to 37°C, shivering occurs. Vasoconstriction develops, along with a hyperdynamic cardiovascular, pulmonary, and metabolic response. Between 33°C and 35°C, the patient becomes confused, ataxic, and amnestic, and shivering becomes more vigorous.

5. What symptoms and physiologic changes occur with moderate hypothermia (30°C to 33°C [86.0°F to 91.4°F])?

The patient develops bradycardia, decreased cardiac output, an irritable myocardium, hypoventilation, "cold diuresis," muscle rigidity, and complex acid–base changes.

6. What symptoms and physiologic changes occur with severe hypothermia (below 31°C [86.0°F])?

There is a progressive loss of consciousness. The muscles begin to relax, and the pupils dilate and become unresponsive to light. Hypotension, hypoperfusion, and acidosis occur, often terminating with ventricular fibrillation, apnea, or asystole.

7. What is the mortality rate associated with hypothermia at a core body temperature of 34°C (93.4°F) and of 32°C (89.6°F) in trauma patients?

The mortality rate for hypothermia is 85% to 100% at 32°C and 14% to 60% at 34°C. The severity of injury also is an important factor in the outcome of these patients, and patients suffering from simple exposure or submersion are more likely to survive.

8. What electrocardiographic changes are indicative of hypothermia?

As core body temperature drops, the rate slows and the P-R and Q-T intervals become prolonged. J waves appear at temperatures less than 35°C and are prominent at 25°C. This J wave is initially seen only as a widened QRS with a slight S-T segment elevation at the J point, but it becomes a pronounced hump that immediately follows the QRS complex.

9. What electrolyte abnormalities must be considered in the hypothermic patient?

Hyperkalemia, hypokalemia, and metabolic acidosis should be considered.

10. What are the causes of the coagulopathy associated with hypothermia?

Dysfunction of enzymatic activity, inhibition of platelet activation, and decreased platelet adherence and aggregation can cause coagulopathy with hypothermia. Because clotting studies, prothrombin and partial thromboplastin times, are normally automatically corrected to 37°C, they do not reflect the prolongation of clotting related to hypothermia.

11. List four factors that cause hypothermia in injured patients.

1. Exposure, as occurs with delayed recovery by the EMS system in a cold environment or even disrobing of the patient in the hospital without providing for warming. Emergency room temperatures are usually 22°C to 25°C (74°F to 76°F).
2. Intravenous infusion of room-temperature fluid.
3. Transfusion of cold blood without warming (4°C to 10°C in the blood bank).
4. The use of general anesthesia markedly inhibits the patient's thermoregulatory responses.

12. How can hypothermia in trauma patients be prevented after arrival in the emergency department?

After patients are disrobed, they should be covered with warm or reflective blankets. All intravenous fluids should be warmed in an incubator or rapid infusion warmer. Blood should always be given through a rapid infusion warmer unless it is very clear that a minimum of replacement will be needed. The ambient air should be kept warm.

13. What additional measures can be taken to avoid or treat hypothermia in the operating room (OR)?

In addition to the measures mentioned previously for the emergency department, warming in the OR should include the use of a forced-air warming blanket over the patient, and a warming blanket that circulates warm water should be placed under the patient. All inspired anesthetic gases should have heated humidification (40°C to 42°C). The OR air should be heated to 26.6°C (80°F) or higher. If the abdominal cavity is open, warm saline (at 40°C) can be used to flood the peritoneal cavity if the temperature falls below 35°C. This fluid is allowed to run into all gutters, into the pelvis, up under the diaphragm, and all around the intestines, and it is allowed to dwell for 2 to 3 minutes. It takes 5 to 10 minutes before core temperature begins to rise, but then rather rapid drops occur. As the irrigation fluid cools, it is removed and replaced with more 40°C saline. If the chest is open, warm saline can be poured around the lungs and heart.

14. What are some disadvantages of surface rewarming?

Surface rewarming may cause vasodilation and may reduce afterload. Additional core cooling may occur because of shifting of cool and acidotic blood from the periphery to the core (i.e., *after drop*).

15. List the methods of "core warming" available to treat the hypothermic trauma patient in the intensive care unit.

The critical care unit environment allows the use of continuous extracorporeal rewarming techniques. The simplest is to use the disposable heat exchanger from the level I rapid infusion blood pump, using an arteriovenous extracorporeal circuit or a venovenous pump (with bubble trap). This circuit can rapidly rewarm patients. Although it is more cumbersome, the standard cardiopulmonary bypass rewarming circuit used for cardiac surgery is often more readily available. Other techniques include warmed pleural cavity, gastric, and bladder irrigation; peritoneal lavage with warmed saline; and the intravenous infusion of superheated fluids (65°C).

16. Which of the available rewarming methods are most effective at heat transfer?

The most effective methods are cardiopulmonary bypass (700 kcal/hr) and extracorporeal rewarming using the disposable level I heat exchanger (100 kcal/hr). Other techniques are, in order of decreasing effectiveness, body cavity lavage (36 kcal/hr), convective warmers (15 to 26 kcal/hr), heating blankets (20 kcal/hr), and airway rewarming using warm humidified gas (8 to 12 kcal/hr).

17. Are there any potential benefits from hypothermia in trauma patients?

Because metabolic rates drop in hypothermic organs, it is postulated that hypothermia may benefit individual organs such as the brain, heart, and kidneys. It is difficult to use this potential benefit clinically without incurring the deleterious effects discussed in Questions 1 through 3. Potentially, total circulatory arrest could be employed along with profound hypothermia to allow repair of otherwise lethal injuries in a bloodless field. This has been studied in laboratory animals but is difficult to translate to the uncontrolled environment in which we encounter such seriously injured trauma patients. Sometimes, when repairing renal or hepatic vascular injuries, surface cooling or even intra-arterial cooling (if organ preservation solutions are available) can markedly extend the safe ischemic interval. Mild hypothermia may be useful in the intensive care unit management of moderate head injuries.

BIBLIOGRAPHY

1. Capone A, Safar P, Radovsky A, et al: Complete recovery after normothermic hemorrhagic shock and profound hypothermic circulatory arrest of 60 minutes in dogs. J Trauma 40:388–395, 1996.
2. Clifton GL, Miller ER, Choi SC, et al: Lack of effect of induction of hypothermia after acute brain injury. N Engl J Med 344:556–563, 2001.
3. Gentilello LM, Cobean RA, Offner PJ, et al: Continuous arteriovenous rewarming: Rapid reversal of hypothermia in critically ill patients. J Trauma 32:316–325, 1992.
4. Gregory JS, Bergstern JM, Aprahamian C: Comparison of three methods of rewarming from hypothermia: Advantages of extracorporal blood warming. J Trauma 31:1247–1251, 1991.
5. Iserson KV, Huestis DW: Blood warming: Current applications and techniques. Transfusion 31:558–571, 1991.
6. Jurkovich GJ, Greisler WB, Luterman A, et al: Hypothermia in trauma victims: An ominous predictor of survivals. J Trauma 27:1019–1024, 1987.
7. Marion DW, Penrod LE, Kelsey SF, et al: Treatment of traumatic brain injury with moderate hypothermia. N Engl J Med 336:540–546, 1997.
8. Romero J, Waxman K: Hypothermia after trauma and surgery. Surg Rounds 2:244–246, 1999.
9. Sheaff CM, Fildes JJ, Keogh P, et al: Safety of 65° intravenous fluid for the treatment of hypothermia. Am J Surg 172:52–55, 1996.
10. Walpoth BH, Walpoth-Aslan BN, Mattle HP, et al: Outcome of survivors of accidental deep hypothermia and circulatory arrest treated with extracorporeal blood warming. N Engl J Med 337:1500–1505, 1997.

38. FAMILY VIOLENCE: CHILD ABUSE, INTIMATE PARTNER VIOLENCE, AND ELDER ABUSE

Deirdre Anglin, M.D., M.P.H., and H. Range Hutson, M.D.

CHILD ABUSE

1. How is child abuse defined?

Child abuse or maltreatment is defined as behavior on the part of the caretaker that is injurious to the child. It may consist of physical abuse, neglect of basic needs, emotional or psychological abuse, and sexual abuse. It may include acts of commission (i.e., physical or sexual abuse) and acts of omission (i.e., failure to provide basic shelter, medical care, or supervision). Child abuse may also be referred to as nonaccidental trauma (NAT).

2. What is the incidence of child abuse in the United States?

The exact incidence of child abuse is unknown because of underreporting. However, there are more than 3 million reports of suspected child abuse and 3000 fatalities attributed to child abuse annually in the United States. It has been estimated that 1.5% of children suffer from neglect and 1% of children are physically abused each year. Two thirds of cases involve children younger than 3 years of age, and one third involve children younger than 1 year of age. Child sexual abuse constitutes 30% to 50% of all confirmed cases of child abuse. Peak ages for sexual abuse are 2 to 6 years and 12 to 16 years.

3. What historical clues suggest child abuse?

- An unexplained injury with no history or a partial history
- A discrepant history between the child and caretakers or between caretakers
- A changing history
- A history not developmentally appropriate for the child
- A history inconsistent with the injury
- A history of previous injuries
- A history of self-inflicted injury
- Delay in seeking medical attention
- Childhood immunizations not up to date
- Presentation for seemingly unrelated symptoms (e.g., irritability, poor feeding)

4. What physical findings suggest child abuse?

- Multiple injuries at different stages of healing
- Injuries to multiple body regions
- Bilateral injuries
- Bruises or welts resembling regular patterns (i.e., shape of a hand, belt, or electric cord)
- Burns (e.g., cigarette burns to the palms or soles; immersion burns to the hands, feet, or buttocks; burns resembling electrical appliances)
- Skull, rib, long-bone, and metaphyseal fractures
- Intra-abdominal injuries
- Abnormal neurologic status
- Retinal hemorrhages
- Munchausen's syndrome by proxy
- Suffocation

- Malnutrition
- Failure to thrive
- Poor hygiene
- Untreated, severe dental caries
- Chemical or substance abuse
- Impaired interpersonal relations (e.g., child's gaze avoidance, passivity, fear, or behavioral changes in the presence of a parent)

5. What radiographic findings suggest child abuse?

Fractures are detected in approximately 30% of abused children. Epiphyseal separation; metaphyseal corner (chip) or bucket-handle fractures; spiral, oblique, and transverse long-bone fractures in nonambulatory children; and periosteal elevation and calcification are lesions pathognomonic of abuse. However, skull fractures and diaphyseal transverse and spiral fractures are more common. Abnormalities highly specific for child abuse include metaphyseal corner or bucket-handle fractures and posterior rib, scapular, spinous process, and sternal fractures. Fractures with moderate specificity for child abuse include multiple fractures at different stages of healing, epiphyseal separations, vertebral body fractures and subluxations, phalangeal fractures of the hands, and complex skull fractures. Fractures that are common but of low specificity include clavicular fractures, long-bone diaphyseal fractures, and linear skull fractures.

Computed tomography (CT) and ultrasound may also demonstrate intra-abdominal injuries from child abuse, including rupture and intramural hematoma of the duodenum and jejunum; mesenteric vascular injury; hepatic lacerations and hematomas; and pancreatic hemorrhage, contusion, or fracture. Intracranial injuries that may be diagnosed by CT or magnetic resonance imaging (MRI) include cerebral edema, cerebral contusions, subdural hematomas, and subarachnoid hemorrhages. Epidural hematomas are uncommon complications of child abuse.

6. Describe the physical and radiographic findings of "shaken baby syndrome."

Shaken baby syndrome typically is diagnosed in children younger than 2 years of age who have been held by the torso and shaken violently, resulting in whiplash-type injuries to the head, neck, and extremities. Physical examination findings may include lethargy, retinal hemorrhages, and evidence of central nervous system or spinal cord dysfunction in the absence of external signs of trauma. Radiographic findings of shaken baby syndrome include CT evidence of subdural or subarachnoid hemorrhages, focal or diffuse brain injury or spinal cord injury, and rib or metaphyseal long-bone fractures.

7. What is a skeletal survey, and when should it be performed?

A skeletal survey, also referred to as a trauma series, is a series of radiographs that includes anteroposterior and lateral views of the skull and chest, anteroposterior views of the extremities, posteroanterior views of the hands, and lateral views of the cervical and lumbar spines. A skeletal survey should be performed for children younger than 5 years of age who are suspected of being victims of child abuse to examine for previous skeletal injuries. Skeletal surveys should be repeated 2 weeks after the initial examination.

8. Name the risk factors for child abuse.

Characteristics that may put a child at risk for injury include premature birth, multiple births (e.g., twins), having disabilities or abnormalities, and having certain behaviors such as persistent crying or hyperactivity. Parental or caretaker characteristics that may be risk factors for abuse include other forms of family violence (e.g., intimate partner violence), substance abuse, caretaker's lack of maturity to care for the child, parental expectations of child's behavior disparate from developmental capabilities, caretaker's lack of support systems, nonbiologic parent (i.e., stepparent), family stresses (e.g., job loss, family death, divorce), and caretakers who were abused as children.

9. List the differential diagnoses for child abuse.

- Trauma related to birth (e.g., cephalohematoma, clavicle fractures)
- Musculoskeletal disorders (e.g., osteogenesis imperfecta, rickets, scurvy, syphilis)
- Bleeding disorders, blood dyscrasias, and vasculitis (e.g., hemophilia, Henoch-Schönlein purpura)
- Folk remedies (e.g., cupping, Cia Gao, coining)
- Bullous skin lesions (e.g., erythema multiforme, staphylococcal scalded-skin syndrome)
- Mongolian spots
- Malabsorption syndromes
- Sudden infant death syndrome (SIDS)
- Cardiopulmonary resuscitation

10. When should child sexual abuse be suspected?

Child sexual abuse should be suspected in children who graphically describe sexual activities. It should be suspected in children who have any of the following findings: physical abuse, vaginal or rectal discharge or bleeding, sexually transmitted diseases, pregnancy in early teens, enuresis, emotional problems in preschool years or adolescence, and suicide attempts.

INTIMATE PARTNER VIOLENCE

11. What is the definition of intimate partner violence?

Intimate partner violence is the threat or infliction of physical harm against past or present adult or adolescent intimate partners. Physical and sexual assault may be accompanied by psychological abuse, intimidation, deprivation, and progressive social isolation. It is a pattern of assaultive and coercive behaviors directed at achieving compliance from and control over the victim. Other terms that may be used interchangeably for intimate partner violence include domestic violence, spouse abuse, battering, and wife beating. The term *intimate partner violence* clearly describes the relationship between victim and perpetrator without specifying the gender of either individual.

12. Describe the epidemiology of intimate partner violence in the United States.

An estimated 12 million women will be victims of physical abuse by their partners during their lives, and 1.5 million women are physically abused annually. However, because intimate partner violence is underreported, these numbers are probably much higher. One third to one half of all women who are murdered annually are murdered by their male intimate partners. Between 1% and 7% of women in the emergency department present because of an acute episode of physical abuse, and as many as 54% of all women who present to the emergency department have been victims of intimate partner violence at some point during their lives.

13. Who is at risk for being victimized by intimate partner violence?

Ninety-five percent of victims of intimate partner violence are women who are abused by men. Intimate abuse also occurs in same-sex relationships and may be perpetrated by women against their male partners. Women of all ages, racial and ethnic origins, socioeconomic states, educational backgrounds, occupations, religions, and personality types are affected by intimate partner violence.

14. Who are the perpetrators of intimate partner violence?

In more than 95% of cases, men are the perpetrators of intimate partner violence. They may be past or present intimate partners. Perpetrators are of all ages, racial and ethnic origins, socioeconomic states, educational backgrounds, occupations, and religions. In the health care setting, perpetrators frequently want to stay with the victim in the examining room and commonly answer questions for the victim. They may even attempt to control the health care provider. They often deny, minimize, and lie about their abusive conduct, blaming others to justify their conduct.

15. What patient population should be screened for intimate partner violence?

Because of the high prevalence of intimate partner violence among women, it is recommended that all female patients be screened by all health care providers in all specialties. Screening for intimate partner violence should be carried out in a safe, private environment after the partner and other family members and friends have been removed from the room. Screening may be performed verbally or using a written questionnaire. Screening may be performed using the following questions:

1. Have you been hit, kicked, punched, or otherwise hurt by someone in the past year? If so, by whom?

2. Do you feel safe in your current relationship? Is there a partner from a previous relationship making you feel unsafe now?

3. Many women with injuries such as yours sustained them when they were hit or hurt by their partner. Is this what happened to you?

4. Has your partner ever forced you to have sex when you didn't want to?

5. Has your partner ever tried to strangle or "choke" you?

16. Describe types of abusive behavior.

- Physical assaults may consist of scratching, biting, pushing, slapping, punching, choking, and using objects (e.g., household objects, firearms, knives).
- Sexual assaults may consist of coerced sex by manipulation or threat, physically forced sex, sexual assault with violence, and forced sex without the use of condoms with a partner positive for human immunodeficiency virus (HIV).
- Psychological abuse may consist of threats of physical harm; attacks against property or pets; verbal attacks and humiliation; isolation; controlling victim's access to money, shelter, food, clothing, transportation, health care, and medications; and the use or abuse of the victim's children (i.e., abusing the children as a way to hurt the victim or using the children to spy on or humiliate the victim).

17. What regions of the body are most frequently injured?

The head, face, neck, and the "bathing suit" region (i.e., breasts, chest, abdomen, buttocks, and genitals) are most frequently injured through intimate partner violence.

18. Name some historical clues that suggest intimate partner violence.

- History inconsistent with the injury
- Delay in seeking medical care
- History of repeated or chronic injuries
- Frequent visits to health care providers
- Noncompliance with medications and medical appointments
- Suicide attempts
- Injuries in pregnancy
- Alcohol or substance abuse
- Child abuse in the same family

19. List some common injuries sustained in intimate partner violence.

Contusions	Ruptured tympanic membranes
Lacerations	Loose and fractured teeth
Fractures (i.e., facial, skull, and extremity)	Hair pulled out
Stab wounds	Neck contusions and cord marks
Gunshot wounds	Grab contusions of the upper arms
Burns (e.g., cigarettes, electrical appliances)	Blunt abdominal trauma in
Blunt head trauma	pregnancy
Subconjunctival hemorrhages	Sexual assault

20. What precautions should be taken when admitting injured victims of intimate partner violence to the hospital?

Patients who are victims of intimate partner violence should be admitted to the hospital as "Jane Doe" or "John Doe." This action prevents further victimization by the batterer during hospitalization. Ward staff should be cautioned not to give out any information concerning the victim over the telephone except to designated individuals.

21. Name complications of intimate partner violence.

Complications of intimate partner violence consist of child abuse, sexual assault, depression, alcohol and substance abuse, suicide, and spousal homicide. In more than 50% of homes where there is ongoing intimate partner violence, there is also ongoing child abuse.

22. What are the complications of battering during pregnancy?

Up to 25% of women seeking routine prenatal care are victims of intimate partner violence. Battering during pregnancy may result in delayed prenatal care, premature labor, premature rupture of membranes, abruption of the placenta, miscarriage and fetal loss, premature delivery, delayed postpartum recovery, impaired bonding, and possibly low-birth-weight babies.

23. What specific referrals should be made for victims of intimate partner violence?

In addition to medical, surgical, and psychiatric referrals that may be indicated, victims of intimate partner violence should be referred to social services, intimate partner violence advocacy services and shelters (including multilingual services and services for gay men and lesbians as needed), a 24-hour hotline, legal assistance, and law enforcement.

24. Why do some victims of intimate partner violence leave their abusive relationships while others do not?

Most victims do leave their abusive relationships; however, they frequently leave temporarily on several occasions before leaving permanently. Women may leave because of increasing severity of abuse, the fear of being killed, if the abuser has abused the children, or on account of interventions of others outside the family. Women may not leave an abusive relationship because of fear of violence and retaliation for leaving, a lack of real options to be safe with her children, low self-esteem, belief in maintaining the family unit at all costs, cultural or religious reasons, a lack of shelters and victims' advocacy programs nationwide, economic hardship, lack of affordable and safe housing, lack of affordable legal assistance, intermittent positive reinforcement, a belief her partner will reform, and a lack of intervention by others outside the family.

25. When is a victim of intimate partner violence at greatest risk for homicide?

A victim of intimate partner violence may be at greatest risk for homicide when she leaves or attempts to leave the relationship. As her health care provider, it is imperative that her risk of lethality be assessed. She should be counseled before discharge about her risk and be advised about precautions she should take to minimize the risk. She should also be assisted in developing a safety plan and plan for a quick escape in case violence erupts at home. She should be advised to keep a bag packed at home or at a friend's house in case of emergency. It should contain copies of important documents and any medications taken routinely.

ELDER ABUSE

26. How is elder abuse defined?

Elder abuse is defined as actions or the omission of actions by a caretaker that result in harm or that threaten harm to the health or welfare of the elderly. Elder abuse includes physical abuse, sexual abuse, neglect, psychological abuse, exploitation, and financial abuse.

27. What is the incidence of elder abuse in the United States?

The rate of elder abuse is estimated at 1.5 million cases in the United States annually. However, elder abuse, like intimate partner violence, is severely underreported. Elder abuse affects approximately 1 of 20 older persons. In one emergency department survey, 2.5% of individuals older than 60 years responded that they were victims of physical abuse.

28. Name risk factors for elder abuse.

Risk factors for elder abuse can be divided into elder characteristics and caretaker or family characteristics.

Elder Characteristics	Caretaker or Family Characteristics
Female gender	Mental or emotional illness
Advanced age	Stress
Dependency	No social support system
Isolation	Overcrowding
Impairment	Economic difficulties
Previous abuse	Abuse as a child
Alcohol abuse	Alcohol or substance abuse
Internalization of blame	
Excessive loyalty to caretaker	

29. Who is the most common perpetrator of elder abuse?

In more than 85% of cases, a relative is the perpetrator of elder abuse, usually an adult child or spouse.

30. What historical clues suggest elder abuse?

- Discrepancies in the history from the patient and caretaker
- Implausible or vague explanations for injuries
- History of previous injuries
- Delays between onset of injury or illness and seeking medical care
- Noncompliance with medications and appointments
- Frequent visits to the emergency department for exacerbations of chronic diseases

31. What physical findings suggest elder abuse?

- Multiple injuries in various stages of healing
- Poor hygiene
- Dehydration
- Malnutrition
- Genital injuries
- Sexually transmitted diseases
- Evidence of improper restraints (e.g., rope marks)
- Undermedication or overmedication

32. What are the health care provider's legal responsibilities in reporting child abuse, intimate partner violence, and elder abuse?

All 50 states require health care providers to report cases that they reasonably suspect or know to involve child abuse. Child protective services should be contacted immediately. The child may be made a ward of the courts if indicated for safety reasons. Mandatory reporting laws requiring health care providers to report known or reasonably suspected elder abuse also been enacted in all states. Fewer than 10 states have mandatory reporting requirements for health care providers to report intimate partner violence. However, some injuries due to intimate partner violence may be reportable to law enforcement under laws regarding assaults resulting in injuries from deadly weapons or other crimes (e.g., firearm, knife). Health care providers should become familiar with the reporting laws of the states in which they practice.

BIBLIOGRAPHY

1. Abbott J, Johnson R, Koziol-McCain J, Lowenstein SR: Domestic violence against women. JAMA 273:1763–1767, 1995.

2. Barnett TM: Child abuse. In Marx JA, Hockberger RS, Walls RM, et al (eds): Rosen's Emergency Medicine: Concepts and Clinical Practice, 5th ed. St. Louis, Mosby, 2002, pp 842–854.
3. Berkowitz DC: Pediatric abuse: New patterns of injury. Emerg Med Clin North Am 13:321–341, 1995.
4. Donald T, Jureidini J: Munchausen syndrome by proxy: Child abuse in the medical system. Arch Pediatr Adolesc Med 150:753–758, 1996.
5. Feldhaus KM, Koziol-McCain J, Amsbury HL, et al: Accuracy of three brief screening questions for detecting partner violence in the emergency department. JAMA 277:1357–1361, 1997.
6. Gazmararian JA, Lazorick S, Spitz AM, et al: Prevalence of violence against pregnant women. JAMA 275:1915–1920, 1996.
7. Houry D, Sachs CJ, Feldhaus KM, et al: Violence-inflicted injuries: Reporting laws in the fifty states. Ann Emerg Med 39:56–60, 2002.
8. Jones JS: Elder abuse and neglect: Responding to a national problem. Ann Emerg Med 23:845–848, 1994.
9. Kleinschmidt KC: Elder abuse: A review. Ann Emerg Med 30:463–472, 1997.
10. Kosberg JI: Preventing elder abuse: Identification of high risk factors before placement decisions. Gerontologist 28:43–50, 1988.
11. Lachs MS, Millemer K: Abuse and neglect of elderly persons. N Engl J Med 332:437–443, 1995.
12. Lachs MS, Williams CS, O'Brien S, et al: Emergency department use by older victims of family violence. Ann Emerg Med 30:448–454, 1997.
13. Muelleman RL, Lenaghan PA, Pakieser RA: Battered women: Injury locations and types. Ann Emerg Med 28:486–492, 1996.
14. Nimkin K, Kleinman PK: Imaging of child abuse. Pediatr Clin North Am 44:615–635, 1997.
15. Wissow LS: Child abuse and neglect. N Engl J Med 332:1425–1431, 1995.

XII. Special Populations

39. PEDIATRIC TRAUMA

Areti Tillou, M.D., and Demetrios Demetriades, M.D., Ph.D.

1. How commonly does trauma affect children?

Injury is the leading cause of death and disability of children older than 1 year of age, exceeding all other causes of death combined. It affects almost one third of children. Unintentional injury deaths account for 65% of all injury deaths in children younger than 19 years of age. For every child who dies of an injury, 40 others are hospitalized, and 1120 are treated in emergency departments.

Motor vehicle accidents are the cause of most deaths, followed by homicide or suicide (predominantly with firearms) and drowning. Falls and vehicular crashes account for 90% of all pediatric injuries. Tragically, home is a common scene for childhood injury. Penetrating injuries are increasing in childhood and adolescence in large cities. The average reported incidence is about 16%, but it is as high as 50% in some series.

2. What main points should be kept in mind when treating pediatric patients?

- Smaller body mass (i.e., greater force applied per unit body area)
- Less body fat (i.e., more intense energy transmission)
- Less connective tissue (i.e., closer proximity to vital organs)
- Larger body surface are to body volume and less fat (i.e., higher thermal energy loss)
- Multisystem injury as a rule in blunt trauma (i.e., requiring thorough multisystem evaluation)
- Emotional instability (i.e., difficult assessment in the emergency department)
- Evolving physiologic growth and phycological development (i.e., posttraumatic distress syndrome symptoms such as phobias, sleep disturbances, rage attacks, and decreased academic performance in more than 50% of children hospitalized after trauma)
- Variations in children's sizes (i.e., Broselow pediatric resuscitation measuring tape used to calculate the weight, tube sizes, and medication doses)

3. What are the three main differences in the pediatric airway?

1. In children, a greater cranium compared with midface and a larger occiput force the cervical spine into a slightly flexed position, obstructing the posterior pharynx. It may be helpful to use a folded blanket or towel to elevate the body of the child and straighten the spine. The face is also slightly more superior and anterior (i.e., sniffing position). A jaw-thrust maneuver is the safest method for improving airway patency.

2. The larynx and vocal cords are higher and slightly more anterior and may be obscured by the large and floppy epiglottis. A straight blade offers better visualization for intubation. The cricoid ring is the narrowest part of the child's airway and forms a natural seal with the endotracheal (ET) tube.

3. Orotracheal intubation with uncuffed tubes is the safest way to secure the airway up to the age of 8 years.

4. What are some specific concerns about obtaining an artificial airway in children?
- Do not use an oral airway unless the child is unconscious.
- Do not twist oral airway by 180 degrees when inserting. It may cause pharyngeal hematoma.
- Choose the appropriate size of ET tube by gauging the diameter of the external nares or the child's little finger. The following formula can be used: 4.0 + (age/4) mm. A 4-year-old child can be intubated using a 4.0 + (4/4) mm = 4.0 + 1 mm = 5.0-mm ET tube.
- Give atropine before any anesthetics or paralytics to prevent bradycardia.
- Beware of a short trachea commonly leading to right mainstem intubation, which occurs in about 17% of emergency intubations (see Figures).
- Do not use nasotracheal intubation in children younger than 12 years of age because of the high incidence of potential complications.
- Never perform cricothyroidotomy in children younger than 11 years of age because of the high risk of permanent stricture, because cricoid cartilage is the only circumferential support to the trachea. In desperate cases, needle cricothyroidotomy with jet insufflation is preferred but may result in hypercarbia.

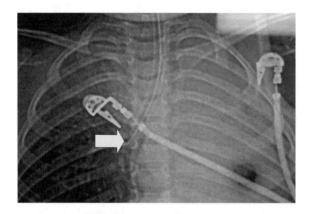

Right mainstem intubation.

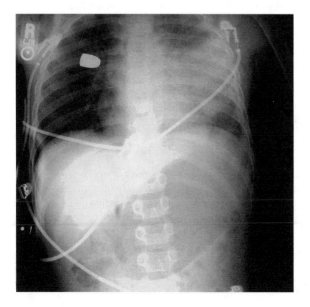

Massive gastric distention.

5. What is the value of prehospital intubation in children?

Prehospital endotracheal intubation of children in an urban setting is not recommended. Attempts at intubation seem to prolong time spent at the injury scene and may increase fatal complications in the subgroups for whom the survival rate is high. Bag-valve ventilation with the appropriate technique provides adequate oxygenation in most cases and is recommended.

6. What should be kept in mind when assessing breathing in children?

- Hypoventilation is the most common cause of cardiac arrest in children.
- Respiratory acidosis is the most common metabolic abnormality.
- When mechanically ventilating, 7 to 10 mL/kg is the recommended tidal volume.
- Use pediatric bag-valve-mask devices to avoid barotrauma to the immature bronchoalveolar tree.

7. What are the important points concerning circulation and fluid resuscitation?

- Approximately 25% of blood loss is required to manifest diminished circulating blood volume. Hypotension is a late deleterious sign that occurs with blood loss of more than 45% of the total blood volume, indicating that all reserves are depleted.
- Tachycardia, poor skin perfusion, and decrease of the pulse pressure by more than 20 mmHg are the initial signs of hypoperfusion. Dulled response to pain can also be a sign of shock.
- In children, blood volume is estimated to be 80 mL/kg, or 9% of their body weight. For initial resuscitation, a bolus of 20 mL/kg of warm crystalloid should be given.
- Up to *three* boluses of 20 mL/kg may be needed to replace a 25% blood loss. Blood transfusion should be considered when starting to use the third bolus. The recommended amount of blood transfusion is 10 mL/kg. Hemodynamically stable children with solid organ injuries can tolerate a decrease in hemoglobin to 7 g/dL without the need for blood transfusion.

8. What are normal vital signs according to age?

Age	Weight (kg)	Heart Rate (beats/min)	Blood Pressure (mmHg)	Respiratory Rate (breaths/min)
Birth to 6 months	3–6	180–160	60–80	60
Infants	12	160	80	40
Preschool	16	120	90	30
Adolescent	35	100	100	20

Adapted from American College of Surgeons Committee on Trauma: Advanced Trauma Life Support Instructors' Manual: Pediatric Trauma. Chicago, American College of Surgeons, 1997, p 361.

9. What are the options for venous access in the pediatric population?

- Peripheral percutaneous venous access (first option)
- Intraosseous infusion (second option, usually in children younger than 6 years)
- Venous cutdown
- Percutaneous femoral line
- Percutaneous subclavian line
- Percutaneous external jugular (EJ) line
- Internal jugular (IJ) line
- Central venous access, sometimes preferred if peripheral intravenous access in the hospital is not feasible and to avoid intraosseous (IO) lines and venous cutdown

10. What are the indications and the proper technique for the insertion of intraosseous lines?

IO lines provide safe and rapid intravenous access in children when peripheral intravenous access cannot be established in a timely manner. Fluids, blood, and drugs can be given through this route.

With the patient in a supine position, the line is placed in a noninjured extremity one finger-breath below the tibial tubercle, away from the epiphyseal plate and toward the foot of the patient. Alternatively, the distal femur approximately 3 cm above the external condyle can be used in cases of tibial fractures. Padding should be placed under the knee to achieve 30-degree flexion. A short, large-caliber, bone marrow aspiration needle or a short, 18-gauge spinal needle is placed through the anterior cortex of the proximal tibia or distal femur into the medullary cavity of the bone.

11. What are specific anatomic characteristics of the cervical spine in children?
  - Only 5% of all spinal cord injuries occur in children. However, pediatric spinal fractures are associated with significant mortality rate compared with those in adults (54.5% versus 20.5%).
  - Interspinous ligaments and joint capsules are more flexible.
  - Vertebral bodies are wedged anteriorly and tend to slide forward with flexion.
  - Facet joints are flat and tend to sublux easier than in adults.
  - Underdeveloped neck musculature and a head that is disproportionately large and heavy compared with the body places the anatomic fulcrum of the spine at the level of the C2 and C3 vertebrae. Subsequently, injuries below the C3 level account for only 30% of pediatric cervical spine injuries.

12. What are some specific radiological findings of interest in pediatric cervical spine films?
  - Pseudosubluxation of C2 on C3 and of C3 on C4 occurs in children younger than 7 years. In some children, the condition is present until the age of 14 years.
  - Increased distance between the dense and the anterior arch of C1 may give the impression of subluxation.
  - Accentuated prevertebral soft tissue space may be seen in children who are agitated and crying, but it should not exceed two thirds of the C2 vertebral body.
  - An absence of normal cervical lordosis may be seen.
  - Basilar synchondrosis of the dense and apical epiphyses may appear as fractures on the plain films.
  - The growth center of the spinous process may appear as a fracture.
  - Up to 20% of children may have spinal cord injury without radiographic abnormality (SCIWRA).

13. What are the specific characteristics of head trauma in pediatric patients?
  - Head injuries are the major cause of death among injured children, and those who survive have a high rate of permanent disability. The central nervous system (CNS) is the most common isolated system injured.
  - The brain size doubles in the first 6 months of life and achieves 80% of the adult size at 2 years of age. Because of its consistency, the cerebral parenchyma is more susceptible to shearing injury.
  - Most head injuries in pediatric population are minor, and full recovery can be expected.
  - Outcome is generally better than for adults, although children are more susceptible to secondary brain injury. However, young children better tolerate intracranial pressure increases because of the open fontanel and mobile cranial suture lines.
  - Children tend to have fewer focal mass lesions than adults, but elevated intracranial pressure due to cerebral edema is more common.
  - A pediatric version of the Glasgow Coma Scale is available for children who cannot speak.
  - Cognitive and behavioral impairments cause some of the most troublesome long-term disabilities, but they are frequently subtle and easily overlooked.

14. What are the signs of increased intracranial pressure in infants?
  - Full fontanel and split sutures

- Altered state of consciousness and paradoxical irritability
- Persistent emesis
- The setting sun sign (i.e., inability to fully open the eyes)
- Typically, infants are late in the development of intracranial hypertension. In older children headache, stiff neck, photophobia, altered level of consciousness, cranial nerve involvement, papilledema, posturing, hypertension with bradycardia (i.e., Cushing's response), hypoventilation, and persistent emesis are common findings.

15. What types of scalp injuries are found in infants and children?

Scalp injuries may manifest in three different forms: *caput secundum,* injury to the connecting tissue itself; *subgaleal hematoma,* injury to the tissue surrounding the skull; and *cephalohematoma,* a collection of blood under the periosteum. Hypotension may occur in infants as a result of head injury because of the potentially large blood loss in the subgaleal or epidural space.

16. What are some characteristics of pediatric chest trauma?

- Rib fractures are rare. Their presence signifies major force and is often associated with underlying intrathoracic injuries.
- Flail chest is rare.
- Lung and myocardial contusions are more common than in adults.
- Aortic rupture is rare in children.

17. What is commotio cordis?

Commotio cordis, a disorder found in the pediatric population, results from a sudden impact to the anterior chest wall (e.g., baseball injuries) that causes cessation of normal cardiac function. Immediate dysrhythmias or ventricular fibrillation may be refractory to resuscitative efforts, resulting in cardiogenic shock and death.

18. What is the incidence of abdominal trauma in the pediatric population?

- Abdominal trauma is the third leading cause of traumatic death following head and thoracic injuries. Thin abdominal wall with poor muscle tone, proportionately larger solid intra-abdominal organs and pliable cartilaginous rib cage increase the risk of intra-abdominal injuries in children.
- In more than 90% of cases, bleeding from an injured spleen, liver, or kidney is generally self-limited, and less than 15% of children require laparotomy.
- Liberal use of computed tomography (CT) is recommended, especially for hemodynamically stable children with probable injuries based on the history, mechanism, and physical examination. Imaging is also strongly recommended in cases of multisystem injury, especially head trauma. In 25% of cases with head trauma and a Glasgow Coma Score of less than 10, the children have significant intra-abdominal injuries.

19. What are some characteristics of abdominal injuries in children?

- Liver and spleen are the most frequently injured organs in the abdomen.
- Duodenal hematomas and blunt pancreatic injuries are commonly caused by blunt trauma from the handlebars of a bicycle, kicks, or impact during contact sports. Most duodenal injuries are not full thickness and result in a submural hematoma that can be managed without an operation. Most pancreatic injuries can also be managed with observation unless there is major pancreatic duct injury.
- Small bowel perforations at or near the ligament of Treitz are typical. Approximately 5% of all children who sustain blunt abdominal trauma have hollow viscus injuries. Children are also more susceptible to Chance fractures in combination with enteric disruption.
- Penetrating injuries to the perineum or straddle injuries often result in intraperitoneal injuries.

20. What are the characteristics of splenic injuries in children?

The spleen is the most commonly injured organ in cases of blunt trauma. More than 90% of splenic injuries can be treated without an operation, compared with about 60% of adult patients.

After traumatic splenectomy, children have a 50-fold increased likelihood of death from septicemia compared with healthy children. In addition to vaccinations against encapsulated organisms, some surgeons recommend daily antimicrobial prophylaxis for most asplenic children, especially those younger than 5 years of age. Others recommend observation and antibiotics on command.

21. Is it important to insert a nasogastric tube?

- Children have a propensity to swallow a large amount of air. Bag-mask ventilation also may result in insufflation of air into the stomach (see lower Figure on page 240).
- Gastric distention may be massive and compromise diaphragmatic excursion, predisposing children to regurgitation and aspiration.
- The tidal volume generated by children depends much more on diaphragmatic function than in adults, and any interference with diaphragmatic excursion, such as gastric distention, can result in respiratory compromise.
- Gastric distention may interfere with the clinical examination of the abdomen.
- Infants are obligate nasal breathers, and an orogastric tube should be placed instead of a nasogastric tube.

22. What should be emphasized concerning extremity fractures?

- Fractures in children may be not seen on initial films.
- Buckle fractures (i.e., bending without fracture lines) and greenstick fractures (i.e., incomplete fractures involving only one cortex) may occur.
- Injury to growth plates may affect normal growth.
- Proportionately more blood is lost from fractures in children than in adults.
- Decreased use of the extremity may be a sign of fracture in a small child who cannot complain of pain.
- Vascular injury rarely leads to ischemia because of extensive collateral circulation and may have an inhibitory effect in normal development.
- Pelvic fractures are unusual, and their presence suggests associated intra-abdominal or genitourinary tract injuries.
- Fractures in children younger than 3 years of age should raise the suspicion of child abuse.

23. What is child abuse?

Child abuse is some form of nonaccidental injury of a child by the parent or guardian. Besides intentional physical abuse, it also refers to sexual and emotional abuse and to child neglect. Almost 1 million children are confirmed victims of physical abuse in a year. All cases of documented or suspected abuse *must* be reported to the appropriate authorities, usually social service agencies or the state's Health and Human Services Department. Approximately 50% of abused children return dead if released to the person who abused them!

24. Under what circumstances should child abuse or neglect be suspected, and what action should be taken?

1. Discrepancy in history and physical findings
2. Repeated visits to various emergency rooms or prolonged time before medical attention is sought
3. Multiple injuries of different ages
4. Recognizable but unusual injuries such as multiple subdural hemorrhages without skull fracture, retinal hemorrhages (in 75% of cases of shaken baby syndrome), perioral and perineal lesions that are unmistakably the result of inflicted trauma

5. All injuries in children of younger than 1 year of age; victims of shaken infant or impact syndrome may present with no external signs of injury

6. Inappropriate parent responses

25. What is the role of injury prevention in pediatric trauma?

Prevention is very important in child injuries. Most injured children succumb before they reach the hospital. Simple measures such as using a bicycle helmet can decrease head injuries by 85%. Similarly, car seats, traffic-calming measures, fire-retardant clothing, and community-based violence prevention programs are examples of effective interventions that can reduce the prevalence of pediatric trauma.

Two important points about the epidemiology of pediatric trauma are that *childhood injury is a preventable disease,* not an accident, and that pediatric trauma care should focus mainly on global outcomes after nonfatal injuries rather than mortality.

BIBLIOGRAPHY

1. American College of Surgeons Committee on Trauma: Advanced Trauma Life Support Course for Physicians, 5th ed. Chicago, American College of Surgeons, 1993, pp 261–281.
2. Arensman RM: Pediatric Trauma. Initial Care of the Injured Child. New York, Raven Press, 1995.
3. Cantor RM, Leaming JM: Contemporary issues in trauma. Evaluation and management of pediatric major trauma. Emerg Med Clin North Am 16:229–256, 1998.
4. Gausche M, Lewis R, Stratton S, et al: Effect of out-of-hospital pediatric endotracheal intubation on survival and neurological outcome: A controlled clinical trial. JAMA 283:783–790, 2000.
5. Knudson MM: Pediatric trauma. In Demetriades D, Asensio J (eds): Trauma Management, 1st ed. Georgetown, TX, Landes Bioscience, 2000, pp 480–491.
6. Sanchez JI, Paidas CN: Childhood trauma: Now and in the new millennium. Surg Clin North Am 79:1503–1535, 1999.

40. TRAUMA DURING PREGNANCY

Edward Newton, M.D.

1. How common is trauma during pregnancy?

Although most pregnancies progress uneventfully, trauma has become an increasingly important cause of fetal and maternal complications. Because of improved treatment of sepsis and hemorrhage, maternal mortality from purely obstetric complications has dramatically decreased over the past five decades. At the same time, trauma has emerged as the leading cause of death in pregnant women, as it is in nonpregnant women between the ages of 15 and 45 years. Overall, 6% to 7% of pregnancies are complicated by trauma. Unsuspected pregnancy is relatively common in reproductive-aged females, and urine pregnancy tests should be routinely obtained for all female patients with reproductive potential.

2. What types of trauma commonly occur during pregnancy?

Blunt trauma primarily due to motor vehicle crashes is the leading cause of major trauma in pregnant women, but there are other causes. As pregnancy progresses, greater bulk and a forward shift in the woman's center of gravity result in more frequent falls and diminished agility in avoiding trauma. Homicide is another leading cause of maternal death, reflecting the epidemic of inner-city violence. Pregnancy is a high-risk state for domestic violence, and this cause must be considered and investigated when treating pregnant trauma victims.

3. How does pregnancy alter the clinical assessment of the trauma patient?

Pregnancy causes major physiologic changes in a woman that affect virtually every organ system. The hemodynamic changes of pregnancy are of primary importance in trauma evaluation. Pregnancy is a high-flow and low-resistance state. Plasma volume expands by 50% by the sixth month, and cardiac output increases by about one third. Blood pressure and central venous pressure fall progressively during pregnancy, and the resting pulse rate increases by up to 20 beats per minute. Consequently, normal pregnancy may mimic hypovolemia with tachycardia and hypotension. These changes make it difficult to rely on vital signs alone to assess hemodynamic status.

Another important change is the physiologic anemia of pregnancy. Because the increase in red blood cell (RBC) mass (18%) is much less than the increase in plasma volume (50%), there is a dilutional effect on the hematocrit, which decreases from 35% to 32% in normal pregnancy. This reinforces the precept that a trend in successive hematocrits is more useful than an isolated value.

As the uterus enlarges, abdominal contents are displaced upward, and diaphragmatic excursion is limited. Apart from gastrointestinal problems, this anatomic change results in a characteristic "hyperventilation of pregnancy" as the respiratory rate increases to compensate for the decrease in tidal volume. Consequently, P_{CO_2} levels are typically low, and the kidney excretes bicarbonate to maintain physiologic pH. The average level of P_{CO_2} is 30 mmHg, and the HCO_3 concentration averages 19 to 22 mEq/L. Tachypnea and low bicarbonate levels may be misconstrued as signs of decompensated shock. The displaced abdominal contents and a higher diaphragm are more susceptible to penetrating injury in the upper abdomen and lower chest.

4. Is prehospital management different for pregnant trauma victims?

In general, the extrication and initial stabilization of pregnant trauma patients is identical to that of nonpregnant patients. The most important difference is that the supine hypotensive syndrome should be avoided. This syndrome occurs when the gravid uterus, which can weigh 10 kg at term, compresses the inferior vena cava and aorta, causing an immediate reduction in venous return to the heart and greatly diminished cardiac output. In a traumatized patient who may already have marginally adequate cardiac output, this syndrome can cause cardiac arrest. Increased venous back pressure may increase the likelihood of placental abruption. Although paramedics are appropriately concerned with immobilizing the patient's spine with a cervical collar and backboard, the supine position should be avoided, and the patient should be transported with the backboard in a 15-degree tilt to the left.

One of the immediate responses to maternal blood loss is that blood flow to the abdominal viscera and uterus are decreased to preserve circulation to the mother's essential organs. Consequently, the patient may appear relatively stable, but the placenta and fetus may be significantly underperfused. To prevent unrecognized fetal hypoperfusion, all pregnant trauma patients should be transported with oxygen flowing and a fluid challenge infusing through a large-bore intravenous line. Because this situation may result in the delivery of a severely premature or traumatized infant, pregnant trauma patients should be transported to a trauma center with appropriate capabilities, such as a neonatal intensive care unit.

5. How does the initial resuscitation of the pregnant trauma victim differ from that of the nonpregnant patient?

Although the patient should be assessed in a slight left lateral position, the primary survey for life-threatening injuries should be conducted as usual. After life-threatening injuries have been addressed, a complete head-to-toe examination should be performed, including assessment of the fetus. Estimating the gestational age of the fetus is essential because much of the algorithmic approach to the pregnant trauma patient hinges on the potential viability of the fetus outside the uterus. Fetal heart tones can be obtained with a Doppler stethoscope by 12 weeks' gestation, and these should be recorded. If the patient is able to provide a history, the date of the last menstrual period (LMP) and estimated date of confinement (EDC) should be determined, as well as any complications during the current and previous pregnancies, presence of contractions, and fetal movements. Measurement of the fundal height can approximate gestational age. Palpation of the fundus at the level of the umbilicus corresponds to a gestational age of 20 weeks, and adding 1 week per additional centimeter beyond the umbilicus provides a reasonable estimate of gestational age. Ultrasound can also provide an accurate measure of gestational age by determining the biparietal diameter of the fetus. Physical examination of the pregnant abdomen is difficult because abdominal organs are displaced by the growing uterus. Chronic stretch of the peritoneum by the expanding pregnancy makes it less sensitive, and peritoneal signs may be subtle or absent.

Pelvic examination is essential. It may reveal vaginal lacerations, rupture of membranes, vaginal bleeding, cervical dilation, presenting fetal parts, and pelvic or sacral fractures that may ultimately make vaginal delivery impossible. The examination must be done under sterile conditions because of the possibility of ruptured membranes.

Crystalloid fluid administration is indicated in all pregnant trauma patients to ensure adequate placental perfusion. If immediate transfusion is indicated, the blood should be Rh negative to avoid isoimmunization of the mother. Indicated radiographs are obtained despite a risk of teratogenesis, although the uterus should be shielded whenever possible. Early consultation with specialists in obstetrics and neonatology is indicated if a potentially viable fetus is found, obstetric complications are present, or delivery is considered imminent.

6. What ancillary methods are useful in evaluating the fetus?

Ultrasound evaluation of the abdomen has become increasingly used as a bedside, noninvasive method to detect organ injury and hemoperitoneum, and it is particularly useful in the pregnant patient. Transabdominal ultrasound can detect the fetal heart rate by 7 to 8 weeks' gestation and provides information on the lie and presentation of the fetus, fetal heart rate, and presence of twin gestations. Occasionally, it can directly detect injuries in the fetus. However, ultrasound is not an accurate method (sensitivity of 40% to 50%) for detecting abruptio placentae, which is the most common cause of fetal death after trauma. Because the clot that forms immediately from abruptio placentae is isodense with the placenta, ultrasound does not reliably detect a fresh hemorrhage, and the placenta may appear to be only somewhat thickened compared with a normal placenta. As the clot liquifies over the next several days, it becomes increasingly sonolucent and consequently easier to detect with ultrasound.

Because there is no reliable method to visualize an acute abruption, fetal heart monitoring is often employed to assess the fetus. This technique simultaneously records fetal heart rate and uterine contractions. There are several characteristic patterns of fetal heart response to a uterine contraction that accurately indicate fetal distress before it becomes apparent clinically.

7. What injuries can occur specifically during pregnancy?

Abruptio placentae. Dissection of blood between the layers of the placenta disrupts the supply of oxygen and nutrients to the fetus. After approximately 50% of the placental surface is disrupted, the fetus cannot survive. Lesser degrees of abruption present as abdominal pain, uterine irritability and contractions, and a variable amount of vaginal bleeding. Characteristic patterns of fetal distress often are seen on fetal heart monitoring. If the fetus is viable (>23 weeks' gestation), a crash cesarean section is indicated. If the fetus is not yet viable, the condition can be managed expectantly but the patient should be monitored for disseminated intravascular coagulation (DIC), which commonly occurs in this setting and may require delivery of a previable fetus. Elevation of the serum D-dimer level may be useful in detecting placental abruption, although it is not specific for this condition.

Uterine rupture. Massive blunt force injures the uterus, which ruptures with explosive force. Most often, the uterus can be palpated as a contracted mass, and fetal parts can be palpated subcutaneously. Because of the forces involved, the fetus usually does not survive, but there are reports of fetal survival in this setting. Treatment generally requires a hysterectomy to control blood loss, but the uterus may be repaired primarily depending on the extent of injury.

Amniotic fluid embolus. After any trauma or surgical manipulation of the pregnant uterus, there is a risk of introducing a bolus of amniotic fluid into the maternal circulation. This causes a devastating condition with a high mortality rate. The diagnosis is suggested by the sudden onset of dyspnea, hypoxemia, and tachypnea that may be followed by adult respiratory distress syndrome (ARDS) and DIC. Treatment is supportive with positive pressure oxygen in an intensive care unit setting, but the maternal mortality rate is approximately 85%.

Fetomaternal hemorrhage. Introduction of only a few milliliters of fetal blood into the maternal circulation causes isosensitization of the patient if there is an Rh mismatch. If the woman is Rh negative and the fetus Rh positive, the woman will form antibodies to the Rh factor. These antibodies attack subsequent Rh-positive fetuses, resulting in erythroblastosis fetalis. Because no tests are sensitive enough to detect such a small amount of fetal blood, it is routine to administer "mini RhoGAM" (50 μg) in the first trimester and regular-dose RhoGAM (300 μg) during the second and third trimesters. This dosage blocks the formation of maternal antibody against the Rh factor. The Kleihauer-Betke test is used to detect the presence of fetal blood cells in a sample of maternal blood and should be obtained whenever fetomaternal transfusion is suspected. However, it is not sensitive enough to detect very small quantities of fetal blood.

Premature labor. Organized uterine contractions are common after trauma to the abdomen. Because abruptio placentae is often associated with contractions, assume it is present when a pregnant trauma victim goes into labor. If the fetus is mature, the labor should be allowed to progress with appropriate fetal monitoring and interventions if distress occurs. The management of a premature fetus is more controversial. Some experts believe that abruptio placentae is the most common cause of premature labor in this setting and that the uterus should not be relaxed with tocolysis because of the risk of increased bleeding. Others feel that labor can safely be arrested with tocolytics. Obstetric consultation is indicated.

Premature rupture of membranes. Occasionally, the placental membranes rupture as a result of increased intrauterine pressure or from direct trauma. The patient may say that her "water broke," or clear fluid is detected on pelvic examination. The fluid can be assessed by Nitrazine paper (vaginal secretions have a pH of 5 to 6, whereas amniotic fluid is generally >7), although this test is inaccurate in the presence of blood. Ferning of the secretions as they are dried on a microscope slide is characteristic of amniotic fluid and may be a more reliable test. The principal risk of premature rupture of the membranes is ascending infection, amnionitis, and fetal loss. Obstetric consultation should be obtained for this complication.

8. How should the pregnancy be managed if the mother has severe injuries?

If the patient has injuries requiring surgery, surgery should never be deferred or delayed because she is pregnant. If the fetus is in no distress and is previable, the uterus should be left alone. If the fetus is at term and stable, cesarean section can be performed after repair of the mother's injuries. If the fetus is viable but in severe distress, emergent cesarean section is indicated if the mother can tolerate this procedure. If the fetus is previable and in severe distress, there are no specific interventions to correct the distress other than optimizing the mother's condition.

9. What is the role of perimortem cesarean section?

Perimortem cesarean section is one of the most dramatic procedures in trauma care. There are numerous reports of successful cesarean delivery and survival of a mature fetus even after the mother has died. In certain conditions, the mother may be declared "brain dead" but maintains normal brainstem function and vital signs. In this case, the fetus can be allowed to mature and be delivered near term. when the woman experiences a cardiac arrest, however, the delivery must be accomplished expeditiously if the fetus is to survive. The procedure should be attempted only when the fetus has some statistical chance for survival (i.e., >23 weeks' gestation); therefore, accurate estimated gestational age and a live fetus are essential. Resuscitation of the mother should continue during the delivery because emptying the uterus is often associated with improvement in the mother's clinical status. After it is determined that the woman is in cardiac arrest, a classic (vertical incision) cesarean section should be started and completed within 5 minutes of the cardiac arrest. Survival of a neurologically intact fetus varies inversely with the delay in accomplishing delivery, and the procedure should probably not be attempted if more than 15 minutes of cardiac arrest has transpired.

10. Can pregnant trauma patients with a normal assessment be discharged home?

Because there is a risk of delayed placental abruption with even relatively minor abdominal trauma, these patients should undergo fetal heart monitoring for at least 4 hours. This period should be extended to 24 hours if the patient develops frequent uterine contractions (>6/hour), vaginal bleeding, abdominal or uterine tenderness, or abnormalities on the fetal heart tracing or if maternal hypovolemia remains uncorrected at 4 hours. Patients should be instructed to return to the emergency department if they develop vaginal bleeding, decreased fetal movements, and increased pain or uterine contractions.

11. Is the management different for penetrating trauma to the pregnant abdomen?

The overall mortality for gunshot wounds of the abdomen is approximately 15%. In contrast, maternal death from a gunshot wound of the pregnant uterus is rare because the uterus and fetus absorb much of the kinetic energy of a bullet. Unfortunately, the incidence of fetal injury is high (60%), and the fetal mortality rate is between 40% and 60%. Nevertheless, several cases of fetal survival with penetrating wounds have been reported.

Penetrating wounds of the lower chest are more likely to involve injury to the hollow viscera and diaphragm, which are displaced upward in advanced pregnancy. Upper abdominal wounds can be explored safely. Pregnancy is often listed as a relative contraindication to peritoneal lavage, but it is safe to perform providing the incision is made above the level of the fundus. A lower threshold (5000 RBC/mL) should be used for considering the lavage positive in lower chest and upper abdominal injuries.

12. What determines the outcome of the pregnancy after trauma?

Many factors influence the outcome of a pregnancy after major trauma, but the overriding principle is that the well-being of the fetus depends almost completely on the well-being of the mother. Consequently, resuscitation of the mother takes first priority. In some studies, no fetuses survived if the mothers died, approximately one half of the fetuses died when the mother arrived in the emergency department in shock, and one fourth died even when the mother had relatively minor injuries. Although severely injured women usually have worse fetal outcomes, a woman may be relatively uninjured while the fetus is in severe distress.

13. Should pregnant women wear seat belts while riding in a motor vehicle?

Few human data are available to answer this question, but some experimental animal data clearly support the use of three-point restraints by pregnant women. The restraints must be worn properly to avoid a lap belt injury to the uterus and fetus. Air bags deploy with explosive force and can also cause maternal injury, particularly in advanced pregnancy, because the abdomen is closer to the point of deployment. Overall, however, both devices save lives, and their use should be encouraged.

BIBLIOGRAPHY

1. Ali J, Yeo A, Gana TJ, et al: Predictors of fetal mortality in pregnant trauma patients. J Trauma 42: 782–785, 1997.
2. Baerga-Varela Y, Zietlow SP, Bannon MP, et al: Trauma in pregnancy. Mayo Clin Proc 75:1243–1248, 2000.
3. Bochiccio GV, Napolitano LM, Haan J, et al: Incidental pregnancy in trauma patients. J Am Coll Surg 192:566–569, 2001.
4. Henderson SO, Mallon WK: Trauma in pregnancy. Emerg Med Clin North Am 16:209–228, 1998.
5. Lavery JP, Staten-McCormick M: Management of moderate to severe trauma in pregnancy. Obstet Gynecol Clin North Am 22:69–90, 1995.
6. Poole GV, Martin JN Jr, Perry KG Jr, et al: Trauma in pregnancy: The role of interpersonal violence. Am J Obstet Gynecol 174:1873–1878, 1996.
7. Rogers FB, Roszyki GS, Osler TM, et al: A multi-institutional study of factors associated with fetal death in injured pregnant patients. Arch Surg 134:1274–1277, 1999.
8. Theodorou DA, Velmahos GC, Souter I, et al: Fetal death after trauma in pregnancy. Am Surg 66:809–812, 2000.
9. Velanziano C: Abdominal trauma in the pregnant trauma victim. Top Emerg Med 15:72–83, 1993.
10. Weiss HB, Songer TJ, Fabio A: Fetal deaths related to maternal injury. JAMA 286:1863–1868, 2001.

41. TRAUMA IN THE ELDERLY

Bradley J. Roth, M.D., and Areti Tillou, M.D.

1. What evaluation should be considered for the elderly patient who falls?

All trauma patients should initially be evaluated using the Advanced Trauma Life Support (ATLS) protocol, but the following studies should also be considered: cardiac monitoring, rapid glucose assessment, complete blood cell count, electrolytes, glucose, calcium, magnesium, phosphorus, electrocardiogram, cardiac enzymes, and head computed tomography.

2. What are the most common causes of accidental death in the elderly patient?

For persons 75 years or older, falling is the primary cause of accidental death, followed by motor vehicle accidents and burns. For those between 65 and 75 years of age, motor vehicle accidents are twice as common as falls. Motor vehicle accidents differ from those involving younger drivers. They usually occur at lower speeds and involve two motor vehicles. Elderly individuals have a higher risk of being struck by a motor vehicle as a pedestrian than younger members of the general population. In 1991, people older than 65 years comprised 12.7% of the population but accounted for 29% of the trauma deaths.

3. In what age group does mortality rate begin to increase for adult trauma patients?

Compared with major trauma patients with similar Injury Severity Scores, the mortality rate begins to increase at 45 years (10.6%) and rises sharply for persons older than 55 years (14.4%). The rate is 15.6% for those between 65 and 74 years. The rate for persons 75 to 84 years of age is more than twice that for patients between 14 and 24 years (20.1% versus 8.9%).

4. How are elderly trauma patients resuscitated?

All trauma patients should be resuscitated using the ATLS protocols. Elderly trauma patients should undergo a streamlined examination, and every effort should be made to begin invasive monitoring early. Hypotensive, acidotic elderly trauma patients have a higher mortality rate than younger patients. In a study of elderly trauma patients, the survival rate was 53% for those who underwent early invasive monitoring (2.3 hours) compared with 7% for the delayed group (5.5 hours).

5. Why does the severely injured elderly patient have a lower than expected cardiac index?

With aging, the beta-adrenergic receptors in the heart decrease in number and become less sensitive to catecholamine stimulation. The sinoatrial node, atrioventricular node, and bundle of His undergo cell loss. The ventricles' walls become less compliant, resulting in decreased stroke volume. Many patients have significant atherosclerotic heart disease or valvular disease. Some patients may be on medications that decrease their cardiac performance.

6. Why is the serum creatinine level commonly near normal limits when renal reserve is usually limited in elderly trauma patients?

The kidney experiences a progressive decrease in function from gradual loss of glomeruli and decreased blood flow. Because of the correlative decrease in muscle mass, the serum creatinine remains unchanged. The kidney has very little reserve with which to respond to stress. Because of a decreased ability to respond to antidiuretic hormone (ADH), the elderly trauma patient may have a decreased ability to concentrate urine, and urinary output is therefore a poor indicator of peripheral profusion.

7. Why does the elderly trauma patient have a limited physiologic reserve?

The process of aging is characterized by progressive loss of individual organ function. The degree of decline is highly variable among different organ systems and individual patients. Elderly patients have a lower cardiac, renal, and respiratory reserve. Age-related osteo-porosis leads to further loss of strength and greater susceptibility to fracture. Progressive de-terioration in cognitive ability, memory loss, and sensory senescence is observed. These pa-tients may have an impaired immune system and mild malnutrition, and glucose intolerance is common.

8. What differences are observed in the elderly blunt thoracic trauma patient compared with patients younger than 65 years?

Elderly patients have similar mechanisms of injury and types of injury. However, in the el-derly population, the ratio of men to women presenting with blunt thoracic trauma approaches 1 (2.7:1 for younger patients versus 1.2:1 in the elderly). The elderly patient is less likely to present in shock but more likely to present without vital signs. Elderly patients also have a higher mor-tality rate (37% versus 18% for younger patients). When comparing elderly patients with car-diopulmonary disease with those without it, the persons with cardiopulmonary disease have a higher mortality rate and longer intensive care unit (ICU) stay. The rapid transfer of elder patients with multiple rib fractures to the ICU and early use of epidural analgesia may be lifesaving in this group.

9. What factors increase the surgical intensive care unit (SICU) mortality rate in the el-derly patient?

The Simplified Acute Physiology Score (SAPS) appears to have more predictive value than age alone when patients are matched for Injury Severity Score (ISS). There was no significant dif-ference in SICU mortality when young and old patients were matched by ISS and SAPS. Elderly patients generally present with a higher SAPS. Hospital mortality after discharge from the SICU appears to increase in the elderly with high SAPS compared with younger patients with similar ISS and SAPS.

10. Is old age alone a reason for early activation of the surgical trauma team?

After trauma, geriatric patients have much higher morbidity and mortality rates. The overall mortality rate for hospitalized geriatric trauma victims is 15% to 30%, compared with 4% to 8% for younger patients. Physiologic response to trauma is frequently absent or blunted in older pa-tients. In the Los Angeles County and University of Southern California Medical Center experi-ence, 63% of geriatric patients with an ISS less than 15 and 25% of patients with an ISS less than 30 did not meet the hypotension or tachycardia criteria for trauma team activation. Modification of the trauma team activation criteria to include age older than 70 years resulted in a significant decrease in the mortality rate for geriatric trauma patients.

11. Compared with children, what is the fatality rate for elderly pedestrians struck by mov-ing vehicles?

Elderly pedestrian trauma patients have the highest population-adjusted mortality rate of all vehicular-pedestrian fatalities. Many of these elderly patients are injured in crosswalks. Some of the effects of aging that hinder their driving ability may also affect their ability to cross busy streets: diminished hearing, sight, muscle strength, and coordination.

12. In elderly trauma patients what predictive value do "normal" presenting vital signs have?

"Normal" presenting vital signs may have very little predictive value for elderly trauma patients. Because of cardiac disease, many elderly trauma patients do not present with the nor-mal tachycardic response to systemic hypoperfusion. This relative bradycardia may be aug-mented by the use of beta-blockers or digoxin. Because of the prevalence of hypertension in the older population a normal-appearing blood pressure may mask a relatively hypotensive state.

BIBLIOGRAPHY

1. Alexander JQ, Gutierrez CJ, Mariano MC, et al: Blunt chest trauma in the elderly patient: How cardiopulmonary disease affects outcome. Am Surg 66:855–857, 2000.
2. Demetriades D, Sava J, Alo K, et al: Old age as a criterion for trauma team activation. J Trauma 51: 754–757, 2001.
3. Finelli FC, Jonsson J, Champion HR, et al: A case-control study for major trauma in geriatric patient. J Trauma 29:541–548, 1989.
4. Johnson CL, Margulies DR, Kearney TJ, et al: Trauma in the elderly: An analysis of outcome based on age. Am Surg 60:899–902, 1994.
5. National Safety Council: Accident Facts, 1992 Edition. Itasca, IL, National Safety Council, 1992.
6. Oreskovich MR, Howard JD, Copass MK, Carrico CJ: J Trauma 24:565–572, 1984.
7. Roth BJ, Velmahos GC, Oder DB, et al: Penetrating trauma in patients older than 55 years: A case-control study. Injury 32:551–554, 2001.
8. Santora TA, Schinco MA, Trooskin SZ: Management of trauma in the elderly. Surg Clin North Am 74: 163–186, 1994.
9. Scalea TM, Kohl L: Geriatric trauma. In Feliciano DV, Moore EE, Mattox KL (eds): Trauma. Stamford, CT, Appleton & Lange, 1996, pp 899–915.
10. Scalea TM, Maltz S, Yelone J, et al: Resuscitation of multiple trauma and head injury: Role of crystalloid fluids and inotropes. Crit Care Med 22:1610–1615, 1994.
11. Scalea TM, Simon HM, Duncan AO, et al: Geriatric blunt multiple trauma: Improved survival with early invasive monitoring. J Trauma 30:129–134, 1990.
12. Schwab CW, Kauder DR: Trauma in the geriatric patient. Arch Surg 127:701–706, 1992.
13. Schwab WC, Shapiro MB, Kauder DR: Geriatric Trauma: Patterns, Care and Outcomes. In Mattox KL, Feliciano DV, Moore EE (eds): Trauma. New York, McGraw-Hill, 2000, pp 1099–1114.
14. Shoemaker WC, Appel PL, Kram HB: Role of oxygen debt in the development of organ failure sepsis, and death in high risk surgery patients. Chest 102:208–215, 1992.
15. Shoemaker WC, Appel PL, Kram HB: Tissue oxygen debt as a determinant of lethal and nonlethal postoperative organ failure. Crit Care Med 16:1117–1120, 1988.
16. Shorr RM, Rodriguez A, Indeck MC, et al: Blunt chest trauma in the elderly. J Trauma 29:234–237, 1989.

42. ALCOHOL AND ACUTE WITHDRAWAL

Gideon P. Naudé, M.B.Ch.B.

1. What is alcoholism?

Alcoholism is a recurring problem associated with the drinking of alcohol that may adversely affect a person's personal life, professional life, education, financial situation, and state of health and may lead to legal problems. Dependence and addiction occur, and if intake is stopped, withdrawal may take place. Denial that alcohol is a problem is common, making the treatment more difficult.

2. Is alcohol dependence (alcoholism) a problem in the United States?

Yes. Along with cancer and heart disease, it is one of the three most common causes of death in the United States. The cost to society is several hundred billion dollars per year, and the cost to the alcoholic and his family in unhappiness and misery is incalculable. About 10% of adult Americans can be classified as alcoholic.

3. Is there a genetic predisposition to alcohol abuse?

It is thought that there is a genetic predisposition to alcoholism in about one half of all alcoholics.

4. What other predisposing factors are there?

A close relationship with an alcoholic, such as a spouse or partner, may lead to problem drinking. Children from dysfunctional families have a higher incidence of alcoholism. About 10% to 20% of alcoholic men have another mental disorder, and depression and preexisting phobias make women more prone to alcoholism. Among the elderly, loneliness and isolation are often causes that lead to problem drinking.

5. Are all people, regardless of sex or race, equally susceptible to the effects of alcohol?

Women become intoxicated sooner and have a higher rate of liver cirrhosis than men. Native Americans, Asians, and Africans become intoxicated earlier than matched drinkers of European descent.

6. Does alcohol have any positive physical or psychological effects?

Taken in moderation (as done by about 60 million Americans), it causes relaxation and mild euphoria and stimulates pleasant social interaction. It may stimulate the appetite if taken preprandially. Moderate alcohol use is beneficial to the cardiovascular system.

7. What are the symptoms of alcohol use?

In modest amounts, alcohol presents no specific symptoms other than slight mood elevation. Mild intoxication is characterized by initial sedation and then relaxation and euphoria. With increased use, this state progresses to inappropriate behavior characterized by loudness, lowered inhibitions, impaired coordination, slurred speech, loss of memory (alcoholics commonly have "blackouts" with memory loss for the period of intoxication), and poor judgment. Labile mood with depression and rage occurs in some drinkers. At higher levels of alcohol intake, nausea and vomiting occur. With further increases, the person becomes obtunded and may progress to drunken stupor or coma. Even higher doses lead to respiratory depression and death.

8. What are the graded effects of acute alcohol intoxication?

Persons not used to alcohol may become intoxicated at levels as low as 40 mg/dL. The average person becomes intoxicated at levels of 100 mg/dL or higher. Alcoholics may develop a tolerance and appear sober with levels of 150 mg/dL. Levels above 400 mg/dL may lead to coma and death.

9. **What is the toxic blood level of alcohol?**

Blood alcohol levels above 400 mg/dL may cause death from respiratory depression or an inability to protect the airway, leading to vomiting and aspiration. Cardiac depression occurs at levels above 1000 mg/dL.

10. **What organs are damaged by alcohol abuse?**
    - Cardiovascular system: hypertension, cardiomyopathy and myocardial infarction
    - Central nervous system: Korsakoff's psychosis, Wernicke's encephalopathy, and early dementia
    - Peripheral nervous system: peripheral neuropathy
    - Oral mucosa: oropharyngeal carcinoma associated with heavy alcoholic intake
    - Esophagus: squamous carcinoma associated with heavy alcohol intake and esophageal varices associated with alcoholic cirrhosis
    - Stomach: gastritis and peptic ulceration
    - Liver: acute alcoholic hepatitis, liver cirrhosis, and liver carcinoma
    - Pancreas: acute and chronic pancreatitis
    - Hematologic effects: macrocytic, megaloblastic, or microcytic anemia; low white blood cell count; and thrombocytopenia
    - Respiratory system: acute respiratory depression with alcohol overdose and a higher incidence of respiratory cancer
    - Unborn children: fetal alcohol syndrome
    - Genital system: testicular atrophy with male impotence
    - General effects: increased likelihood of trauma (i.e., accidental and intentional, spouse and child abuse), drowning, fire hazard, and freezing and cold damage

11. **What occurs in chronic alcohol use?**

Continuous alcohol use damages target organs. Dietary insufficiency makes alcohol-induced organ damage worse. Additional harmful habits such as smoking and drug addiction hasten the harmful effects of alcohol.

12. **Does improvement take place if alcohol intake is stopped?**

Yes. Rapid improvement occurs in the fluid and electrolyte balance, hematologic picture, hypertension, and the malabsorption state of the small intestine. Slow to improve are chronic pancreatitis, liver cirrhosis, and neurologic (particularly cognitive) deficit.

13. **How is an intoxicated trauma patient treated?**

In addition to the injuries, the effects of alcohol itself may further lower the level of consciousness, increasing the danger of vomiting and aspiration, which should mandate control of the airway with intubation.

Very high levels of alcohol may require ventilatory assistance if significant respiratory depression has occurred. It may also be necessary to pass a gastric tube to remove alcohol in the stomach that has not been absorbed yet. An intoxicated patient needing urgent surgery may require very small amounts of an anesthetic agent to reach surgical anesthesia.

14. **What are the signs of acute alcohol withdrawal?**

After a period of consistent and heavy drinking, a person usually experiences withdrawal when alcohol consumption is stopped or slowed down after being admitted to the hospital or incarcerated in prison. Then, one or more of the following reactions occur:
    - Tremors that start about 12 hours after stopping drinking and become severe in 24 to 36 hours
    - Withdrawal seizures occurring 8 to 24 hours after alcohol cessation

- Alcoholic hallucinations (frequently within the first 2 days) that usually last less than a week and that are usually visual (typically insects, snakes, or other small animals) but may be auditory in the form of threatening or mocking voices or a combination of the two
- Delirium tremens occur 2 to 14 days after drinking cessation and is a late manifestation. Clouding of the consciousness, inattentiveness that leads to abnormal perception, and frequently bizarre and inappropriate behavior are characteristic. Hallucinations and violent behavior may occur.

15. What are the effects of maternal alcohol abuse on the fetus?

The fetal alcohol syndrome occurs if the pregnant woman consumes alcohol. The severity of the abnormality is dose dependent, manifesting with more severe abnormalities if higher doses of alcohol were taken. The syndrome is characterized by low fetal birth weight, physical abnormalities, and mental impairment. It can be avoided if the woman does not ingest alcohol during pregnancy.

16. Are there special problems associated with alcoholism in women?

Alcoholism may go unrecognized in women because they tend to drink more covertly, sometimes do not have to hold down a job, and if at home, may have alcohol easily available all the time. Alcoholism is more prevalent among women who are unmarried, divorced, or unemployed. Female alcoholics have a higher incidence of being married to alcoholics. Liver disease, suicide, and trauma are more common in women than men, and the average life expectancy of a female alcoholic is almost 15 years less than that of women who are not alcoholics.

17. What legal and associated problems are strong indicators of alcoholism?

A prison record or a history of spousal and child abuse suggests alcoholism. Statistics indicate that a person with one arrest for drunken driving has a 70% chance of being an alcoholic, two arrests indicate a 90% chance, and three arrests indicate a 100% chance. Alcohol or other drugs are involved in more than one half of all serious trauma.

18. What is alcohol idiosyncratic intoxication?

Idiosyncratic intoxication is behavior that is not typical of the person when not drinking. This usually takes the form of aggressive or violent behavior while under the influence of alcohol, followed by a return to normal behavior and amnesia of the event.

19. Is alcoholism a treatable condition?

Yes. With prolonged treatment, more than 60% of alcoholics can be cured and rehabilitated to become useful members of society. Left to their own devices, fewer than 20% of alcoholics can remain "dry."

20. What is the treatment of delirium tremens (DTs)?
- Hospitalization in a quiet, restful environment.
- Hydration is achieved with intravenous fluids if the patient has not been drinking water or has been vomiting.
- Adequate nutrition is important because many of these patients are chronically malnourished.
- Vitamins such as B-complex, folate (1 mg/day), and thiamine (at least 100 mg/day) should be given as supplements to the diet.
- Sedation can be achieved with a benzodiazepine (e.g., diazepam, chlordiazepoxide, oxazepam, lorazepam).
- Seizures can be prevented by administering phenytoin (Dilantin), 300 mg/day for 5 days.

21. Are the DTs dangerous or just bothersome?

Untreated, DTs are associated with a significant mortality rate, reported to be as high as 15% in some series.

BIBLIOGRAPHY

1. Barker LR, Burton JR, Zieve PD: Ambulatory Medicine, 4th ed. Baltimore, Williams & Wilkins, 1995.
2. Blume SB: Women and alcohol. JAMA 256:1467, 1986.
3. Fein R: Alcohol in America: The Price We Pay. Newport Beach, CA, Care Institute, 1984.
4. Goodwin DW: Is Alcoholism Hereditary? New York, Oxford University Press, 1974.
5. Skinner HA, Hold S, Schuller R, et al: Identification of alcohol abuse using laboratory tests and a history of trauma. Ann Intern Med 101:847, 1984.
6. Way LW: Current Surgical Diagnosis and Treatment, 10th ed. Norwalk, CT, Appleton & Lange, 1994.

XIII. Diagnostic Modalities

43. COMPUTED TOMOGRAPHY, MAGNETIC RESONANCE IMAGING, AND PERITONEAL LAVAGE IN INJURIES

Patricia Eubanks May, M.D.

1. What is a diagnostic peritoneal lavage (DPL), and how is it performed?

A DPL is the placement of a catheter into the abdomen to assess for intra-abdominal injury. A DPL is performed by either an open or closed technique by making a small incision in the infraumbilical midline and placing a plastic catheter into the pelvis. Initial aspiration is performed. If this returns no blood, then 1 L of normal saline is infused. After infusion, the fluid is drained out of the abdomen by gravity (by placing the IV bag to the floor) and sent to the laboratory.

2. Which is preferred: the open or closed technique of DPL?

The open technique. In the open technique, a small incision is made in the fascia and peritoneum through which the catheter is inserted under direct visualization. The closed technique involves making a small incision and puncturing the fascia with a needle over which the catheter is advanced (using the Seldinger technique). This technique is not done commonly because of the risk of injury to the viscera or other intra-abdominal structures with insertion of the catheter.

3. What constitutes a "positive" DPL?

If 10–20 ml of gross blood or intestinal contents are obtained, no further tests are performed. The patient is taken directly to the operating room. If the fluid drained from the lavage contains $>100,000$ RBC/mm^3, > 500 WBC/mm^3, any food material or bacteria, or an amylase > 20 IU, the tap is considered positive.

4. How do you perform a DPL if a pelvic fracture is present?

The incision is made *above* the umbilicus and the catheter directed away from the pelvic hematoma. Consideration should be made for computed tomography (CT) scan in this setting if the patient is stable.

5. Which patients should undergo DPL?

DPL is indicated in unstable trauma patients in whom you suspect abdominal injury. DPL is rapid and sensitive; however, it is *not* specific. The most useful application of DPL is in patients with other serious injuries, particularly cranial injuries resulting in altered level of consciousness. Equivocal physical findings, intoxication with drugs or alcohol, or the need for other immediate operations (such as craniotomy) are indications for DPL in the unstable patient.

6. When was DPL first introduced to diagnose hemoperitoneum?

H. D. Root first introduced DPL in 1965.

7. What accounts for false-negative DPLs?

An injury to a hollow viscus resulting in minimal or no contamination to the peritoneal cavity at the time of DPL or a retroperitoneal injury account for the majority of false-negative DPLs. Additionally, placement of the catheter into the properitoneal fat (more common in obese patients) or intra-abdominal adhesions that prevent blood from mixing with the lavage fluid may account for false-negative DPLs.

8. What accounts for false-positive DPLs?

Bleeding from the incision or catheter injuries of the omentum or mesentery may result in a false-positive DPL. The presence of a pelvic or retroperitoneal hematoma may also cause a false-positive test. Of note, 15–25% of patients taken to surgery for a positive DPL will have trivial injuries that do not require surgical repair.

9. What are relative contraindications to DPL?

Previous abdominal surgery and pregnancy are considered contraindications.

10. When is abdominal CT scanning indicated in trauma?

In the *stable* patient in whom you suspect intra-abdominal injury, a CT scan is useful. CT scanning is used in patients with altered mental status, spinal injuries, or pelvic or extremity fractures.

11. What are the advantages of the CT scan over DPL?

The CT scan is more specific than DPL in diagnosing the site of injury. It is particularly useful in diagnosing solid organ injuries. Additionally, the CT scan is able to more accurately diagnose retroperitoneal injuries. Thus, CT scan lowers the rate of nontherapeutic laparotomies when compared with DPL.

12. What area of injury does the abdominal CT scan underdiagnose?

CT scanning can miss enteric injuries if there has been minimal spillage. Therefore, a negative CT scan does not rule out a bowel injury. The patient should be observed with serial physical examinations. If the patient's mental status does not facilitate reliable physical examination, then consideration should be made for DPL or follow-up CT scanning if the patient's condition deteriorates.

13. How is the trauma abdominal CT scan performed?

The patient is given IV contrast and possibly a small bolus of oral contrast (not always necessary), and axial images are obtained from the lower thorax through the pelvis. The addition of a small amount of oral contrast can help define duodenal or pancreatic injuries.

14. What are considered positive CT scan findings?

Fluid around the liver or in the pelvis is considered positive. Liver, spleen, or any other organs visualized to be lacerated or disrupted are positive findings. Nonperfusion of the kidneys after the administration of intravenous contrast dye is suggestive of renal artery thrombosis or injury. Additionally, the CT scan is particularly useful in diagnosing pelvic fractures. Extravasation of dye after the administration of IV contrast can diagnose renal parenchymal or collecting system injuries. Bladder injuries can be diagnosed if the Foley catheter is kept clamped after giving IV contrast to allow distention of the bladder. Spinal column injuries and vascular injuries can be demonstrated as well.

15. Does a positive CT scan finding necessitate a laparatomy?

No. Solid organ injuries can often be managed nonoperatively. This conservative management strategy was first proven successful in the pediatric population and has subsequently been extended to adults.

16. What is the grading system used to stratify liver injuries?

Grade I: subcapsular, nonexpanding hematoma < 10% surface area; laceration that is non-bleeding and < 1 cm parenchymal depth.

Grade II: subcapsular, nonexpanding hematoma 10–50% surface area, or intraparenchymal hematoma < 10 cm; capsular tear with active bleeding, 1–3 cm parenchymal laceration, < 10 cm in length.

Grade III: subcapsular, > 50% surface area or expanding; ruptured subcapsular parenchymal hematoma; intraparenchymal hematoma > 10 cm or expanding; > 3 cm parenchymal laceration.

Grade IV: ruptured intraparenchymal hematoma with active bleeding; parenchymal laceration involving 25–75% of hepatic lobe.

Grade V: parenchymal disruption involving > 75% of hepatic lobe; juxtahepatic venous injuries (retrohepatic vena cava or major hepatic veins).

Grade VI: hepatic avulsion.

17. What are the criteria for nonoperative management of hepatic injuries?
1. Hemodynamic stability.
2. CT scan identifies the site of injury.
3. No peritoneal signs.
4. No associated enteric or other injuries requiring operation.
5. Small requirement for blood transfusions.

Nonoperative management is generally reserved for grade I–III injuries; however, successful nonoperative management of grade IV and V injuries is increasingly reported.

18. What do you do if the CT scan shows free peritoneal fluid or fluid in the pelvis without any identifiable solid organ injury?

Free peritoneal fluid without solid organ injury or pelvic fracture is suggestive of enteric perforation or mesenteric bleeding and warrants exploratory laparatomy.

19. What is the grading system for splenic injuries?

Grade I: minimal capsular tear; no bleeding.

Grade II: minor capsular or parenchymal disruption with bleeding.

Grade III: major parenchymal fracture.

Grade IV: crushing or major parenchymal disruption localized to one area.

Grade V: diffuse parenchymal fractures; hilar injuries.

20. What are the criteria for nonoperative management of splenic trauma?

The same general requirements for nonoperative management of liver injuries apply to splenic injuries. Grades I–III can be managed conservatively. However, unlike liver injuries, nonoperative management has been successfully extended to higher grades of splenic injuries.

21. What role does CT have in the evaluation of head trauma?

CT scanning is the modality of choice in the evaluation of patients with acute head injury. Early detection of intracerebral blood or epidural and subdural hematomas is easily accomplished with CT scanning. Certain changes such as mild edema, subdural hematomas, or minimal parenchymal bleeding may not be evident on the initial CT scan. Thus, follow-up scanning several hours later may be used to enhance detection of intracranial injuries.

22. What kind of CT scan of the head is performed for trauma?

A noncontrast head CT with bone windows is performed. This test is rapid and sensitive.

23. What constitutes mediastinal widening, and how do I work it up?

A mediastinal width greater than 8 cm at the level of the aortic knob on an anteroposterior (AP) chest x-ray is considered mediastinal widening. This finding is suspicious for thoracic aortic rupture and warrants further radiographic studies. The gold standard for diagnosing aortic injury from blunt trauma is an arch aortogram.

24. Is CT scan able to accurately and reliably diagnose great vessel injury?

This is controversial:

For: The thoracic CT scan can demonstrate mediastinal hemorrhage and aortic contour abnormalities. CT can be valuable in determining the need for arteriography in those patients with mediastinal widening after blunt decelerating trauma. Thus, a normal CT scan in a patient with a widened mediastinum can preclude aortography.

Against: Thoracic CT findings are nonspecific. In most prospective and retrospective studies performed to date, an abnormal CT scan prompted subsequent aortography to define the injury. Thus, in those patients in whom your index of suspicion is high, aortography has the best sensitivity. CT scanning is unnecessary, expensive, and can waste valuable time.

25. Is CT scan sensitive in diagnosing other blunt thoracic injuries?

The CT scan can detect pulmonary consolidation or contusion, hemothorax, pneumothorax, and pneumomediastinum easily. In general, CT scanning cannot specifically diagnose esophageal rupture or injury. If esophageal rupture is suspected, a Gastrografin esophagram followed by barium contrast, if the Gastrografin study is negative, is the study of choice.

26. What are the indications for cervical spine CT scanning?

Equivocal findings on plain radiography

Unexplained focal neck pain

Neurologic findings or pain referable to the cervical spinal cord without radiographic findings

A patient who cannot be cleared radiographically

Cervical injuries to assist with treatment planning

27. Is MRI useful in the setting of trauma?

No. While MRI may be more sensitive than CT scan in detecting neurologic injury and many types of craniocerebral trauma, it is not performed for trauma because it takes longer than CT scanning, it requires patient cooperation, and access to the patient in the magnet is difficult (to maintain support and monitoring devices). Improvements in the newer generations of MRI may shorten the procedure and may more easily accommodate support equipment and personnel.

BIBLIOGRAPHY

1. Feliciano DV, Moore EE, Mattox KL (eds): Trauma, 3rd ed. Stamford, CT, Appleton & Lange, 1996.
2. Mattox KL (ed): Complications of Trauma. New York, Churchill Livingstone, 1994.
3. Mirvis SE, Young JWR (eds): Imaging in Trauma and Critical Care. Baltimore, Williams & Wilkins, 1992.
4. Pacter HL, Feliciano DV: Complex hepatic injuries. Surg Clin North Am 76:763–782, 1996.
5. Pretre R, Chilcott M: Blunt trauma to the heart and great vessels. N Engl J Med 336:626–632, 1997.
6. Root HD, Hauser CW, McKinley CR, et al:Diagnostic peritoneal lavage. Surgery 57:633, 1965.

44. ULTRASOUND IN TRAUMA

M. Margaret Knudson, M.D.

1. What is ultrasound?

Ultrasound is sound with a frequency above the human threshold for hearing, which is 20,000 cycles per second or 20 kilohertz (kHz). In medical ultrasound, a transducer that contains a piezoelectric crystal generates the sound wave. When the transducer is placed on the skin surface, it causes the molecules in the tissue to vibrate and sets up the sound wave. As the sound wave travels through the tissue, it contacts interfaces (such as the liver, bone, etc.) and part of the sound-wave signal is reflected back toward the transducer, thus creating an image on the screen. The rest of the sound wave is either reflected away from the transducer or is absorbed by the tissue (a process called attenuation). The speed of the ultrasound wave through the tissue varies; for example, the velocity through air is 330 m/sec, through lung is 600 m/sec, through the liver is 1,555 m/sec, and through the skull is 4,000 m/sec. The pictures created on the screen result from these differences among tissues (i.e., finding the window to distinguish one organ from another).

2. What transducer would you choose to use in the trauma patient?

Diagnostic ultrasound frequencies range from 2 megahertz (MHz) to 10 MHz. In general, the higher the ultrasound frequency, the better the image resolution, but the poorer the penetration. Therefore, if one would like to examine the abdomen or chest of a trauma patient, the examiner will sacrifice resolution for penetration and choose a general purpose probe with deep penetration, such as a 3.5 MHz probe. In contrast, for examining relatively superficial blood vessels, a small-parts probe with good resolution (5.0 or 7.5 MHz) is preferred.

3. What do you need to know to get a high-quality image on your ultrasound screen?

The following are the important steps in performing a good ultrasound exam:

1. You must know how to turn on the machine! Most machines used in training programs have the capability to record the exam in real time on VCR, so it is important to turn on the VCR and insert the tape as you begin your exam. These videotapes can be reviewed later as part of the educational and quality-assurance programs.

2. Choose the appropriate probe (3.5 MHz for most patients) and orient it properly. Most probes have a dot or line marking the up-position. This up-position should be oriented toward the patient's head for longitudinal scans. With this orientation, the cephalic portion of the patient's body will be toward the left side of the screen (as you face the screen). When you are scanning in transverse, the dot or line on the transducer should be directed toward the patient's right side; thus, the right side of the patient will be on the left side of the screen (i.e., as you face the screen, the liver will appear on your left side).

3. Once you have oriented the probe, find the acoustic transmission gel and be liberal with its use. You can apply it directly to the probe, to the patient's skin, or to both surfaces. If your images are "all dark" you have probably not applied enough gel. When examining the trauma patient, it is wise to use a plastic cover over the probe so that there is no risk of transmission of blood from one patient to the next. Be sure to apply this plastic cover tightly, however, so that there is no air under it (remember that air will scatter the beam).

4. Adjust the gain on the machine. The gain is the amplification (the brightness) of the received signal. Most machines allow you to adjust not only the overall gain (usually a dial on the machine), but also the time gain compensation (TGC) in the focal zone (usually several slide keys on the machine). TGC is used to adjust for signals with time and depth, and allow for an image that is balanced in the near field (close to the probe), far field, and in the area of interest, the focal zone.

4. Can you explain the term *echogenicity*?

When you first look at ultrasound images, they appear to be all gray and white. However, as you practice and train your eye, you will learn to distinguish different tissues by their ultrasound images (i.e., their degree of echogenicity). For example, the diaphragm reflects back virtually all of the ultrasound waves and appears white or *hyperechoic* on the screen. In contrast, blood in the abdomen or pericardial sac readily transmits the ultrasound wave and thus appears black (*anechoic* or *echolucent*).

5. What does the term *duplex* refer to in ultrasound?

Ultrasound machines with duplex capabilities are capable of providing simultaneous real time and Doppler images. Remember from your physics days that a Doppler shift is a change in frequency of a reflected wave owing to the relative motion between the reflector and the transducer (Remember the old train whistle approaching the station?). Color flow Doppler (CFD) machines permit instantaneous detection of the Doppler shift frequencies by superimposing colors over the normal range of cross-sectional image (red coming toward the probe, blue going away from the probe). CFD exams are essential in vascular imaging.

6. Name five applications for ultrasound in trauma.

1. The use of echocardiography to evaluate the pericardium for blood after chest trauma
2. The use of abdominal ultrasound to evaluate for fluid or blood after blunt trauma
3. The use of duplex imaging to evaluate peripheral blood vessels after penetrating trauma to the extremities or neck
4. The use of transesophageal echocardiography to evaluate the aorta in a patient with a widened mediastinum
5. The use of duplex venous imaging to evaluate for venous patency or clot after trauma

7. What is the FAST exam for trauma?

The FAST exam, or **f**ocused **a**bdominal **s**onogram for **t**rauma, is designed to detect fluid (i.e., blood) in the pericardium or abdomen after trauma. Performing FAST is fast, generally done in 2–3 minutes by experienced examiners, and involves looking at four areas in the supine trauma patient (see Figure): (1) the sagittal view in the subxiphoid area examines the heart and pericar-

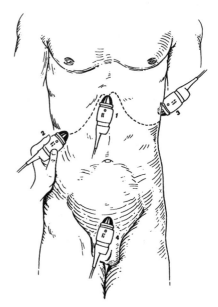

Schematic drawing of the four transducer positions for the FAST exam. (From Rozycki GS, Ochsner MG, Schmidt JA, et al: A prospective study of surgeon-performed ultrasound as the primary adjuvant modality for injured-patient assessment. J Trauma 39:492, 1995, with permission.)

dial sac for fluid; (2) a sagittal view obtained in the right midaxillary line between the 11th and 12th ribs to examine for blood in Morison's pouch; (3) a sagittal view obtained in the left mid-axillary line between the 10th and 11th ribs to visualize the spleen and kidney and to look for blood in the splenorenal recess and in the subdiaphragmatic space; and (4) a transverse (coronal) section superior to the symphysis pubis to look for fluid in the pelvis. Note: With this last view, the bladder should be full!

8. How can the FAST exam be incorporated into the initial trauma evaluation?

The FAST exam should be performed during the secondary survey, after the initial stabilization of the trauma patient. It should be considered an alternative to diagnostic peritoneal lavage for the detection of blood in the abdomen, and it has been demonstrated to be useful in determining the need for laparotomy in unstable patients and for thoracotomy in patients with penetrating chest trauma.

9. What are the applications of ultrasound in pediatric trauma patients and in injured pregnant patients?

Ultrasound is painless, noninvasive, and portable, all features making it attractive in the evaluation of the pediatric patient. Because of their small size, children are relatively easy to image by ultrasound (although you might choose to use a higher frequency probe, such as a 5 MHz), and this exam is better tolerated than a CT scan, which often requires sedation in order to obtain satisfactory images. In the pregnant patient, ultrasound has been used not only to examine the mother for injury, but also to assess the age of the fetus and the presence of fetal heart sounds or fetal movement, and to examine for uterine rupture and placental lacerations, both potential complications of trauma during pregnancy.

10. Is there any role for ultrasound in trauma outside of the emergency setting?

As surgeons get comfortable performing and interpreting ultrasound exams, the uses of ultrasound continue to expand. Ultrasound can be used to follow blunt injuries to the spleen, liver, and kidney that are being managed nonoperatively. It can be used to detect pleural fluid in patients in the ICU. Serial duplex venous imaging has been used to follow patients who are at high-risk for developing deep venous thrombosis. Central venous line placement can be facilitated by ultrasound. Repeat abdominal sonography is indicated in evaluating a trauma patient with an unexplained drop in hematocrit. Repeat echocardiography may be useful in the postthoracotomy patient. Color-flow duplex exams can be used to evaluate an arterial or venous anastomosis in the postoperative period.

11. How does one become proficient in the use of ultrasound in trauma?

First, take an accredited course. For example, the American College of Surgeons is currently sponsoring semiannual courses in conjunction with its regular spring and fall meetings. Many of these courses include instructions on other uses of ultrasound, including vascular, breast, laparoscopic, and intraoperative ultrasound. The courses include both didactic and hands-on practice sessions. Second, one must be supervised by an experienced sonographer for the initial exams. Some data suggest that the amateur sonographer needs 100 supervised scans before being considered proficient in performing and interpreting trauma ultrasound exams.

CONTROVERSIES

12. Why not leave ultrasound to the radiologists who can undoubtedly perform ultrasound exams with higher accuracy than the surgeons?

First, the trauma surgeon is standing at the bedside when the patient arrives and has the opportunity to perform the FAST exam in the most timely manner. There is no reason to wait until a radiologist or a radiology technician is available. Second, for the surgeon, the anatomy of intra-abdominal organs is second nature, thus making it relatively easy for surgeons to understand ultrasound images. Third, several studies have demonstrated that surgeons can perform FAST exams with a sensitivity of 90.8%, a specificity of 99.2%, and an accuracy of 97.8% compared with radiologists.

13. Is ultrasound in trauma a cost-effective method of detecting injuries?

When incorporated into a clinical algorithm, ultrasound has been demonstrated to be a cost-effective method of evaluating injured patients (see Figure). This may be particularly true in evaluating patients with penetrating chest trauma, where other methods of assessing for cardiac injuries are indirect and costly. While formerly, the initial investment in ultrasound equipment was prohibitive, high-quality machines are now available for as little as $20,000.

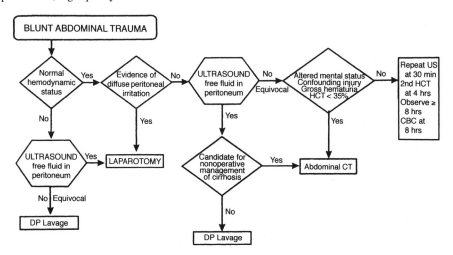

Clinical pathway incorporating ultrasound in trauma evaluation. (From Branney SW, Moore EE, Cantrill SV, et al: Ultrasound-based key clinical pathway reduces the use of hospital resources for the evaluation of blunt abdominal trauma. J Trauma 42:1086–1090, 1997, with permission.)

14. Will ultrasound replace CT scanning in the evaluation of blunt abdominal trauma?

CT scanning is still superior to ultrasound in detecting a solid organ injury and in grading its severity. In most surgeons' hands, ultrasound is limited to detecting abdominal fluid but is not particularly accurate in demonstrating which organ is injured. Currently, ultrasound should be considered an alternative to diagnostic peritoneal lavage in the evaluation of blunt abdominal trauma.

15. Most cardiac injuries are obvious; why bother with ultrasound?

About 10–20% of cardiac injuries are initially occult. This is particularly true in patients with blunt trauma who have other reasons for hypotension and in patients with penetrating chest trauma where the pericardial injury is large enough to relieve tamponade. These cardiac injuries are easily detected by an experienced echocardiographer.

16. What is the role for transesophageal echocardiography (TEE) versus angiography in patients with a widened mediastinum?

Although there was initial enthusiasm for the use of TEE in the evaluation of the patient with a widened mediastinum after blunt chest trauma, most studies have found that TEE misses both aortic and other major vascular injuries in the chest. Biplanar TEE improves the accuracy of this technique, but spiral CT scanning is also evolving as a less-invasive method of evaluating the thoracic aorta. Currently, angiography is still considered the most accurate and cost-effective method of detecting a thoracic aortic injury, but TEE may be useful in unstable patients who cannot be transported to the angiography suite or in patients who are in the operating room for other life-threatening injuries and in whom there is a concern for an aortic injury.

BIBLIOGRAPHY

1. Ben-Menachem Y: Assessment of blunt aortic-brachiocephalic trauma: Should angiography be supplanted by transesophageal echocardiography? J Trauma 42:969–972, 1997.
2. Bode PJ, Niezen RA, van Vugt AB, et al: Abdominal ultrasound as a reliable indicator for conclusive laparotomy in blunt abdominal trauma. J Trauma 34:27–31, 1993.
3. Branney SW, Moore EE, Cantrill SV, et al: Ultrasound-based key clinical pathway reduces the use of hospital resources for the evaluation of blunt abdominal trauma. J Trauma 42:1086–1090, 1997.
4. Forster R, Pillasch J, Zielke A, et al: Ultrasonography in blunt abdominal trauma: Influence of the investigators' experience. J Trauma 34:264–269, 1993.
5. Han DC, Rozycki GS, Schmidt JA, et al: Ultrasound training during ATLS: An early start for surgical interns. J Trauma 41:208–213, 1996.
6. Healy MA, Simons RK, Winchell RJ, et al: A prospective evaluation of abdominal ultrasound in blunt trauma: Is it useful? J Trauma 40:875–883, 1996.
7. Kearney PA, Smith DW, Johnson SB, et al: Use of transesophageal echocardiography in the evaluation of traumatic aortic injury. J Trauma 34:696–701, 1993.
8. Knudson MM, Lewis FR, Atkinson K, Neuhaus A: The role of duplex ultrasound arterial imaging in patients with penetrating extremity trauma. Arch Surg 128:1033–1037, 1993.
9. Luks FI, Lemire A, St. Vil D, et al: Blunt abdominal trauma in children: The practical value of ultrasonography. J Trauma 34:607–610, 1993.
10. McKenney M, Lentz K, Nunez D, et al: Can ultrasound replace diagnostic peritoneal lavage in the assessment of blunt trauma? J Trauma 37:439–441, 1994.
11. Minard G, Schurr M, Croce MA, et al: A prospective analysis of transesophageal echocardiography in the diagnosis of traumatic disruption of the aorta. J Trauma 40:225–230, 1996.
12. Rozycki GS, Feliciano DV, Schmidt JA, et al: The role of the surgeon-performed ultrasound in patients with possible cardiac wounds. Ann Surg 223:737–744, 1996.
13. Rozycki GS, Ochsner MG, Schmidt JA, et al: A prospective study of surgeon-performed ultrasound as the primary adjuvant modality for injured-patient assessment. J Trauma 39:492–498, 1995.
14. Rozycki GS, Shackford SR: Ultrasound, what every trauma surgeon should know. J Trauma 40:1–4, 1996.
15. Staren ED (ed): Ultrasound for the Surgeon. Philadelphia, Lippincott-Raven, 1997.

45. WOUND EXPLORATION AND PRECAUTIONS IN THE MANAGEMENT OF TRAUMA PATIENTS

Gideon P. Naudé, M.B.Ch.B.

WOUND EXPLORATION

1. What is the purpose of wound exploration?

Wound exploration differentiates injuries that are superficial, requiring simple wound toilet and suture in the emergency room or office, from injuries that are penetrating and cause injury to underlying vital structures, requiring more extensive repair in the operating room. The viability of nerves, muscles, and underlying blood vessels is evaluated, and obvious foreign bodies are removed.

2. When is wound exploration carried out?

It is performed on wounds caused by penetrating injuries.

3. Should all penetrating wounds be explored?

No. If the patient requires a procedure such as a laparotomy, thoracotomy, or exploration of a neck injury based on clinical findings or imaging studies, the wound is not explored in the emergency department but managed as part of the patient's surgery in the operating room.

4. What precautions are taken during exploration?

Injuries close to major vessels should not be explored in the office, because a brisk bleed from a large artery or vein is best managed in the operating room.

5. How is wound exploration carried out?

With good lighting and assistance to achieve adequate exposure, the area is first prepared with a disinfectant and draped in a sterile fashion. Local anesthesia is used, and the wound is explored to ascertain the complete depth and course. If it is found to be blind ending, having caused no injury to underlying deep structures, only wound management is carried out. If found to be penetrating, further diagnostic modalities are used, including exploratory surgery.

6. Is wound exploration of value for stab wounds of the back?

Yes. If the wound tract is blind ending, local wound care is all that is needed. If, because of the thickness of the muscles, the end of the tract cannot be visualized, other diagnostic modalities will be needed.

7. Is blind probing of the wound of value?

No. Frequently, it is misleading because a wound tract is not always straight, and probing may give the false impression of a blind-ending tract. Probing in the vicinity of injured blood vessels may cause bleeding that could be difficult to manage in the office or emergency department.

PRECAUTIONS IN THE MANAGEMENT OF TRAUMA PATIENTS

8. How do we know which trauma patients have conditions such as tuberculosis, hepatitis, or acquired immunodeficiency syndrome (AIDS)?

We do not. Unlike elective surgical patients who may have a complete workup before surgery and in which case precautions can be taken by the health care workers, trauma patients arrive with injuries requiring immediate attention. Time is not available in these emergency situations to test the patients before physical contact and surgery. We therefore must manage all patients as if they were infected.

9. What precautions should be taken by the emergency medical personnel when dealing with these patients?

- Protection from body fluids (e.g., blood, saliva) should be used during examination and intubation.
- A protective gown and gloves should be worn.
- Eye protection in the form of goggles or a visor is worn.
- A mask should be worn to protect the face, mouth, and nose from blood splashes.
- Safety needles with protective sheaths to prevent needle sticks are used.
- When a "sharp," such as a scalpel, is handed to the physician, it should be placed in a container (e.g., a kidney dish), and the container is held out to the physician who then removes the scalpel. When the scalpel is no longer needed, it is placed back in the container, which the nurse or operating room technician then takes back. This method prevents injuries to the surgeon and staff.

10. Are vaccinations available to reduce the risk of infection in high-risk personnel?

Hepatitis B vaccination is available. However, no effective vaccine is available for other strains of hepatitis or the human immunodeficiency virus (HIV), and we are awaiting the development of effective measures.

11. What is done after exposure to body fluids?

Splashing of the eyes, mouth, and nose requires immediate washing of the area with copious amounts of water. Splashing of areas of skin damage, such as sores, requires washing and the application of a disinfectant. Scratches or cuts from contaminated blades or needles also require washing and disinfection. Needle sticks should be cleaned as well as possible. The health worker and the patient are then tested for HIV and hepatitis virus strains. If the patient tests positive for hepatitis B, the health worker will require gamma-globulin and, later, vaccination if no adequate antibodies to the virus are present. The HIV-positive status of the patient must be documented, and the health care worker must be tested repeatedly—at 6 weeks, 3 months, 6 months, and 1 year. The antiretroviral drug AZT can be administered, even though no proof of the efficacy of this form of prophylaxis is available. Newer drugs show more promise. The health care worker is advised to practice safety precautions (including sexual precautions) until it is known whether infection has occurred.

In the case of tuberculosis, the purified protein derivative (PPD) is administered after a contact. If positive, further investigations are performed and treatment instituted, if necessary.

BIBLIOGRAPHY

1. Civetta JM, Taylor RW, Kirby RR (eds): Critical Care, 2nd ed. Philadelphia, Lippincott-Raven, 1992.
2. McCarthy MC, Lowdermilk GA, Canal DF, Broadie TA: Prediction of injury caused by penetrating wounds to the abdomen, flank, and back. Arch Surg 126:962–965, 1991.
3. Thal ER: Evaluation of peritoneal lavage and local exploration in lower chest and abdominal stab wounds. J Trauma 17:642–648, 1977.
4. Way LW (ed): Current Surgical Diagnosis and Treatment, 10th ed. Norwalk, CT, Appleton & Lange, 1994.

XIV. Psychiatric Aspects of Trauma

46. PSYCHIATRIC ASPECTS OF TRAUMA

Barbara A. Silver, M.D.

ANXIETY DISORDERS

1. What are the primary symptoms of posttraumatic stress disorder (PTSD)?
- Persistent re-experiencing of the traumatic event
- Emotional numbing and avoidance of stimuli associated with the trauma
- Persistent symptoms of increased autonomic arousal

2. How is acute stress disorder (ASD) differentiated from PTSD with regard to symptomatology and with regard to time course?
Dissociative symptoms are seen in ASD either during or after the trauma, but they are not always seen in PTSD. Symptoms of ASD must begin within 1 month of the trauma and last less than 1 month, while symptoms of PTSD may begin at any time and must last more than 1 month.

DELIRIUM

3. What are possible causes of delirium?
Remember the mnemonic I WATCH DEATH:
Infections
Withdrawal
Acute metabolic
Trauma
CNS pathology
Hypoxia
Deficiencies
Endocrinopathies
Acute vascular
Toxins/drugs
Heavy metals

4. What factors may contribute to the development of delirium in a burn patient?
Acute metabolic changes, infections, and use of narcotic analgesics may contribute to the development of delirium in a burn patient. A burn patient who has a history of drug abuse, alcohol abuse, or dementia is at higher risk of developing delirium.

5. What are the mental status findings in delirium with regard to (1) orientation and (2) perceptual abnormalities?
1. Disorientation to time and place are seen in delirium.
2. Visual hallucinations, auditory hallucinations, and illusions are commonly seen in delirium.

6. What class of psychotropic agents is considered the pharmacologic treatment of choice for delirium (other than delirium related to alcohol withdrawal), and what neurologic side effects can occur with this class of psychotropic agents?

High-potency neuroleptics are considered the treatment of choice for delirium. Potential neurologic side effects include acute dystonic reactions (sustained contractions of the muscles of the mouth, neck, tongue, or eyes), parkinsonism (tremor, rigidity, and bradykinesia), and akathisia (motor restlessness and agitation).

7. The synthetic narcotic meperidine (Demerol) can be associated with central nervous system (CNS) agitation, tremulousness, delirium, and seizures. What is the mechanism by which this occurs?

The metabolite of meperidine, normeperidine, is CNS excitatory and toxic, causing the agitation and the delirium. Because normeperidine has a much longer half-life than meperidine, normeperidine levels increase with repeated dosing of meperidine, leading to the symptoms of toxicity. This is particularly problematic in patients who are narcotic tolerant and require large doses of meperidine. It can also be more problematic in patients with renal failure, because normeperidine excretion is decreased in renal failure.

ALCOHOL AND SUBSTANCE RELATED DISORDERS

8. What physical findings (including vital signs) are seen with alcohol withdrawal?
Hypertension
Tachycardia
Diaphoresis
Tremulousness

9. What is the treatment for alcohol withdrawal?
A benzodiazepine, such as lorazepam, diazepam or chlordiazepoxide, should be administered to prevent and treat the symptoms of withdrawal. Multivitamins, thiamine (100 mg/day), and folic acid (1 mg/day) should be administered to correct nutritional deficiencies.

10. What is Wernicke-Korsakoff syndrome?
Wernicke's encephalopathy is an acute syndrome that consists of the triad of confusion, ataxia, and cranial nerve palsy. Korsakoff's syndrome is a chronic amnestic syndrome that usually follows Wernicke's encephalopathy. Anterograde amnesia (impaired ability to learn new information) is more severe than retrograde amnesia (impaired memory of material learned before and the onset of symptoms). The Korsakoff patient is alert and responsive and no longer displays symptoms of encephalopathy.

11. What are the symptoms of opioid withdrawal syndrome?
Hypertension, tachycardia, temperature dysregulation, piloerection, pupillary dilation, restlessness, insomnia, chills, opioid craving, muscle aches, nausea, vomiting, and diarrhea can all be seen with opioid withdrawal.

12. What agent can be used to treat the autonomic symptoms of the opioid withdrawal syndrome, and how does it work?
Clonidine, an alpha-2 adrenergic agonist acts on presynaptic noradrenergic nerve endings in the locus ceruleus and blocks the adrenergic discharge produced by opioid withdrawal. This blocks the autonomic symptoms of opioid withdrawal but not the subjective discomfort and craving.

SUICIDE

13. What is the SAD PERSONS scale?
This suicide risk assessment mnemonic stands for:
Sex
Age

Depression
Previous attempt
Ethanol abuse
Rational thinking loss
Social supports lacking
Organized plan
No spouse
Sickness

14. What are the demographic risk factors for suicide, with regard to sex, age, race, and marital status?

Male sex, older age, Caucasian ethnicity, and unmarried status are risk factors for suicide.

15. What neurotransmitter abnormalities have been lin ked to suicide?

Serotonergic dysfunction, including low levels of the serotonin metabolite 5-hydroxyindoleacetic acid (5HIAA) in the cerebrospinal fluid (CSF), has been linked to suicide, particularly suicide by violent means.

16. How do men and women differ with regard to the method used for suicide?

Men are more likely to use violent means, such as firearms, hanging, or jumping. Women are more likely to overdose on medications or take poison.

PERSONALITY DISORDERS

17. What are some problems that intensive care unit (ICU) staff may encounter in working with a patient with a dependent personality disorder (1) facing a choice of amputation versus attempted salvage of a leg and (2) coping with the postoperative course if the patient decides to have the amputation?

1. A patient with dependent personality disorder might display difficulty with the choice of amputation versus attempted salvage. The patient also would try to elicit excess reassurance from staff about the decision.

2. Postoperatively, the patient may display excessive need for assistance with tasks that the patient is physically able to do and may have difficulty dealing with the transfer from the ICU to a regular ward.

18. What are some problems that hospital staff may encounter in dealing with a patient with a borderline personality disorder hospitalized after a motor vehicle accident with regard to (1) staff relationships with the patient and (2) pain control?

1. A patient with borderline personality disorder may display intense and unstable relationships with staff: idealizing staff at times and devaluing staff at other times.

2. Pain control may be difficult if the patient has a substance abuse history.

DEFENSE MECHANISMS

19. How would the defense mechanisms of denial, regression, and intellectualization be demonstrated in a patient with traumatic paraplegia?

- A patient in **denial** might say that his inability to walk is only temporary and that, as soon as his pain recedes, he will be able to walk again.
- A **regressive** patient would display immature behavior, wanting excess assistance from family and staff.
- A patient using **intellectualization** as a defense mechanism would study his condition, requesting detailed medical information from his physicians, without displaying emotions.

LEGAL ISSUES

20. What is "informed consent" for surgical treatment?

Prior to consenting to surgical treatment, the patient or patient's guardian must understand:

- The nature of the problem for which surgery is recommended
- The proposed surgical treatment
- The benefits of the treatment versus any alternative treatments versus no treatment
- The risks of the treatment versus any alternative treatments versus no treatment
- That consent is voluntary

21. Who can provide informed consent for surgical treatment?

- A competent adult (all adults are considered competent unless declared incompetent by the court)
- A parent of a minor
- An emancipated minor (a minor who has a child or who is married, in military service, or declared emancipated by the court)
- An adult designated by the patient to exercise his or her durable power of attorney for health care

22. When is informed consent not necessary?

- Emergencies—Informed consent is not necessary when treatment is necessary before a full explanation can be given or before consent can be obtained.
- Incompetency—An incompetent patient cannot provide informed consent. This protects incompetent patients from foregoing treatment.
- Waiver—A patient can waive the right to information to the physician.
- Therapeutic privilege—The physician may believe that the information would be deleterious to the patient.

PSYCHOPHARMACOLOGY

23. Name two risks of treating a traumatic brain injury patient with a tricyclic antidepressant (TCA).

TCAs lower the seizure threshold, increasing the risk of seizures in a patient with traumatic brain injury. The anticholinergic effects of TCAs interfere with cognition and memory.

24. What complication can occur if a patient being treated with codeine is also treated with a selective serotonin reuptake inhibitor (SSRI) such as fluoxetine (Prozac) or paroxetine (Paxil)?

Fluoxetine and paroxetine are potent inhibitors of the hepatic cytochrome P4502D6 enzyme. This enzyme is necessary for the metabolic conversion of codeine to morphine, the active metabolite. Concomitant administration of the SSRI and codeine will thus compromise the analgesic effect of codeine.

25. What complications may arise in treating the traumatic brain injury patient with a benzodiazepine?

Benzodiazepines can:

- Produce amnesia, worsening memory problems
- Exacerbate problems with balance, ataxia, and coordination
- Produce sedation, decreasing psychosocial function
- Lead to dependence

BIBLIOGRAPHY

1. Andreason NC, Black DW (eds): Introductory Textbook of Psychiatry, 3rd ed. Washington, DC, American Psychiatric Association Press, 2001.

2. Ereshefsky L, Alfaro CL, Lam YWF: Treating depression: Potential drug interactions. Psych Annals 27: 244–258, 1997.
3. Kaplan HI, Sadock BJ (eds): Synopsis of Psychiatry. Baltimore, Williams & Wilkins, 1998.
4. Robinson DJ: Disordered Personalities—A Primer. London, Ontario, Rapid Psychler Press, 1996.
5. Rundell JR, Wise MG (eds): Textbook of Consultation–Liaison Psychiatry, 2nd ed.. Washington, DC, American Psychiatric Association Press, 2002.
6. Schatzberg AF, Cole JO, DeBattista C (eds): Manual of Clinical Psychopharmacology, 4th ed. Washington, DC, American Psychiatric Association Press, 2002.
7. Sederer LI, Rothschild AJ (eds): Acute Care Psychiatry. Baltimore, Williams & Wilkins, 1997.
8. Silver JF, Yudofsky SC, Hales RE (eds): Neuropsychiatry of Traumatic Brain Injury. Washington, DC, American Psychiatric Association Press, 1994.
9. Stoudemire A (ed): Clinical Psychiatry for Medical Students, 3rd ed. Philadelphia, J.B. Lippincott, 2002.
10. Wyszynski AA, Wyszynski B: A Case Approach to Medical–Psychiatric Practice. Washington, DC, American Psychiatric Association Press, 1996.

XV. Miscellaneous

47. CONTRIBUTIONS OF THE MEDICAL EXAMINER OR CORONER IN TRAUMA CARE: PHYSICAL DIAGNOSIS, FOREIGN BODIES, AND EVIDENCE

Thomas T. Noguchi, M.D., Lakshmanan Sathyavagiswaran, M.D.

1. When should I report a death to the medical examiner or the coroner? What does the medical examiner's office or coroner's office need?

Each state has laws on which sudden and unexpected deaths, including traumatic deaths or deaths by violence, accident, suicide, and homicide or by any suspicious means, are reportable to the medical examiner or coroner's office. Physicians are also required to report any death suspected of being caused by a contagious disease constituting public hazards and report deaths during work. In California, deaths occurring within 24 hours after therapeutic or diagnostic procedures are also reportable.

2. What does the medical examiner or coroner's office need?
- A complete copy of all medical records, including all culture and toxicology reports, should be submitted.
- Specimens include admission blood, gastric lavage samples, and blood from the cranial cavity (subdural and epidural) in cases of head trauma needing neurosurgical intervention.
- All clothing should be retained.
- All appliances (e.g., endotracheal tube, casts, intravenous lines) should be left with the body.
- After death, the body should not be disturbed (e.g., cleaning).
- In the case of an injured pregnant mother, when stillbirth or a perinatal death occurs, the placenta is important for assessment of the cause and effect relationship. The placenta should be saved and should be submitted to the medical examiner or coroner's office with the fetus or deceased newborn baby.
- At the time of reporting to the medical examiner or coroner's office, if the autopsy has already been done at the hospital, the autopsy report should be typed on a priority basis and submitted at the same time the body is transferred to the office.
- For tissue harvesting from a case falling under the medical examiner or coroner's jurisdiction, clearance by the medical examiner or coroner is required.

3. How can a surgeon or emergency department physician assist in future medicolegal proceedings?
- Document evanescent findings caused by drying, washing, or other causes (e.g., foam in the nose, soot in gunshot wound cases).
- Eyes should be examined for conjunctival petechial hemorrhages, because such hemorrhages are observed in cases of asphyxiation.
- The operating room nurse should be instructed to properly label all samples and evidence

taken during surgery. It is the ultimate responsibility of the physician to ensure the specimens are properly labeled. The submitted specimen may not be admissible in court if there is any suspicion of error in identification.

- Document iatrogenic damage by invasive procedures or surgery and the amount of blood loss. Properly describe the wound (e.g., size, shape, regularity of edges), including anatomic location; take photographs; and quantify internal hemorrhages. After death, no additional incision should be made.

4. Lawyers often talk about evidence. What is evidence?

Evidence has been defined by previous rulings as any pertinent information, witness account, written or recorded document, photographs, x-ray films, laboratory test results, or other documentation for the purpose of inducing belief in the minds of court and juries about the contention. The evidence can be presented by the act of parties and through the medium of witnesses, records, documents, and concrete objects.

5. Could any foreign body or material be evidence?

Yes. In a case of an assault, any matter that is transferred from the object or the assailant that could indicate the assailant was at the crime scene at the time of the event is evidence. It could tie the assailant to the criminal event. Any foreign body could be evidence. A forensic expert's opinion, based on the examination of such evidence, has progressively been relied on by the judges and juries as reliable evidence in recent years.

6. Do I need to save a paint chip found in the laceration of a comatose patient of a motor vehicular accident? Why?

Yes. In a case of a hit-and-run victim, a piece of paint may be the sole evidence that ties the victim to the car that was driven by the assailant. A hit-and-run driver, by leaving the scene of an injured victim, has committed a crime of felony punishable by state law for a prescribed term in a state prison.

7. How do I save the paint chip for use as evidence?

Each medical center should have a written procedure that all personnel are required to follow, and they should maintain a log for saving evidence. The procedure must include documentation so that the attorney can prove that the foreign body or material that the surgeon had taken during the examination or operation is the same material that produced as evidence in the court. This is known as *the chain of custody of the evidence*. In the case of a high-profile trial, the evidence often becomes the key deciding factor of guilt or innocence.

8. What happens if we cannot produce any documentation?

The proof that the evidence was taken from the specific patient is called *the chain of custody*. The record or documentation should be able to produce an unbroken chain of custody for all evidence taken. When this is not done, the chain of evidence is declared broken. Without a documented chain of custody, the report on the examination of such evidence is not allowed to be mentioned in court, nor can the existence of such evidence (e.g., paint chip) be mentioned during the court procedure. The judge will rule the evidence as "not admissible," and as far as the jury is concerned, this evidence does not exist.

9. What should be done with the patient's clothing, which is bloody and soiled?

The clothing should be kept and preserved. The clothing may contain physical evidence that can be used to persuade the court or jury for or against the proposed theory of what happened. In traffic accident cases, the soiled clothing may contain faint tire marks or oil stains that could be matched to a certain automobile. Other materials that may be on the clothing, such as hair, fibers, blood stains, stain patterns, soil, fragments of glass, paint chips, and vegetation material, can all be useful evidence.

10. What about partially burned clothing in burn cases?

Save it. In a case of arson, the partially burned clothing can serve as evidence. The clothing may be contaminated with a flammable material that can be identified as to the type of chemical and additives present.

11. Should a blood-soaked T-shirt and jacket be folded and placed in a plastic bag to save?

No. Blood patterns on the clothing may be important evidence that should be preserved. A plastic bag may cause decomposition of the blood and promote bacterial growth, making it difficult to conduct detailed forensic examination. The clothing should be hung up and dried first and then wrapped in butcher paper or placed in a brown paper bag, not a plastic bag. Minute hair, fibers, dust, and other particles might have been transferred from the assailant to the patient's clothing while they were in contact. Care should be taken in preserving all such evidence. The local police agency should work with the hospital personnel in establishing the procedure to save all potential evidence.

12. Would a gunshot wound be considered evidence?

Yes. It is evidence that needs to be properly documented or preserved. A photograph taken of the wound could be used as evidence. A detailed description of the wound in the patient's medical records would also be regarded as evidence.

13. What does a lawyer want to know about a wound? What features of the wound are important in a criminal or civil trial?

- The age of the wound (i.e., fresh or old), when a wound was inflicted
- Type of instrument or weapon used and how it was used (e.g., cutting action, gouging, blunt force)
- Direction of force
- Amount of force involved
- The shape of the wound, documented by accurate measurements and photographs, for identifying and matching any weapons found at the scene or later elsewhere

14. How can I tell the type of instrument used to cause the wound?

The clues may be subtle. In the case of a hit-and-run injury, there is often a partial imprint of a tire mark on the skin or clothing surface. Photographs should be taken with a ruler and victim-identifying information. A coat hanger can leave a wire pattern on the skin. A hammer blow leaves a circular or semicircular wound. Bruises on the prominent areas of the body with underlying bone (e.g., back of head, shoulder-blade area, elbow, hips, knees, ankles) may indicate a typical pattern of a fall on a level surface.

15. If the patient had been hit by a police baton, would you expect a single line of bruising on the skin?

No. Two parallel, dark red stretch makings are seen. The baton forces the skin to stretch to either side of the baton, resulting in two markings.

16. Are bite marks considered evidence?

Yes. They can be vital evidence. An assailant may be identified by the detailed examination of the bite marks compared with dental exemplars from a suspect taken by a forensic odontologist. Bite marks are often found in cases of rape, sexual assault, and domestic violence. Photographs should be taken of any bite marks seen on the victim. A special sexual assault kit should be available and used by trained personnel, such as forensic nurses, to collect evidence.

17. How would I remove a fragment of bullet lodged in the soft tissue?

Ideally, the bullet should be removed without distorting the rifling striations on the bullet. The preferred method is to use a rubber catheter—tipped, metal instrument such a Kelly forceps. The striations on the bullet are vital evidence for identifying the gun from which the bullet was shot.

18. What should I do with the bullet once I have removed it?

The bullet should be rinsed and placed in a container that prevents accidental sticking. The container or envelope should be clearly labeled with the identification of the patient, the date and time of removal from the patient, and a brief description of the degree of deformity. If more than one bullet is removed from the patient, each bullet should be placed in a separate envelope with information on the anatomic location where each bullet was found. Two bullets could have been fired from different guns, and two defendants may stand trial.

19. How should the bullet be identified and recorded?

Notation should be made about location, the specific structure involved, and the date and time of removal. The identification label should be completed by the surgeon who removed the bullet. If the surgeon removed the bullet and gave it to a nurse, who placed it in an envelope, labeled the envelope, and signed the containers, the nurse will become a part of the chain of custody and may have to testify as well as the surgeon who removed the bullet. It is best to keep the chain as short as possible, because everyone involved in the chain may be required to testify.

20. Should I attempt to determine which is an entrance wound and which is an exit wound?

It is not always easy for treating physicians or surgeons to determine from the surface wound characteristics which is an entrance or exit wound. A lawyer can use differences of opinion to imply there exists uncertainty. Keep it mind that the jury will be instructed that the evidence must be beyond reasonable doubt. In a living patient, the wound will heal and wipe out any distinguishing characteristics, so it is best to include a detailed description of the wound as observed the first time. The information should be noted in the patient's chart. It may be best not to guess which is an entrance or exit wound, but instead provide detailed descriptions of the wounds. If the patient dies, the forensic pathologist faces the difficult task of assessing the wound that is often distorted by tissue changes caused by surgical intervention or the healing process. Photographs with a ruler and patient identification are additional evidence.

21. Should a surgical incision be made through a gunshot wound in the head, or should cutting through the wound be avoided to preserve the evidence?

As vital evidence, it is preferred that the wound be preserved and a photograph be taken before surgical intervention and distortion by the healing process takes place. Surgeons should avoid removal of wounds, incising them, or inserting tubes through the wounds, if possible.

22. A woman slashed her wrist with a razor blade at least 10 times. The wounds were jagged. Many wounds were deep; a few were shallow. Would these wounds be described as multiple lacerations or incised wounds?

Regardless of the gross appearance, any wound caused by a sharp-edged cutting instrument is an incisional wound. Laceration means the wound was caused by a blunt force tearing the skin and soft tissue over bony prominences. Lacerations could, for example, be inflicted by the blunt force of a hammer, rock, or falling on the edge of a sidewalk.

23. In a case of child abuse, evidence of frequent abuse is manifested by bruises in different stages of healing. How do I tell which is an old and which a new injury?

Careful observation at the time of initial examination is essential. Very recent injuries appear red-purple. As the injury ages, the color gradually becomes indistinct red-brown or dark brown, and the margins begin to fade to light yellow. There may be tissue swelling that gradually goes down. The bruise may have a central abrasion that heals with predictable changes and scab formation. The injuries may also show pattern similar to the class characteristics of an instrument that may have been used, such as a looped electrical cord. These observations should be recorded in detail.

24. For trauma quality assessment purposes, we use the Injury Severity Score (ISS) and Trauma and Injury Severity Score (TRISS). Autopsy findings are needed to evaluate the effectiveness of treatment. How can we obtain the autopsy report from the medical examiner's or coroner's office in a timely fashion?

In some jurisdictions, there is ongoing feedback of collaborative information. The prompt submission of the autopsy report or the provisional autopsy findings by the medical examiner's or coroner's office is essential for the effective operation of the trauma quality assessment committee. There is need for closer cooperation.

The principal duties and responsibilities of the medical examiner are to determine the cause and manner of death, and the quality assessment issues are not always kept in mind by the departmental pathologists at the time of autopsy. The director of the trauma service should meet with the administrative heads of the medical examiner's or coroner's office to establish an ongoing, cooperative procedure for information exchange. In the County of Los Angeles, the coroner's office regularly provides copies of autopsy reports to the trauma centers. There is also innovative cooperation with the pathology departments of the medical centers in the county. The coroner's office has allowed certain teaching medical centers to conduct selected coroner's autopsies by board-certified hospital pathologists who are also deputized by the coroner's office. The direct communication and information obtainable from the hospital pathologist in trauma cases provide invaluable assistance to the trauma centers for maintaining effective trauma service and critical care to the community. Deputized pathologists are required to maintain their credentials at the coroner's office and to attend the regular update meetings at the coroner's office. For judicial reasons, all homicide cases are still handled in the Los Angeles Forensic Science Center of the Coroner's Office, and a forensic pathologist is appointed as Chair of the Combined Trauma Death Review Committee in one of the medical centers.

48. ALCOHOL AND ILLICIT DRUGS

Javier Romero, M.D., and Howard Belzberg, M.D.

1. What is the extent of alcohol and illicit drug use in the United States?

More than 9 million Americans are thought to be alcoholic, and more than 30 million have experimented with cocaine, with approximately 5 million regular users and 0.5 million addicted to opioids.

2. What percentage of trauma patients has a positive blood alcohol concentration on presentation to the emergency room?

Several studies have reported that 40% to 70% of trauma patients were positive for high blood alcohol concentrations. Evidence of combined alcohol and other drugs was found in 20% to 35% of the tested trauma population.

3. Alcohol is involved in what percentage of fatal motor vehicle accidents annually?

Alcohol is associated with more than 50% of all motor vehicle fatalities. Several studies have shown that alcohol use carries a higher morbidity rate for admitted trauma patients.

4. What are some of the impairments seen with alcohol intoxication?
- Poor judgment
- Decreased reaction time
- Lowered vigilance
- Decreased visual acuity
- Feeling of omnipotence
- Increased willingness to engage in risky behaviors

5. What are some of the physiologic responses to alcohol?
- Cardiac depression
- Respiratory depression
- Decreased level of consciousness
- Osmotic diuresis
- Decreased immunity
- Blunting of catecholamine response
- Hypothermia due to vasodilatation

6. What is the cellular response to alcohol?

Alcohol acts in part by altering the lipid matrix of the cell membrane and by interacting with the inhibitory neurotransmitter gamma-aminobutyric acid (GABA) receptor complex, resulting in an alteration of the ion fluxes through chloride channels.

7. What is a BAL?

Blood alcohol concentrations (BALs) are measured in milligrams of alcohol per deciliter of blood. This figure is converted to a percentage (100 mg/dL = 0.1%).

8. At what blood alcohol level does impairment begin?

Impairment begins at 50 mg/dL for most adult males, but in women and elderly persons, impairment may begin at lower levels. The probability that an automobile collision will occur starts increasing at a level of 40 mg/dL and rises sharply at 100 mg/dL of blood alcohol.

9. What is the blood alcohol level that most states define as the legal limit for driving under the influence?

The legal level is 100 mg/dL or 0.1% in most states. Some states have lower levels.

10. What screening tests are available to assess for "alcohol problems"?

The Michigan Alcohol Screening Test (MAST), a structured interview consisting of 25 questions, is one of the most commonly used screens to detect alcohol problems. MAST has been extensively validated for the use with trauma patients. The Short Michigan Alcohol Screening Test (SMAT), a revised and shorter screening test, has similar reliability. The CAGE test (i.e., cut down, annoyed by criticism, guilty about drinking, eye-opener drinks), with a sensitivity of 85% and a specificity of 90%, is a four-question test that has been used for assessing chronic alcohol problems.

11. Does a positive blood alcohol test result increase the possibility of future injuries?

One study followed 2500 trauma patients for 18 months after their injuries. Those who were intoxicated at the time of the initial injury were 2.5 times more likely than other patients in the group to sustain a second injury during the 18-month period.

12. At what rate is alcohol cleared from the bloodstream of the average patient?

The rate of alcohol metabolism is fairly consistent at 15 to 20mg/dL per hour. A trauma patient who initially has a blood alcohol level of 100 mg/dL will test at 60 to 70 mg/dL in 2 hours.

13. What electrolyte deficiency is most often seen with chronic alcohol consumption?

Magnesium deficiency is common in the alcoholic trauma patient, often requiring major replacement. Although serum magnesium levels are widely available, the intracellular nature of the ion leads to difficulty in evaluating total body levels. Low serum levels of magnesium (<2 mg/dL) are likely to be associated with hypomagnesemia. Conversely, normal serum levels do not ensure adequate magnesium stores.

14. What are the signs of alcohol withdrawal?
- Tremor
- Anxiety
- Agitation
- Insomnia
- Tachycardia
- Hypertension
- Diaphoresis
- Hallucination
- Seizure
- Delirium

15. What is the mortality of delirium tremens (DTs)?

Although, DTs occur in 5% of alcohol-withdrawal cases, it carries a mortality rate of 10% to 15%. Typically, trauma patients exhibit DTs within 48 hours after injury, but this may be delayed for 4 or 5 days or more.

16. Who should be screened for alcohol?

The U.S. Department of Health and Human Services recommends that blood alcohol levels and urine drug screening tests be obtained routinely for all hospitalized trauma patients who are 14 years of age or older at the time of admission to the emergency room or trauma center.

17. Are there any modalities to decrease alcohol consumption by trauma patients?

A randomized, prospective, controlled trail at a level I trauma center demonstrated that, with a single in-house motivational intervention, a significant decrease in alcohol consumption was seen at the 12 month follow-up compared with controls. Moreover, the intervention group had a 47% reduction in recurrent injury episodes requiring medical care.

18. What is the treatment for alcohol withdrawal?

Early treatment involves standard supportive measures and intensive care unit monitoring. Careful monitoring of fluid status and electrolyte replacement should constitute initial treatment. Intravenous administration of 100 mg of thiamine and 50 g of glucose should be given to prevent Wernicke's encephalopathy. Benzodiazepines are the mainstay for treatment of acute alcohol withdrawal. Benzodiazepines act on the GABA receptors, are cross-tolerant with ethanol, and therefore function as a replacement drug for alcohol. An effective treatment modality is an alcohol intravenous drip that can be titrated to clinical effect.

19. What two drugs are responsible for most positive drug screens in the trauma population?

Cocaine and opiates were the drugs identified in more than 90% of the cases in a study done in a level I trauma center.

20. List some physiologic effects of cocaine.

Neurological. Cocaine stimulates dopamine release, stimulates the sympathetic nervous system, blockades serotonin reuptake, and affects local anesthesia caused by sodium channel inhibition. It also lowers the seizure threshold.

Cardiovascular. Initial effects are vagogenic, including a transient bradycardia. The vagolytic episode is rapidly replaced by a sympathetic stimulation induced by reduced reuptake of catecholamines. This often manifests with severe hypertension, tachycardia, arrhythmias, and chest pain. Young trauma patients often suffer acute myocardial infarction from the cocaine-associated coronary vasoconstriction. An alpha-adrenergic blocking agent (phentolamine) may aid in the prevention of acute myocardial infarction.

Respiratory. Bronchiolitis obliterans with organizing pneumonia and interstitial pneumonitis are seen with cocaine use, which can be occasionally associated with respiratory arrest.

21. What are some of the clinical manifestations of cocaine withdrawal?

When ingestion of cocaine ceases, dopamine depletion becomes evident in the following forms:
- Fatigue
- Hypersomnolence
- Hunger
- Anxiety
- Paranoid behavior
- Hyperreflexia
- Depression

22. List the treatment options for acute cocaine intoxication.

Agitation is the most common presenting problem. It may be treated with benzodiazepines. Beta-blockers should be avoided because of the possibility of rebound hypertension due to the unopposed alpha effects. Nitrates are effective in lowering the blood pressure, reducing cardiac ischemia, and limiting the size of the cardiac infarct. Arrhythmias are best controlled with calcium channel blockers.

23. What are some of the clinical manifestations of opiate intoxication?

Opioids act through the central nervous system receptors (i.e., mu and kappa). Patients present with the following effects:
- Miosis
- Bradycardia
- Dysphoria

- Ventilatory depression
- Sedation
- Hallucination
- Analgesia

24. What is the treatment for acute opiate intoxication?

Acute opiate intoxication is the most life-threatening complication with this category of drug. The respiratory compromise may progress to cardiopulmonary arrest. Naloxone is the specific antidote for opiate intoxication. Naloxone treatment must be titrated to ensure three effects:

Dosage. Most patients respond to 0.8 to 1.2 mg of naloxone given intravenously, but larger or repeated doses may be required

Duration. Typically, naloxone has duration of action of 1 to 2 hours. However, many opiate preparations have durations of action exceeding 4 hours. In these cases, a continuous intravenous infusion may be required.

Withdrawal. The use of naloxone may induce an acute episode of withdrawal. The withdrawal syndrome consists of nausea, vomiting, and anxiety. Care must be taken to avoid aspiration during these attacks.

25. List the general approach to acute drug and alcohol toxicity.

- Protect the airway
- Ventilatory support
- Support circulation with volume
- Control hypotension with dopamine
- Control agitation with benzodiazepines
- Control hypertension with calcium channel blockers
- When in doubt, try naloxone

BIBLIOGRAPHY

1. Cornwell EE III, Belzberg H, Velmahos G, et al: The prevalence and effects of alcohol and drug abuse on cohort-matched critically injured patients. Am Surg 64:461–465, 1998.
2. Jenkins DH: Substance abuse and withdrawal in the intensive care unit. Surg Clin North Am 80:1033–1053, 2000.
3. O'Connor PG, Sammet JH, Stein MD: Management of hospitalized intravenous drug users: Role of the internist. Am J Med 96:551–558, 1994.
4. Soderstrom CA, Cole FJ, Porter JM: Injury in America: The role of alcohol and other drugs. An EAST position paper prepared by the Injury Control and Violence Prevention Committee. J Trauma 50:1–12, 2001.
5. Spies CD, Dubisz N, Neumann T, et al: Therapy of alcohol withdrawal syndrome in intensive care unit patients following trauma: Results of a prospective, randomized trial. Crit Care Med 24:414–422, 1996.
6. Spies CD, Rommelspacher H: Alcohol withdrawal in the surgical patient: Prevention and treatment. Anesth Analg 88:946–954, 1999.
7. U.S. Department of Health and Human Services, Substance Abuse and Mental Health Services Administration: Alcohol and Other Screening of Hospitalized Trauma Patients. Treatment Improvements Protocol (TIP) Series 16, 1995.

49. A POTPOURRI OF TRAUMA QUESTIONS

Edward E. Cornwell III, M.D.

1. What anatomic consideration allows for different management of gunshot injuries to the left versus right renal vein?

Renal vein injuries requiring ligation to control life-threatening hemorrhage will also require a nephrectomy on the right side because of inadequate venous drainage and subsequent congestion and ischemia of the right kidney. On the other hand, since the left gonadal vein drains into the left renal vein, injuries to the left renal vein between the junction of the gonadal vein and the inferior vena cava can be managed with ligation without left nephrectomy.

2. What is the normal serum fibrinogen level (with units)?

Zero (gotcha). Serum, by definition, has no fibrinogen. Plasma is whole blood minus the red cells, and serum is the plasma minus the clotting factors.

3. Describe your management of a patient with a gunshot wound to the stomach, tail of the pancreas, small bowel injuries × 6, and through-and-through injury of the descending colon requiring resection.

This question encompasses the evolution of thought in the management of colon injuries since World War II, when it was thought that virtually all penetrating colon injuries mandated colostomy rather than primary repair. Surgical thinking has evolved, however, and most trauma surgeons now manage many, if not most, colon injuries by primary repair or resection and primary anastomosis. While the likelihood of postoperative septic complications appears to be related to the severity of the associated intra-abdominal injuries (as expressed by the numeric Penetrating Abdominal Trauma Index, it does not appear that performing a colostomy decreases that operative risk. While performing a colostomy avoids the presence of a colon anastomotic line, colonic anastomotic leak is the least common (1–2%) of all septic complications (wound infection, intra-abdominal abscess, peritonitis, fascial dehiscence) seen after the surgical management of penetrating colon injuries. The prospective randomized trials that have been done on patients with penetrating colon injuries would suggest that performing a colostomy does not decrease the septic complication risk, but adds a subsequent mandatory operation for colostomy closure and its inherent morbidity.

4. A patient with an abdominal gunshot wound has a left renal vascular injury and left kidney injury. You are considering left nephrectomy, but want to be sure that the right kidney (which is palpable) is functioning. Describe how this can be done.

Place an atraumatic clamp on the ureter of the kidney that you are contemplating removing (left kidney in this example). If the patient has a functioning kidney on the other side, an intravenous ampule of methylene blue should lead to blue coloring of the urine in the Foley bag within a few minutes. This is more convenient and less time-consuming than an intraoperative intravenous pyelogram.

5. One hour after an operation for a gunshot wound to the abdomen, your patient is in the recovery room and is cyanotic and tachycardic. His hematocrit at the end of the operation was 30. Is this patient more likely to be experiencing hypoxemia, major hemorrhage, or both?

Most likely, severe hypoxemia. Consider that 5 gm/dl of deoxygenated hemoglobin in the venous system are required to produce cyanosis. A patient with a total hemoglobin of 10 (hematocrit of 30) would have to have to have 50% of his blood desaturated to produce cyanosis. Major postoperative hemorrhage as the cause of this patient's problem (for example, rapid bleeding to a hemoglobin of 7 and hematocrit of 21) would require an even higher oxygen extraction ratio and, therefore, a lower venous saturation (lower than 30% saturation and greater than 70% desaturation of the venous blood) in order to produce the requisite 5 gm/dl of deoxygenated hemoglobin to produce cyanosis. The patient described is more likely to have a stable hemoglobin of 10 and an extremely low (but much more possible) venous saturation of 50%. This explains why pallor rather than cyanosis is the more common manifestation in the bleeding (but still living) trauma surgery patient. Cyanosis is much more common on the medical services, where hypoxemia secondary to cardiopulmonary dysfunction and a relatively normal hematocrit is a relatively common clinical presentation.

6. A 70-kg patient presenting to the emergency department with a gunshot wound to the abdomen has a blood pressure (BP) of 70 and a pulse of 140. How much blood must this patient have lost to produce this clinical picture?

About 1500 cc. In order to make this clinical assessment, one must keep in mind the amount of circulating blood volume in a healthy, pretraumatized patient. That figure is approximately 70 cc/kg, or 5 L in a 70 kg patient. Hemorrhage is classified into 4 grades:

Class I: 0–15% circulating blood volume lost; minimal change in vital signs.

Class II: 15–30% circulating blood volume lost; slight tachycardia, narrow pulse pressure, slight decrease in stroke volume.

Class III: 30–40% circulating blood volume lost; typically, the minimal amount of loss necessary to produce gross hypotension (30% of 5 L = 1500 cc).

Class IV: > 40% circulating blood volume lost; these patients are in extreme hemorrhagic shock and are on the verge of cardiopulmonary arrest.

7. A 25-year-old motorcyclist who is unconscious and in profound shock (BP 60/40, pulse = 135) has good rectal tone and moves his legs on noxious stimuli. He is likely to have what complex of injuries?

Major head injury and **ongoing hemorrhage.** The major head injury is indicated by the unconscious state, with no eye-opening and a Glasgow Coma Score of 8 or less. It is critical not to attribute hypotension to head injury, because intracranial bleeding would be insufficient to explain the volume of blood lost necessary to produce this clinical picture. Cervical spine injury is a less likely explanation, owing to the adequate rectal tone and the leg movement. It is unlikely that sepsis appears this early after admission, and pericardial tamponade is possible but less commonly seen after blunt trauma. Tension pneumothorax secondary to broken ribs and pulmonary laceration is a possibility and may prompt the clinician to place chest tubes, but the safe assumption—and one that must direct vigorous fluid and blood resuscitation—is that this patient is in hypovolemic hemorrhagic shock from bleeding into either the chest or abdominal cavity.

8. A 23-year-old patient with a stab wound to the right chest is admitted to the emergency room with a blood pressure of 124/80, a pulse of 85, and respirations of 20. After 2 L of crystalloid resuscitation, the patient develops dyspnea, cyanosis, tachypnea, and a blood pressure of 90 with a pulse of 120. What is the next appropriate step?

Place a right chest tube. This patient most likely has a tension pneumothorax rather than hemorrhagic shock. Rapid blood loss to produce this hypotension would be extremely unlikely, even with extreme desaturation, to have a high enough unsaturated hemoglobin circulating (5 gm/dl) to produce cyanosis. Similarly, distended neck veins would be unlikely in such an extremely hypovolemic patient. Therefore, this patient's severe respiratory distress, combined with distended neck veins and hypotension, suggests a mechanical cause and impaired venous return to the heart due to loss of most of the right lung volume secondary to a tension pneumothorax. A chest tube rather than rapid transfusion will be life-saving in this patient.

9. How can sampling error in obtaining mixed venous gases give the mistaken clinical impression of sepsis?

Vigorous withdrawal of this blood sample from the pulmonary artery port of the Swan-Ganz catheter will lead to a partially oxygenated specimen and mimic the oxygen transport values of sepsis. Artificially raising the mixed venous saturation to 80% in a patient with 100% arterial saturation and an hemoglobin (Hgb) level of 10 gm/dl will artificially raise the mixed venous oxygen content (Hgb $\times$ 1.34 $\times$ % sat [venous]) to about 10.7 ml/dl. Given an arterial oxygen content of 13.4 (Hgb $\times$ 1.34 $\times$ art O_2 sat), the AVO$_2$ difference (arterial O_2 content minus venous O_2 content) will artificially be narrowed to 2.7 ml/dl. This will artificially decrease the value for the extraction ratio (O_2 consumption/O_2 delivery). Therefore, the entire O_2 transport picture of sepsis (high venous O_2 content, low AVO$_2$ difference, relatively low O_2 consumption, and low extraction ratio) is created by an error in obtaining the sample.

10. How can chronic cocaine abuse in a heavily intoxicated trauma patient mimic a cervical spine injury?

Like the patient with a cervical spine injury, the intoxicated chronic cocaine user may manifest no motion, low blood pressure, *and* absence of the compensatory tachycardic response.

11. What are the critical concepts of aminoglycoside therapy in septic ICU patients?

Success of therapy relies on early therapeutic serum drug levels. There has been enthusiasm for employing doses ranging from 3 mg/kg every 8 hrs to 7–11 mg/kg every 24 hrs to achieve this. Although these regimens, combined with careful monitoring of serum drug levels, have not increased the toxicity, some clinicians are reluctant to employ these large doses. These clinicians are better off prescribing another drug, as suboptimal drug levels benefit nobody.

12. Name four common nosocomial pathogens that are directly related to prolonged prior use of antibiotics.

Candida species, vancomycin-resistant *Enterococcus, Enterobacter cloacae,* and methicillin-resistant *Staphylococcus aureus.*

13. What duration of antibiotic therapy does the literature support for a patient with a gunshot wound to the (1) stomach; (2) stomach and small bowel × 4; (3) transverse colon and pancreas; and (4) transverse colon, pancreas, retroperitoneum, and requiring 10 units of blood?

Twenty-four (24) hours in each situation. Although clinicians commonly employ longer durations in patients — such as (3) and (4), with more severe injuries — the current literature provides no basis for this practice. Although there are patients who can be identified to be at high risk for postoperative septic complications, prolonging antibiotic therapy has not been shown to decrease that risk. It does, however, increase risk of resistant organisms.

14. How does heroin abuse cause thrombocytopenia?

"Street pushers" commonly "cut" the drug with quinine. Quinine serves as a hapten in a complement-mediated antigen–antibody reaction against platelets.

BIBLIOGRAPHY

1. Chappius CW, Frey DJ, Dietzen CD, et al: Management of penetrating colon injuries: A prospective randomized trial. Ann Surg 213:492–498, 1991.
2. Gonzales RP, Merlotti GJ, Holevar MR: Colostomy in penetrating colon injury: Is it necessary? J Trauma 41:271–275, 1996.
3. Moore EE, Dunn EL, Moore JB, Thompson JS: Penetrating abdominal trauma index. J Trauma 21:439–445, 1981.
4. Nelken N, Lewis F: The influence of injury severity on complication rates after primary closure of colostomy for penetrating colon trauma. Ann Surg 209:439–447, 1989.
5. Stone HH, Fabian TC: Management of perforating colon trauma: Randomization between primary closure and exteriorization. Ann Surg 190:430–433, 1979.

INDEX

Page numbers in **boldface type** indicate complete chapters; f = figures, t = tables.

Modified abbreviated injury severity scale (MISS), 154
Modular diets, 204
Monitoring, of severe head injury, 55
Moraxella catarrhalis, in ventilator-associated pneumonia, 49
Morphine, for intracranial hypertension, 54
Mortality, after trauma, causes of, 172
Motor vehicle accidents, history-taking on, 7
Multiple victim incidents, field management of, 1
Muscle, healing of, 190
Musculoskeletal trauma, electrical exposure and, 218
Myocardial contusion, diagnosis of, 97–98
Myocardial trauma, blunt, evaluation of, 98
Myrdriasis, causes of, 69
Myxedema coma
    management of, 180
    manifestations of, 180

Nail bed trauma
    distal phalanx fracture with, 197
    evaluation of, 197
    repair of, 197–198
Nasal fractures, 64
    effects of, 75
    repair of, 75
Nasoethmoid complex fracture
    definition of, 75
    treatment of, 75
Nasogastric intubation
    in children, 244
    indications for, 204
    timing of, 108
Nasojejunal tubes, indications for, 204
Nasomaxillary buttress, 66
Near-infrared spectroscopy (NIRS)
    advantages of, 226
    mechanism of, 226
Neck
    anatomy of, 77
    bleeding from, management of, 78
    zones of, 71–72, 77, 163f, 164, 168
Neck trauma
    electrical exposure and, 218
    management of, 71
    penetrating, **77–83**
        definition of, 165
        evaluation of, in hemodynamically stable patients, 78
        exploration of, indications for, 78
        resuscitation in, 78
        structures associated with, 168
        surgical management of, 79
    plastic surgery for, 194–195
    vascular, **168–171**
        diagnosis of, 168–169
        findings in, 77
        management of, 169
Necrotic tissue, versus living tissue, in electrical burns, 221
Needle cricothyrotomy, 4
Needlestick injuries, prevention of, 268

Needle thoracostomy, field, indications for, 5
Neisseria meningitides, in postsplenectomy sepsis, 123
Nerve, palsies of, 155
Nerves, peripheral, healing of, 190–191
Neurogenic shock, 30
    definition of, 87
Neuroleptics, for delirium, 270
Neurological examination, in head injury, 52
Neurologic findings, in carotid artery injuries, 168
    and management, 170
Neurologic trauma, electrical exposure and, 218
Neuromuscular blockade, for intracranial hypertension, 54
Neurotransmitter abnormalities, and suicide, 271
Nitrazine paper, for chemical burns to eye, 68–69
Nonlethal weapons, effects of, 37
Nonunion, factors affecting, 200
Nose trauma, **71–76**
Nosocomial pathogens, 285
Nutrition
    in burn patient, 209
    initiation of, 201
    with pancreatic trauma, 136–137
    surgical, **201–205**
        cessation of, 205
        results, assessment of, 204–205

Ocular forced duction test, 61
Odontoid fracture, types of, 84
Ohm's law, 42
Open-bite deformity, causes of, 63
Open fractures
    closure of, 152
        timing of, 152
    debridements of, 151
    Gustilo-Anderson grading of, 151
Open reduction and internal fixation (ORIF), 154–155
Ophthalmologic trauma, **68–70**
    referral for, 69–70
Opiates
    intoxication
        manifestations of, 281–282
        treatment of, 282
    and positive drug screen, 281
Opioid withdrawal syndrome
    symptoms of, 270
    treatment of, 270
Oral feeding, 204
Orbit
    architecture of, 194f
    bones of, 60
    depth of, 60
Orbital apex syndrome, versus superior orbital fissure syndrome, 62
Orbital blow-out fracture
    definition of, 60
    most common orbital wall in, 60
    signs and symptoms of, 69
    signs of, 60
    treatment of, 194